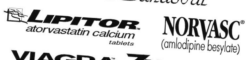
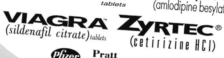
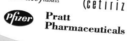

INTRAVASCULAR ULTRASOUND

INTRAVASCULAR ULTRASOUND

Edited by

Raimund Erbel MD FACC FESC
Professor of Medicine and Cardiology and Director
Department of Cardiology
University of Essen
Essen, Germany

Jos R T C Roelandt MD FACC FESC
Professor of Cardiology and Head
Department of Cardiology
Thoraxcentre
University Hospital Rotterdam and Erasmus University
Rotterdam, The Netherlands

Junbo Ge MD
Director
Intravascular Ultrasound Laboratory
Consultant Cardiologist
Department of Cardiology
University of Essen
Essen, Germany

Günter Görge MD
Consultant Cardiologist
Department of Cardiology
University of Essen
Essen, Germany

MARTIN DUNITZ

© Martin Dunitz 1998

First published in the United Kingdom in 1998 by
Martin Dunitz Limited
The Livery House
7–9 Pratt Street
London NW1 0AE

A CIP record for this book is available from the British Library.

ISBN 1–85317–315–0

Composition by Scribe Design, Gillingham, Kent, United Kingdom
Originated by Bright Arts, Hong Kong
Printed and bound in Singapore by Imago

Contents

List of Contributors

Mahmoud Ashry MD
Research Fellow, Department of Cardiology,
University of Essen, D-45122·Essen, Germany.

Dietrich Baumgart MD
Research Fellow, Department of Cardiology,
University of Essen, D-45122 Essen, Germany.

Nicolas Bom MSC PhD
Erasmus University, Medical School, 3015 GD
Rotterdam, The Netherlands.

Nico Bruining BSC
Technical Scientific Programmer, Department of
Cardiology, Thoraxcentre, University Hospital –
Dijkzigt, 3015 GD Rotterdam, The Netherlands.

Thomas Buck MD
Research Fellow, Department of Cardiology,
University of Essen, D-45122 Essen, Germany.

Luigi Campolo MD
Director, Catheterization Laboratory, Department of
Cardiology, Ospedale Niguarda Ca Granda, Milano,
Italy.

Gan Bapptistta Danzi MD
Cardiologist, Catheterization Laboratory,
Department of Cardiology, Ospedale Niguarda Ca
Granda, Milano, Italy.

Bernard de Bruyne MD PhD
Co-Director, Cardiovascular Center, Onze Lieve
Vrouw Ziekenhuis, Aalst, Belgium.

Pim de Feyter MD PhD FESC
Cardiac Catheterization Laboratory, Department of
Cardiology, Thoraxcentre, University Hospital –
Dijkzigt, 3015 GD Rotterdam, The Netherlands.

Lucia Di Francesco PhD
Centro Cuoro Columbus, 20145 Milano, Italy.

Carlo Di Mario MD PhD FESC FACC
Director of Clinical Research, Centro Cuoro
Columbus, 20145 Milano, Italy.

Hakan Emanuelsson MD
Chief of Interventional Cardiology, Division of
Cardiology, Sahlgrenska University Hospital,
Gothenburg, Sweden.

Raimund Erbel MD FACC FESC
Professor of Medicine and Cardiology and Director,
Department of Cardiology, University of Essen,
D-45122 Essen, Germany.

Eckart Fleck MD FESC
Professor and Director, Department of Internal
Medicine/Cardiology, Virchow-Klinikum,
Humboldt Universität, Berlin, D-13353 Germany.

Junbo Ge MD
Director, Intravascular Ultrasound Laboratory and
Consultant Cardiologist, Department of Cardiology,
University of Essen, D-45122 Essen, Germany.

Herbert J Geschwind MD FESC
Professor, Unité d'Hemodynamique et de
Cardologie, Hopital Henri Mondor, 94010 Créteil,
France.

Robert Gil
Department of Cardiology, Pomeranian Medical
Academy, 70–111 Szczecin, Poland.

Günter Görge MD
Consultant Cardiologist, Department of Cardiology,
University of Essen, D-45122 Essen, Germany.

Olivier Gurné MD
Cardiologist, Catheterization Laboratory,
Department of Cardiology, University of Louvain,
Mont-Godinne Hospital, Yvoir, Belgium.

Claude Hanet MD
Cardiologist, Catheterization Laboratory,
Department of Cardiology, University of Louvain,
St Luc Hospital, Brussels, Belgium.

Michael Haude MD
Head, Catheterization Laboratory, Department of
Cardiology, University of Essen, D-45122 Essen,
Germany.

Guy Heyndrickx MD PhD FESC
Head, Catheterization Laboratory, and Co-Director, Cardiovascular Center, Onze Lieve Vrouw Ziekenhuis, Aalst, B-9300 Belgium.

Akira Itoh MD
National Cardiovascular Centre, Osaka, Japan.

Peter Kearney MD MRCPI
Consultant Cardiologist, Cork University Hospital, Wilton, Cork, Eire.

Morton J Kern MD
Professor of Medicine, and Director, J G Mudd Cardiac Catheterization Laboratory, St. Louis University Health Sciences Center, St. Louis MO 63110–0250, USA

Lothar Koch PhD
Physicist, IMM Institut für Mikrotechnik GmbH, D-55129 Mainz-Hechtsteim, Germany.

Fengqi Liu MD
Cardiologist, Department of Cardiology, University of Essen, D-45122 Essen, Germany.

Volker Mühlberger MD
Chief of Interventional Cardiology, Department of Medicine, University of Innsbruck, Tirol, Austria.

Antonino Nicosia MD
Research Fellow, Cardiac Catheterization and Intracoronary Imaging Laboratory, Thoraxcenter, Erasmus Universiteit Rotterdam, 3000 DR Rotterdam, The Netherlands.

Joj Peels MD
Interventional Cardiologist, Department of Cardiology, University Hospital Groningen, Groningen, The Netherlands.

Jan Piek MD
Department of Cardiology, Academic Medical Centre, Amsterdam, The Netherlands.

Gerold Porenta MD
Cardiologist, Department of Cardiology, University of Vienna School of Medicine, Allgemeines Krankenhaus, Wien, Austria.

Francesco Prati MD
Cardiologist, Department of Cardiology, Ospedali di S Camillo, I-00152 Roma, Italy.

Peter Probst MD FESC
Professor and Director, Catheterization Laboratory, Department of Cardiology, University of Vienna School of Medicine, Allgemeines Krankenhaus, Wien, Austria.

Paulina Ramo MD PhD
Honorary Senior Registrar and Research Fellow, Department of Cardiology, Western General Hospital, Edinburgh EH4 2XU, UK.

Jos R T C Roelandt MD PhD FACC FESC
Head, Division of Cardiology, Thoraxcentre, University Hospital – Dijkzigt, 3015 GD Rotterdam, The Netherlands.

Thomas Roth PhD
Biologist, IMM Institut für Mikrotechnik GmbH, D-55129 Mainz-Hechtsteim, Germany

Erwin Schroeder PhD
Head, Department of Interventional Cardiology, University of Louvain, Mont-Godinne Hospital, Yvoir, Belgium

Patrick W Serruys MD PhD FESC FACC
Professor of Interventional Cardiology, Cardiac Catheterization Laboratory, Division of Cardiology, Thoraxcentre, Academic Hospital – Dijkzigt 3015 GD Rotterdam, The Netherlands.

Vijay T Shah MD
Department of Cardiology, University of Essen, D-45122 Essen, Germany.

Timothy Spencer PhD
Physicist, Department of Medical Physics, Western General Hospital, University of Edinburgh, Edinburgh EH4 2XU, UK.

Madoka Sunamura MD
Research Fellow, Thoraxcentre, University Hospital – Dijkzigt, 3015 GD Rotterdam, The Netherlands.

Eduardo Verna MD
Chief of Interventional Cardiology, Department of Nuclear Medicine, Ospedale Regionale, I-21100 Varese, Italy.

Clemens von Birgelen MD
Clinical and Research Fellow, Cardiac Catheterization and Intracoronary Imaging Laboratory, Thoraxcentre, University Hospital – Dijkzigt, 3015 GD Rotterdam, The Netherlands.

Vasilis Voudris MD FESC
Cardiology Department, Onassis Cardiac Surgery Center, Athens, Greece.

Christian Vrints MD PhD
Acting Head, Department of Cardiology, University Hospital of Antwerp, Antwerp, Belgium.

Ernst Wellnhofer MD
Cardiologist, Department of Internal Medicine/Cardiology, Virchow-Klinikum, Humboldt Universität, Berlin, D-13353 Germany.

Preface

Intravascular ultrasound was introduced a decade ago. It provides detailed information about the pathology of the arterial wall. Guide wire based Doppler techniques provide further information on intravascular bloodflow. The techniques are therefore complementary and have contributed considerably to our understanding of the pathophysiology of vascular atherosclerosis and the practice of interventional procedures. *Intravascular Ultrasound* presents a complete overview of currently available technologies for intravascular assessment and their clinical applications. It is based mainly on the extensive experience of The Thoraxcentre, Erasmus Medical Centre, Rotterdam, The Netherlands and the Cardiovascular Centre, University – Gesamthochschule, Essen, Germany.

The newest developments including tissue characterization, three-dimensional reconstruction and quantitative analysis are dealt with in detail and experimental applications, such as in pulmonary and aortic disorders, are also discussed, along with future applications.

The editors are thankful for the great support by Alan Burgess and Tanya Wheatley of Martin Dunitz Limited. The editors also want to thank all technicians who have been involved in the IVUS-studies in both catheterization and interventional laboratories in Rotterdam and Essen. We thank also all physicians who have participated and supported our efforts.

JRTC Roelandt
R Erbel
G Görge
J Ge

1 Introduction

Raimund Erbel and Junbo Ge

Coronary imaging techniques

Heart catheterization is, despite new, promising, noninvasive techniques—transthoracic and transesophageal echocardiography, magnetic resonance imaging, positron emission tomography—still the most important diagnostic tool in cardiology for clinical decision-making. According to a European survey, 675 760 catheterizations were performed in 1993. The number increased within one year to 808 861 cases. Per million inhabitants in Europe, 1825 catheterizations were performed, ranging from 83 in Romania to 4398 in Germany.[1]

In the early days of catheterization congenital and acquired valvular heart diseases were the primary indications, as the ongoing progress of cardiac surgery provided new forms of therapy. Coronary angiography was not widely accepted before the new therapeutic interventions—aortic coronary bypass surgery in 1968 and percutaneous transluminal coronary angioplasty (PTCA) in 1977—were introduced. It was Sones and co-workers in Cleveland who introduced, in 1959, selective coronary angiography.[2] The development of the transfemoral approach, with specially designed catheters, by Judkins (1967) was very important for its integration into clinical routine.[3] Most patients seen in heart catheterization and open heart surgery nowadays are patients with coronary artery disease.

Coronary angiography was believed to be the 'gold-standard' for coronary artery imaging. As no other method was available, discrepancies found by comparison of pathologic–anatomic studies and coronary angiography were nearly always neglected.[4–7] In main-stem disease this had particular important clinical consequences.[4] Coronary angiography is a contour method. Information about the cross-sectional structure of the vessel lumen is not available. Area stenoses cannot be determined directly, only indirectly, by measuring the diameter

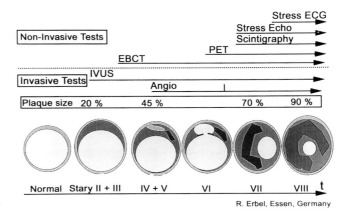

Figure 1.1. Time sequence of diagnostic tests for detection of coronary artery disease in relation to plaque development (gray area within vessel)[11] and calcium deposits (black area). Vessel area enlargement demonstrates coronary artery remodeling. ECG, electrocardiogram; PET, positron emission tomography; EBCT, electron beam computed tomography; Angio, coronary angiography.

within the lesion and a reference segment. In the early stages of coronary arteriosclerosis remodeling occurs.[6–9] It compensates for coronary luminal narrowing until the plaque size increases to a level of 40–45%, or the total vessel area increases by more than 80%.[8–10] The early stages of coronary artery disease cannot be detected (Fig. 1.1).[6–9] The reference segment itself is often involved in the disease process, leading to underestimation of the stenosis severity.

After the introduction of digital subtraction angiography, it was hoped that this technique would allow coronary artery visualization after intravenous contrast injection. But up to now, the results have been disappointing.[11,12]

The latest development is the introduction of the synchrotron technique in Brookhaven, USA, and Hamburg, Germany. Hamm et al.[13] demonstrated that synchrotron visualization of the coronary arteries is very promising. The patient remains in a sitting position. After intravenous injection of contrast material the coronary arteries are visualized in a similar way to conventional coronary angiography. Of course, limitations exist and we are still far from widespread use. But it can be regarded as one of the most interesting developments in noninvasive coronary visualization, similar to established coronary angiography but also with all its limitations.

Using electron beam tomography (= electron computed tomography = ultrafast computed tomography) and contrast injection, a three-dimensional coronary imaging technique has been developed in Erlangen, Germany.[14] These authors have applied this technique in order to evaluate the effects of coronary angioplasty and believe that this technique can be used after interventions in order to detect restenoses noninvasively and thus reserve invasive coronary angiography for those with pathologic results. Limitations are present in visualizing the distal right and left circumflex coronary arteries. But it can be expected that technical progress will eliminate some of these limitations.

In many respects magnetic resonance imaging has increased the diagnostic capabilities of noninvasive cardiology. With regard to coronary artery imaging, great steps forward have been demonstrated by van der Wall et al.[15] and Scheidegger et al.[16] Not only before but also after intervention the imaging allows the visualization of lesions of the proximal parts of the left and right coronary artery. With electrocardiography (ECG) and respiration-triggering, and using new software programs, the time necessary to do a complete study has dramatically decreased. Further improvement can be expected but limitations are still present in visualizing the arterial wall. However, enthusiasm for this technique has diminished and the number of publications on the topic is decreasing, according to the Medline survey.

Magnetic resonance imaging, synchrotron coronary angiography and electron beam tomography angiography will have the same limitations as conventional coronary angiography, as they are all visualizing the coronary lumen and not the arterial wall. Their main advantage is, however, that they are noninvasive techniques. A breakthrough can be anticipated when they will be able to demonstrate not only the lumen, but also the arterial wall, as has been shown for electron beam tomography.[17]

As the history of intravascular ultrasound chapter by Roelandt demonstrates, the idea of using ultrasound-equipped catheters in order to image organs from inside the body is quite old. But only the development of new catheterization techniques such as guiding catheters, guide wires and the use of interventional techniques stimulated the progress of intravascular ultrasound.

Intracoronary ultrasound

Intracoronary ultrasound is an invasive but important new technique for imaging coronary arteries, as not only the lumen but also the coronary artery vessel wall can be visualized (Fig. 1.1). The architecture of the wall, its components, size, shape, surface and consistency can be analyzed. Even a semiquantitative tissue characterization is possible, with high sensitivity for detection of calcification, and lower but still clinically useful sensitivity for characterization of lipid pools and fibrotic tissue.[18] Recent attempts to use pathologic anatomic recommendations for the description of arteriosclerosis by intracoronary ultrasound have been successful.[19,20] The method is invasive, and not all parts of the coronary artery tree can be scanned, but ICUS appears to be the new gold-standard which can detect coronary artery disease earlier than any other clinically available method (Fig. 1.1).

Coronary interventions and the future potential role of intracoronary ultrasound

The main limitations for coronary interventions have been acute complications, with coronary dissection and thrombus formation leading to urgent bypass surgery, combined with a high rate of myocardial infarction and high mortality. In addition, balloon angioplasty still has a restenosis rate of 30–40%, which increases in patients with unstable angina and after myocardial infarction to 60%. Every change in the technique, or the use of additional medication, was unsuccessful in reducing these limitations. The introduction of coronary stenting by Puel and Sigwart,[21,22] Roubin[23] and Schatz[24] significantly affected the world of interventions. At the same time, new interventional techniques such as coronary atherectomy by Simpson[25] and rotational coronary angioplasty by Fourrier et al.[26] and Erbel et al.[27] resulted in improvement of the acute success rate, reduction of acute complication rate and reduction of restenosis rate.

Coronary stenting

Coronary stenting in particular was very promising, but limited by new complications: subacute coronary thrombosis leading to emergency situations due to acute myocardial infarction. Thus the application was limited to a few centers because subacute thromboses were observed in up to 30% of the patients with acute coronary syndromes.[28] The first improvement was attained by the introduction of the determination of prothrombin fragments 1 and 2, that is, by better monitoring of anticoagulation. But the major progress was due to the technique of Colombo in Milan, Italy.[29] He demonstrated by intravascular ultrasound that, using regular balloons and conventional pressures of 6–8 atm, it was not possible to attach the stent struts to the vessel wall. Using higher pressures, and larger balloons, as had already been suggested by Schatz, the subacute thrombosis rate could be reduced dramatically. This was further supported by the introduction of ticlopidin as an adjunctive therapy to acetylsalicyclic acid. Anticoagulation was no longer necessary.[30]

The use of larger balloons and higher pressures was accompanied by an increasing number of coronary perforations.[31] This was followed by the advice not to use large balloons. But this demonstrates also that a knowledge of details of the physics involved was lacking. In-vitro studies have reported that the true size of coronary vessels can be underestimated by up to 25% due to technical problems.[32] This means that the true size of coronary arteries which are imaged is underestimated and the balloons which are selected do not fit the coronary artery because they exceed the vessel size. The thesis 'the bigger, the better' is no longer valid when the ratio of the balloon to the coronary artery diameter is more than 1.3.[33]

Coronary flow reserve assessment by intracoronary Doppler

For a long time it was observed that, after coronary angioplasty, coronary flow reserve was improved[34,35] but only rarely normalized. It was suggested that it would improve during follow-up and that coronary flow reserve only rarely normalizes acutely due to microvascular disease or pathological coronary vascular tone. Coronary flow reserve measurements after PTCA with intracoronary ultrasound Doppler demonstrated that the flow is increased and, after stenting, even normalized in up to 90% of patients.[36]

These results were confirmed by myocardial flow reserve estimation by densitometry.[37] But it was the introduction of the Doppler flow guide wire with an ultrasound crystal at the tip which brought the breakthrough for the Doppler technique as, in addition, fast Fourrier transformation analysis was available in a compact system with the estimation of mean and peak flow velocities, enabling the calculation of coronary flow reserve velocity after injection of vasodilators such as adenosine and papaverine. Using this technique, multiple centers confirmed the results concerning stenting.[38–40] As a result of these findings, coronary stenting will not only be used in a ratio of 30–40% for reduction of restenosis,[41] but also to increase the functional result of the intervention. The percentage of stented patients will further increase in the future.

Intravascular ultrasound techniques

During the last 8 years intravascular ultrasound catheter size has continuously decreased from 6 F. to, currently, 2.9 F. and already ultrasound guide wires have been developed. In order to avoid nonuniform rotation, to reduce friction in the coronary artery and to reduce damage to the vessel wall, ultrasound transducers are nowadays used within sheaths (MicroView/Spycatheters, Boston Scientific, MA, USA). They are ideal in order to obtain continuous pullbacks with reduced friction, more constant speed and more uniform rotation.

Whereas previously pullbacks were performed using hand-held techniques, nowadays step motors are used to obtain motorized pullbacks with a variety of speeds between 0.25 and 1.0 mm. Not only mechanical but also electronic systems are now available, providing images with high resolution. The progress of resolution is shown in Fig. 1.2, comparing images from 1990 and 1996. The new techniques, better computerized image acquisition and postprocessing, as well as increased transducer frequency from 10 to 30 MHz, enable the better delineation of structures with a higher resolution. It can be anticipated that the increase in resolution by using ultrasound catheters of up to 50 MHz will give even further insight into the vessel wall architecture.[42]

Tissue characterization is one of the big advantages of intravascular ultrasound in visualizing the coronary artery. Nowadays a calcification can be differentiated from a noncalcified lesion and already first attempts to perform a classification recommended by the American Heart Association[19,20] have been made. Many efforts are currently being made

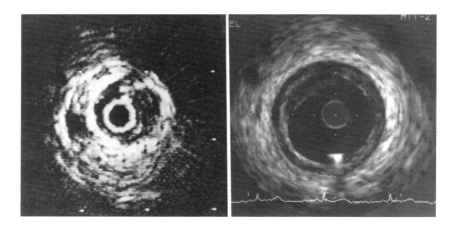

Figure 1.2. Comparison of intracoronary ultrasound images. The left panel is an image from 1990; the right panel is an image from 1996. The image quality and resolution improved greatly as the development of software and design of ultrasound catheters progressed.

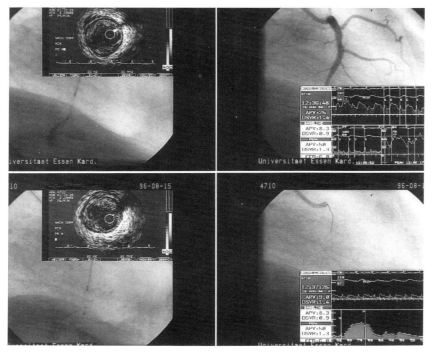

Figure 1.3. The Echomap system integrated angiographic images with intravascular ultrasound (HP Sonos Intravascular, Andover, MA, USA, left panels) and intracoronary Doppler flow mapping (Cardiometric FloMap, Mountain View, CA, USA, right panels). The site where the image was obtained can be documented very precisely on X-ray film.

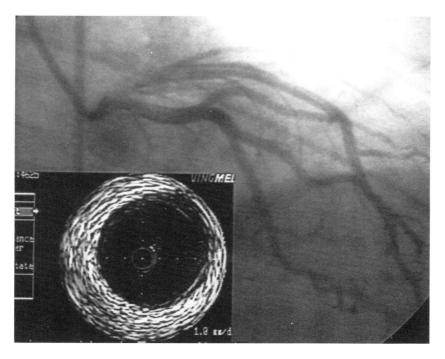

Figure 1.4. Echomap combining IVUS image obtained with Vingmed system (Sonotron, Horten, Norway) and a normal angiogram. Intimal thickening is shown on IVUS image.

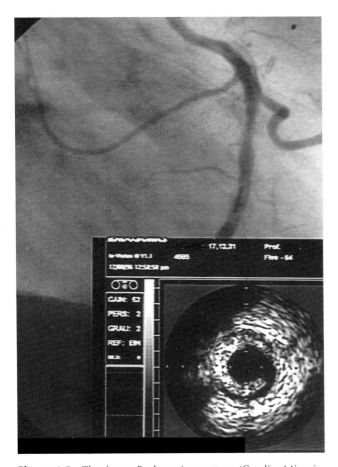

in order to be able to obtain deeper insight into tissue characterization.[43–45] At the moment these are still in the research stages.

Intravascular ultrasound is also able to analyze the pulsation of the coronary artery. Normal values have already been established.[46] In patients with hypertension, and particularly in patients with coronary artery disease, pulsation is reduced, resulting in a reduced shape change of the artery. Coronary pressure depicted by guide wires which are already available or, in the future, wires combined with intracoronary Doppler, will allow the analysis of pressure dimension curves. The compliance of the vessels can be estimated.[47] As was suspected, the change in the compliance of the coronary artery is an earlier event than the morphological change. This technique has important implications for the future because scientists are interested in the influence of drugs on coronary vascular compliance.

A great step forward is the introduction of the frame-in-frame system (Echomap) integrated in the catheterization laboratory by Siemens (Erlangen, Germany) (Figs 1.3–1.5). In one frame the position of the catheter is visible with the intracoronary image enhancing the reproducibility. Storage is digital rather than analog. As Doppler flow information can also be shown, coronary flow reserve and not only flow reserve velocity can easily be assessed with high resolution (Fig. 1.6).

Figure 1.5. The latest Endosonics system (Cordis, Miami, FL, USA) demonstrated an intimal dissection which was not detected by coronary angiography after PTCA of a right coronary artery.

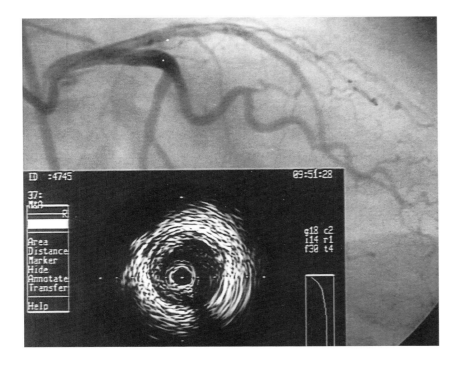

Figure 1.6. Echomap emerging CVIS (Scimed, Boston Scientific, Natick, MA, USA) intracoronary ultrasound image and coronary angiogram in a patient with angiographically normal coronary arteries. IVUS shows eccentric plaque formation.

Combined imaging and interventional systems: the route to sophisticated interventions

Usually intracoronary and intravascular ultrasound catheters are used as stand-alone systems and multiple changes of the catheters over the wires are necessary. The introduction of combined catheters—balloon and ultrasound—were the first attempts at a combination system.[48] Intravascular ultrasound allows immediate pre- and postimaging of lesions, which are treated by the balloon. The problem is that any change of the balloon size will also limit this advantage. In addition, no imaging during the procedure is possible as the transducer is located proximally to the balloon. The solution may be attempted by imaging guide wires.

Yock et al. suggested using coronary atherectomy catheters in combination with intracoronary ultrasound in order to image the vessel wall and to direct the interventional device.[49] This technique is already used in experiments and the first patients have been treated. The main limitation is that the ultrasound crystal is fixed on the rotating knife. Thus, the artery cannot be imaged before the cutting procedure commences without damaging the wall. Therefore Erbel et al. introduced vision-guided coronary atherectomy, combining atherectomy devices with lasers instead of mechanical systems and allowing angioscopic and intravascular ultrasound guidance of the intervention (Fig. 1.7).[50] Forward-looking catheters were developed in order particularly to penetrate coronary occlusions.[51,52] Combined or stand-alone systems will be used. All these ideas are based on the argument for 'sophisticated intervention': seeing and treating is the aim.

Micromotor-based intravascular ultrasound

The next step in miniaturization will be the introduction of micromotors for intravascular ultrasound.[53] The main advantage will be the avoidance of nonuniform rotation and the combination with therapeutic and interventional systems. After development by Lancée et al.,[53] the first three patients were imaged in the iliac artery in 1995, in Essen, Germany. The first use of micromotors in man was by Serruys and Erbel.[54]

Future developments

Another limitation of intravascular ultrasound is that the catheters are running over guide wires. Thus only parts of the vessel in given angles are imaged. The aim should be, however, to guide the tip independently and to be able to steer the tip of the catheter. The steering capability is the major factor necessary before vision-guided interventions or the guiding of ultrasound without X-ray can be applied.[55] Once steerability is present the catheters will be able to be moved in the aorta or in the pulmonary artery as well as other organs without X-ray, as the anatomy is known and any advancement of the catheter can be controlled by side or forward viewing. It may even be possible then to use intravascular ultrasound or intraluminal ultrasound in the emergency room.

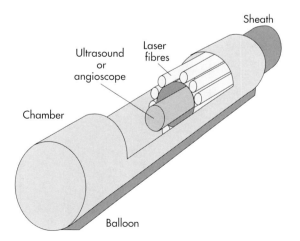

Figure 1.7. Schematic drawing of the vision-guided atherectomy catheter developed by Erbel et al.[50]

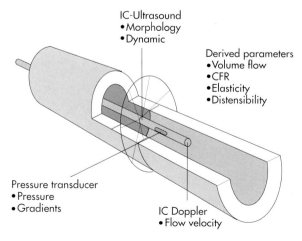

Figure 1.8. Schematic drawing of future development of combined intravascular diagnostic catheter.

Future diagnostic catheters should provide not only morphologic information, but also information concerning the coronary function, such as pressure parameters, flow parameters and the compliance of the vessel (Fig. 1.8). In addition, future development should be aimed at combining diagnostic and therapeutic catheters as proposed by Erbel et al., that is, vision-guided coronary intervention.

Conclusion

This book aims to offer an insight into the current use of intravascular and intracoronary ultrasound, providing information about the technical aspects of intravascular ultrasound, normal values, the diagnostic role of intravascular ultrasound in coronary artery disease as well as aortic and pulmonary artery diseases, and demonstrating their application in intracoronary interventions. In addition, aspects of peripheral arteries and imaging of the aorta and the pulmonary artery are provided, as well as new developments such as 3D reconstruction or the use of intravascular ultrasound probes to image the aorta by the transesophageal approach, that is, lighthouse transesophageal echocardiography (TEE).[56]

References

1 Unger F. European survey on cardiac interventions open heart surgery PTCA cardiac catheterisation 1994. *Ann Acad Sci Artium Europ* 1995; **12**: 1–59.

2 Sones FM, Shirey EK, Proudfit WL, Westcott RN. Cine coronary arteriography. *Circulation* 1959; **20**: 773–4.

3 Judkins MP. Selective coronary arteriography. IA percutaneous transfemoral technique. *Radiology* 1967; **89**: 815–24.

4 Isner JM, Kishel J, Kent KM, Ronan JA, Ross AM, Roberts WC. Accuracy of angiographic determination of left main coronary arterial narrowing. Angiographic histologic correlative analysis in 28 patients. *Circulation* 1981; **63**: 1056–64.

5 Freudenberg H, Lichtlen PR. The normal wall segment in coronary stenoses—a postmortem study. *Z. Kardiol* 1981; **70**: 863–9.

6 Stiel G, Stiel LSG, Schofer J, Donath K, Mathey DG. Impact of compensatory enlargement of atherosclerotic coronary arteries on angiographic assessment of coronary artery disease. *Circulation* 1989; **80**: 1603–9.

7 Hutchins GM, Bulkley BH, Ridolfi RL, Griffith LSC, Lohr FT, Piasio MA. Correlation of coronary arteriograms and left ventriculograms with postmortem studies. *Circulation* 1977; **56**: 32–7.

8 Glagov S, Weisenberg E, Zarins CK, Stankunavicius R, Kolettis GJ. Compensatory enlargement of human atherosclerotic coronary arteries. *N Engl J Med* 1987; **316**: 1371–5.

9 Zarins CK, Weisenberg E, Kolettis G, Stankunavicius R, Glagov S. Differential enlargement of artery segments in response to enlarging atherosclerotic plaques. *J Vasc Surg* 1988; **7**: 386–94.

10 Ge J, Erbel R, Zamorano J et al. Coronary artery remodelling in atherosclerotic disease: an intravascular ultrasonic study in vivo. *Coron Artery Dis* 1993; **4**: 981–6.

11 Peppler WW, Kudva B, Dobbins JT et al. A digitally controlled beam attenuator. *Proc SPIE* 1982; **347**: 106.

12 Ross AM, Johnson RA, Katz RJ et al. Diagnosis of coronary disease by aortic digital subtraction angiography. *Circulation* 1983; **63**: III43.

13 Hamm CW, Meinertz T, Dix WR et al. Intravenous coronary angiography with dichromography using synchrotron radiation. *Herz* 1996; **21**: 1–5.

14 Achenbach S, Moshage W, Bachmann K. Coronary angiography by electron beam tomography. *Herz* 1996; **21**: 1–13.

15 van der Wall EE, Vliegen HW, de Roos A, Bruschke AVG. Magnetic resonance imaging in coronary artery disease. *Circulation* 1995; **92**: 2723–39.

16 Scheidegger MB, Stuber M, Boesiger P, Hess OM. Coronary artery imaging by magnetic resonance. *Herz* 1996; **21**: 1–7.

17 Schmermund A, Baumgart D, Görge G, Seibel R, Grönemeyer D, Erbel R. Non-invasive visualization of coronary arteries with and without calcification by electron beam computed tomography. *Herz* 1996; **21**: 118–26.

18 .Di Mario C, The SHK, Madretsma S et al. Detection and characterization of vascular lesions by intravascular ultrasound. An in vivo study correlated with histology. *J Am Soc Echocardiogr* 1992; **5**: 135–46.

19 Stary HC, Chandler AB, Dinsmore RE et al. A definition of advanced types of atherosclerotic lesions and a histological classification of atherosclerosis. *Circulation* 1995; **92**: 1355–74.

20 Erbel R, Ge J, Görge G et al. Intravaskuläre Sonographie bei koronarer Herzkrankheit. *Dtsch Med Wschr* 1995; **120**: 847–54.

21 Sigwart U, Puel J, Mirkovitch V, Joffre F, Kappenberger L. Intravascular stents to prevent occlusion and restenosis after transluminal angioplasty. *N Engl J Med* 1987; **316**: 701–6.

22 Sigwart U, Urban P, Golf S et al. Emergency stenting for acute occlusion after coronary balloon angioplasty. *Circulation* 1988; **78**: 1121–7.

23 Roubin GS, Cannon AD, Agrawal SK et al. Intracoronary stenting for acute and threatened closure complicating percutaneous transluminal coronary angioplasty. *Circulation* 1992; **85**: 916–27.

24 Schatz RA, Baim DS, Leon M et al. Clinical experience with the Palmaz–Schatz coronary stent: initial results of a multicenter study. *Circulation* 1991; **83**: 148–61.

25 Simpson JB, Selmon MR, Robertson GC et al. Transluminal atherectomy for occlusive peripheral vascular disease. *Am J Cardiol* 1988; **61**: 96G–101G.

26 Fourrier JL, Auth DC, Lablanche JM, Brunetaud JM, Gomeaux A, Bertrand ME. Human percutaneous coronary rotational atherectomy. Preliminary results. *Circulation* 1988; **78**: II82 (abst).

27 Erbel R, O'Neill W, Auth D et al. Hochfrequenz-Rotationsatherektomie bei koronarer Herzkrankheit. *Dtsch Med Wschr* 1989; **114**: 487–95.

28 Haude M, Erbel R, Issa H, Meyer J. Quantitative analysis of elastic recoil after balloon angioplasty and after intracoronary implantation of balloon expandable Palmaz–Schatz stents. *J Am Coll Cardiol* 1993; **21**: 26–34.

29 Colombo A, Hall P, Nakamura S et al. Intracoronary stenting without anticoagulation accomplished with intravascular ultrasound guidance. *Circulation* 1995; **91**: 1676–88.

30 Morice MC. Advances in post stenting medication protocol. *J Intervent Cardiol* 1995; **7**: 32A–35A.

31 Colombo A, Hall P, Itoh A et al. The optimal pressure for stent implantation. In: Sigwart U, ed. *Endoluminal Stenting.* (London: WB Saunders, 1996): 280–8.

32 Stähr P, Rupprecht HJ, Voigtländer T, Koch L, Kearney P, Brennecke R. Validation of diameter and lumen area measurements of intracoronary ultrasound. *Circulation* 1994; **90**: I163.

33 Schmitz HJ, Erbel R, Meyer J, von Essen R. Influence of vessel dilatation on restenosis after successful percutaneous transluminal coronary angioplasty. *Heart J* 1996; **131**: 884–91.

34 Zijlstra F, Reiber JC, Juilliere Y et al. Normalization of coronary flow reserve by percutaneous transluminal coronary angioplasty. *Am J Cardiol* 1988; **61**: 55–60.

35 Wilson RF, Johnson MR, Marcus ML et al. The effect of coronary angioplasty on coronary flow reserve. *Circulation* 1988; **77**: 873–85.

36 Rupprecht HJ, Erbel R, Kooymann C, Schmitz A, Görge G. Stent implantation: cosmetics or functional improvement? *Circulation* 1991; **84**: II196.

37 Haude M, Lang M, Issa H, Renneisen U, Brennecke R. Additional improvement of stenosis dimensions and coronary flow after intracoronary implantation of Palmaz–Schatz stents. *Circulation* 1991; **84**: II196.

38 Ge J, Erbel R, Zamorano J et al. Improvement of coronary morphology and blood flow after stenting: assessment by intravascular ultrasound and intracoronary Doppler. *Int J Card Imaging* 1995; **11**: 81–7.

39 Kosa I, Blasini R, Schneider-Eicke J et al. Assessment of coronary flow reserve after stent implantation using positron emission tomography. *J Am Coll Cardiol* 1996; **27**: 49A.

40 Bowers TR, Safian RD, Steward RE, Shoukfeh MM, Benzuly KH, O'Neil WW. Normalization of coronary flow reserve immediately after stenting but not after PTCA. *J Am Coll Cardiol* 1996; **27**: 19A.

41 Haude M, Baumgart D, Caspari G, Görge G, Ge J, Erbel R. Relation between minimal luminal dimensions and myocardial perfusion reserve immediately after stenting and at 6 months follow-up. *J Am Coll Cardiol* 1996; **27**: 391A.

42 Lockwood GR, Ryan LK, Gotlieb AI et al. In vitro high resolution intravascular imaging in muscular and elastic arteries. *J Am Coll Cardiol* 1992; **20**: 153–60.

43 Fitzgerald PJ, Cogburn MA, Wing K et al. Determination of arterial wall components using intravascular backscatter analysis. *Circulation* 1990; III458 (abst).

44 Ramo MP, Spencer T, Kearney P et al. Can ultrasound texture analysis distinguish between red and white thrombi: a comparative study of intravascular videodensitometric and radiofrequency data. *J Am Coll Cardiol* 1996; **27**: 199A.

45 Roth T, Koch R, Ge J et al. Automatische Erkennung von Gefäßwandmorphologien auf der Basis der Analyse hochfrequenter IVUS-Ultraschallsignale. *Biomed Tech* 1996; **1**: 41–2.

46 Ge J, Erbel R, Gerber Th et al. Intravascular ultrasound imaging of angiographically normal coronary arteries: a prospective study in vivo. *Br Heart J* 1994; **71**: 572–8.

47 The SHK, Gussenhoven EJ, Wenguang L et al. Intravascular ultrasound assessment of lumen geometry and distensibility of the angiographically normal artery: a correlation with quantitative angiography. *Echocardiography* 1992; **9**: 133–9.

48 Hodgson MC, Graham SP, Savakus AD et al. Clinical percutaneous imaging of coronary anatomy using an over-the-wire ultrasound catheter system. *Int J Card Imaging* 1989; **4**: 187–93.

49   Yock PJ, Fitzgerald PJ, Sudhir K et al. Intravascular ultrasound imaging for guidance of atherectomy and other plaque removal techniques. *Int J Card Imaging* 1991; **6**: 179–89.

50   Erbel R, Roth T, Koch L, Ge J, Haude M. The precision-guided directional laser atherectomy catheter: a new approach to percutaneous coronary revascularization. *J Am Coll Cardiol* 1995; **25**: 268A.

51   Liang DH, Hu BS. A novel forward viewing intravascular ultrasound catheter. *Echocardiography* 1995; **12**: 275–81.

52   Evans JL, Ng KH, Vonesh MJ et al. Arterial imaging with a new forward-viewing intravascular ultrasound catheter. I: initial studies. *Circulation* 1994; **89**: 712–17.

53   Lancée CT, Bom N, Roelandt J. Future directions in intravascular ultrasound: from micro-motors to imaging guidewire systems. *Echocardiography* 1995; **12**: 275–81.

54   Erbel R, Roth Th, Koch L et al. IVUS of micromotors for cardiovascular imaging. *MITAT* 1997 (in press).

55   Görge G, Ge J, Haude M, Baumgart D, Buck Th, Erbel R. Initial experience with a steerable intravascular ultrasound catheter in the aorta and pulmonary artery. *Am J Card Imaging* 1995; **9**: 180–4.

56   Görge G, Erbel R. Intravascular ultrasound catheters for transoesophageal echocardiography: lighthouse transoesophageal echocardiography. *Eur Heart J* 1994; **15**: 101.

2 The history of intravascular ultrasound

Jos R T C Roelandt and Nicolas Bom

Contrast arteriography has been the principal method for assessment of the presence and severity of both peripheral and coronary artery disease and most cardiovascular imaging experience has been gained with this imaging technique. With this method, however, both the extent and severity of arterial atherosclerotic disease are underestimated and it has been impossible to provide information about wall morphology. In addition, the large intra- and inter-observer variability limits the quantitative assessment of therapeutic interventions.[1,2] Noninvasive ultrasound imaging provides cross-sectional images of accessible but limited portions of the peripheral arterial system.[3,4] Resolution is limited and the typical three-layered structure of muscular arteries is rarely appreciated. Precordial cross-sectional echocardiography allows the visualization of proximal parts of the coronary arteries but the success rate is low and the image quality insufficient for clinical decision-making in patients with coronary artery disease.[5] Intraoperative epicoronary echocardiography has confirmed the abnormal findings of earlier pathologic studies and further corroborated the insensitivity of coronary arteriography in appraising the extent and distribution of atherosclerotic wall involvement.[6] Fiberoptic angioscopy allows visualization of the endothelial surface of the arterial wall and has significantly added to our understanding of the mechanisms of acute ischemic syndromes.[7,8] The method has practical limitations (it requires complete replacement of blood by large volumes of translucent liquid) and, as with contrast arteriography, no information on the arterial wall under the endothelial surface is obtained.

The rapid progress in interventional cardiology and, more particularly, the introduction of techniques such as mechanical atherectomy and laser, have stimulated the development of an imaging method for characterizing and locating pathology under the endothelial surface. Intravascular ultrasound offers this potential and has fundamental advantages over all other presently available imaging techniques. Thus, many research groups have directed their efforts to developing catheter ultrasonic imaging devices allowing circumferential imaging through the blood of the arterial wall under the endothelial surface.

Intracoronary ultrasound has been developed over a short period of time, and a variety of catheter systems is now available to the interventionist.

Early developments

The first approaches towards the use of intracardiac ultrasound were for diameter measurement. In 1956, Cieszynski[9] built an ultrasonic catheter and obtained good echoes from the endocardial surface of the right and left ventricles in dogs. He speculated about the potential of the method for cardiac diagnosis in men and stressed the absence of any adverse effects. Ten years later, Kossoff[10] described a catheter tip transducer of 2 mm diameter and operating frequency of 8 MHz for measuring intracardiac septal and ventricular wall thickness with an accuracy of up to 0.1 mm. He mentioned the movement of the catheter in the cardiac chamber as one of the problems. Peronneau[11] pointed out that the cavity to be measured does not generally have the form of a 'surface of revolution', and that two opposite acoustic elements instead of one should be mounted at the tip of the catheter. Carleton and co-workers[12,13] applied a 2.5 MHz cylindrical element of 3.1 mm outer diameter and radiating through a 360° arc. He distinguished two echoes, from the distances of the shortest and longest elements to the cardiac chamber wall from which he derived the chamber diameter in experiments in dogs. He suggested the need for adding a forward-looking echo element.

In 1969, Stegall et al.[14] introduced two transducers (0.7 × 1.5 mm) mounted at the end of a catheter-carried 'feeler gage' to determine intra-aortic and intracarotid diameter. It was a transit-time system operating at around 5 MHz. Another technique proposed by Kardon et al.[15] involved ultrasonic transit-time measurement between two elements mounted at a distance on a catheter. The catheter had to be manipulated so that it came to rest in a predetermined loop inside the ventricle.

The principle of a transducer mounted at the tip of a catheter from which the beam scans structures which are aligned perpendicularly to it offers the simplest approach to cross-sectional imaging with ultrasound. If the transducer rotates in synchrony with a display time-base, radial scanning produces cross-sectional images perpendicular to the catheter. This rotational technique was already used by Wild and Reid[16] for transrectal scanning of the prostate. Omoto[17] used an intravenous probe with a guide wire tip to study cardiac structures, and Ebina et al.[18] described in 1967 a miniature concave transducer for rotation inside a rubber cuff positioned in the esophagus. In 1966 Wells[19] proposed the first design of a practical intravenous probe with mechanical rotation and a flexible shaft for rotational real-time cross-sectional scanning: 'The probe must be of sufficiently small dimensions to permit easy insertion into the vein... .' Eggleton et al.[20] approximated a cardiac cross-section by rotating a four-element catheter. Results of their system depended on a stable condition of the heart since data had to be accumulated over many beats for reconstruction of a cardiac cross-section. All these early attempts proved to be of limited diagnostic use. The stiffness of the catheter and the size of the transducer assembly, the poor image quality, the long transmission pulse which blurs the near field structures and the slow acquisition time all impaired their practical implementation. As early as 1969 Bom et al.[21] initiated a research program to develop invasive real-time and cross-sectional ultrasonic imaging using state-of-the-art technology. A 32-element circular phased array with an outer diameter of 3.2 mm mounted at the tip of a 9 F. catheter was constructed. As pointed out in the original paper, the array design was a compromise between the optimal design and the limitations imposed by technological constraints. The final design was chosen to operate at 5.6 MHz with a narrow main beam. With this catheter, in 1975, real-time intraluminal images such as left ventricular cross-sections were recorded in animal experiments. A serious limitation in the images originated from the grating lobes in the directivity pattern, and the catheter size and its steerability.

Recent developments

Intravascular and, more particularly, intracoronary ultrasound require both a small transducer assembly

and a catheter delivery system with optimal steerability and flexibility. Different approaches have been used.

Electronic multielement systems

A multielement phased array with an integrated circuit for initial echo-data processing at the catheter tip was described in 1989.[22] This design allows a reduction in the number of electrical wires and thus a smaller-size catheter with better flexibility. The introduction of a movable guide wire would offer advantages during catheterization.

The main problem inherent in phased-array technology is that it is both complicated and relatively expensive. Lack of resolution and a dead zone for imaging as a result of the 'ringdown' artefact in the near field put limitations on circular phased-array systems for imaging of smaller diameter vessels and critical stenoses. However, considerable improvements to the image quality have been made over the years, mainly by replacing the synthetic transducer material by piezoelectric crystals.

Mechanical single-element systems

Circumferential scanning with a single transducer remains the simplest approach to cross-sectional imaging. Based on this principle several investigators followed Wells[19] and have designed and constructed an ultrasonic catheter for real-time intravascular imaging.[23–27] When the transducer is mounted in the axis of a catheter, the ultrasound beam can be swept around in a plane perpendicular to the catheter's long axis either by rotating the transducer or rotating an acoustic mirror in front of it (in a manner similar to the display of light from a lighthouse) to obtain a 360° display of the arterial cross-section. The center frequencies used for catheter-tip imaging range between 20 and 40 MHz.

Despite the greater attenuation with distance of the higher-frequency ultrasound, these catheters are suitable for imaging of small arteries, such as coronary arteries, and both the catheter and transducer assembly are sufficiently small to allow catheterization of small arteries. The cross-sectional lumen area which can be visualized is only limited by the catheter size but the need for a drive shaft restricts both the steerability and flexibility. This problem could be solved by positioning a micromotor at the distal end of the catheter. Prototypes of a motor with 1 mm outer diameter have been constructed, driving a small acoustic mirror in saline at uniform rotational speed.[28]

Table 2.1 Characteristics and relative advantages of different intravascular ultrasonic imaging techniques.

Property	I	II	III	IV
Frame rate	+	+	++	+++
Signal-to-noise ratio	++	+++	+++	+++
Near-field beam definition	—	+	++	++
Far-field beam definition	++	++	+	+
Focusing applicable	+++	+	++	++
Size transducer assembly	+	+	++	+
Catheter shaft size	+++	+	++	+++
Combined imaging/ therapeutic procedure	++	—	+	++
Scanning position control	+++	—	—	++
Combination with Doppler	++	—	—	++

I: Electronic multielement; II: rotating single element; III: rotating mirror, static element; IV: motor driven mirror, static element.

It is not clear which of these approaches will ultimately prove to become the optimal design, but it may well be that each of these systems may have advantages for a specific application. Characteristics of the different intravascular scanning techniques are shown in Table 2.1. The study of larger arteries and intracardiac imaging will require lower-frequency transducers to be used than those intended for detailed coronary artery studies. The data presented in this volume indicate that intravascular ultrasound imaging is feasible, safe, and provides useful clinical information.

Intravascular Doppler techniques

The frequency shift in reflected ultrasound waves allows us to measure blood velocity. A number of approaches have been described where Doppler methods were carried out through catheter mounting of the transducers.

Stegall described in 1967[29] a continuous-wave Doppler catheter which was used for instantaneous phasic coronary blood velocity measurement. A pulsed Doppler catheter tip version was introduced by Reid and co-workers in 1974.[30] The echo part could be inserted down the center of a 7 F. catheter.

Measurements were made in coronary and femoral arteries in dogs. Smaller sizes of catheter such as 5 F. and high-frequency (20 MHz) ultrasound were introduced by Hartley and Cole[31] in 1974. They suggested an annular element. This paved the way for Sibley et al.[32] to combine this with a guide wire 12 years later.

Although mechanical rotation for imaging was introduced earlier, Gichard and Auth[33] first described in 1975 a catheter construction with a rotating echo element mounted on a rotating flexible shaft for Doppler purposes. The diameter of the probe was 3 mm. This paved the way towards mechanically rotating catheter tip imaging devices.

Further concepts included work by Martin et al.[34] to combine a forward-sampling Doppler (at 15 MHz) with transverse vessel area measurement in order to calculate blood flow. They also described an echo tip assembly with the possibility of using an inflatable balloon. All currently clinically utilized Doppler flow velocity catheters make use of range-gated principles sampling blood flow velocity a short distance distal from the crystal at a frequency of 20 MHz.

Doppler catheters provide measurement of blood flow velocity only in the longer coronary arteries and are sensitive to any changes in lumen area, flow velocity profile and angulation. Because of their size relative to the size of the arteries and stenoses, they cause significant flow disturbances. Recently a low-profile (0.018 and 0.014 inch) Doppler angioplasty guide wire (175 cm long) with a 12 MHz or 15 MHz ultrasound transducer integrated onto its tip and with a real-time spectral analysis system has been introduced.[35]

New ideas have appeared to use the speckle changes in the cross-sectional image of an intravascular imaging catheter to calculate blood flow. Rapid changes occur in areas with high blood velocity and slow changes in areas with slow blood flow. All this information integrated over the entire cross-section might result in a measurement of volume flow.

Combination techniques

Given the great interest in on-line guiding and monitoring of intravascular interventions, there has been a great impetus to develop ultrasound imaging and therapeutic catheter hybrids.

A combination of forward-looking echo elements with laser ablation through a central fiber was described by Webster.[36] Another ultrasound-guided laser angioplasty system was described by Angelsen and Linker.[37] Crowley et al.[38] have also described a prototype photo-acoustic ablation catheter.

The combination of ultrasound imaging with atherectomy was suggested by Yock.[39] A mechanically rotating transducer and a rotating cutting element are incorporated in a catheter with an added guiding tip. An inflatable balloon can be used to press the atherectomy cutter towards the arterial obstruction.

Slager and colleagues[40] described a recanalization method based on spark erosion. This can be used in a selective way to evaporate atherosclerotic plaque and other obstructions. They suggested a number of combinations with echo. The transducer and the rotating beam-deflecting mirror create the cross-sectional image. On the opposite side of the rotating tip a spark electrode can be positioned. Thus spark electrode and visualized obstruction are almost in the same plane. A number of hybrid catheters combining intravascular ultrasound imaging and balloon percutaneous transluminal coronary angioplasty (PTCA) systems have also been described.[41] There is now a combined balloon dilatation and ultrasound imaging catheter commercially available (Endosonics Corp., Pleasanton, CA) but the assembly does not allow imaging of the vessel wall through the balloon. Since directly imaging through the balloon would have many advantages, transparent balloon material is being searched for. Other combination devices include the echo Doppler tip with a PTCA balloon catheter as described by Serruys et al.[42]

References

1   Fisher LD, Judkins MP, Lesperance J et al. Reproducibility of coronary arteriographic reading in the coronary artery surgery study (CASS). *Cathet Cardiovasc Diag* 1982; **8**: 565–75.

2   Siegel RJ, Swan K, Edwalds G, Fishbein MC. Limitations of post-mortem assessment of human coronary artery size and luminal narrowing: differential effects of tissue fixation and processing on vessels with different degrees of atherosclerosis. *J Am Coll Cardiol* 1985; **5**: 342–6.

3   Pignoli P, Tremoli HE, Poli A, Oreste P, Paoletti R. Intimal plus medial thickness of the arterial wall: a direct measurement with ultrasound imaging. *Circulation* 1986; **74**: 1399–406.

4   Blankenhorn DH, Chin HP, Conover DJ, Nessim SA. Ultrasound observation on pulsation in human carotid artery lesions. *Ultrasound Med Biol* 1988; **14**: 583–7.

5   Taams MA, Gussenhoven EJ, Cornel JH et al. Detection of left coronary artery stenosis by transesophageal echocardiography. *Eur Heart J* 1988; **9**:1162–6.

6   McPherson DD, Hiratzka LF, Lamberth WC et al. Delineation of the extent of coronary atheroclerosis by high-frequency epicardial. *N Engl J Med* 1987; **316**: 304–9.

7   Forrester JS, Litvack F, Grundfest W, Hickey AI. A perspective of coronary disease seen through the arteries of living man. *Circulation* 1987; **75**: 505–13.

8   Forrester JS, Litvack F, Grundfest W, Segalowitz J, Hickey AI. Cardiac angioscopy in acute ischemic syndromes. *Am J Card Imaging* 1988; **2**:178–84.

9   Cieszynski T. Intracardiac method for the investigation of structure of the heart with the aid of ultrasonics. *Arch Immun Ter Dow* 1960; **8**: 551–7.

10   Kossoff G. Diagnostic applications of ultrasound in cardiology. *Australas Radiol* 1966; **X**: 101–6.

11   Peronneau P. Catheter with piezoelectric transducer. US Patent no. 3 542 014, 1970.

12   Carleton RA, Sessions RW, Graettinger JS. Diameter of heart measured by intracavitary ultrasound. *Med Res Eng* 1969; May/June: 28–32.

13 Carleton RA, Clark JG. Measurement of left ventricular diameter in the dog by cardiac catheterization. Validation and physiologic meaningfulness of an ultrasonic technique. *Circ Res* 1968; **22**: 545–58.

14 Stegall HF, Pratt JR, Moser PF. Carotid mechanics in situ. *Fed Proc* 1969; **28**: 585.

15 Kardon MB, O'Rourke RA, Bishop VS. Measurement of left ventricular internal diameter by catheterization. *J Appl Physiol* 1971; **31**: 613–15.

16 Wild JJ, Reid JM. Progress in techniques of soft tissue examination by MC pulsed ultrasound. In: Kelly E, ed. *Ultrasound in Medicine and Biology* (Washington: American Institute of Biological Sciences, 1950): 30.

17 Omoto R. Intracardiac scanning of the heart with the aid of ultrasonic intravenous probe. *Jpn Heart J* 1967; **8**: 569–81.

18 Ebina T, Oka S, Tanaka M et al. The diagnostic application of ultrasound to the disease in mediastinal organs. Ultrasono-tomography for the heart and great vessels. *Sci Rep Res Inst Tohoku Univ* 1965; **12**: 199–212.

19 Wells PNT. Developments in medical ultrasonics. *World Medical Electronics* 1966; **66,4**: 272–7.

20 Eggleton RC, Townsend C, Kossoff G et al. Computerized ultrasonic visualization of dynamic ventricular configurations. *Proceedings of the eighth ICMBE, July 1969* (Chicago: Palmer House): 87.

21 Bom N, Lancée CT, van Egmond FC. An ultrasonic intracardiac scanner. *Ultrasonics* 1972; **10**: 72–6, and US Patent no. 1 402 192, 1973.

22 Hodgson J McB, Graham SD, Savakus AD et al. Clinical percutaneous imaging of coronary anatomy using an over-the-wire ultrasound catheter system. *Int J Card Imaging* 1989; **4**: 187-93.

23 Mallery JA, Gregory K, Morcos NC et al. Evaluation of an ultrasound balloon dilatation imaging catheter. *Circulation* 1987; **76**: IV371 (abst).

24 Yock PG, Linker DT, Thapliyal HV et al. Real-time, two-dimensional catheter ultrasound: a new technique for high-resolution intravascular imaging. *J Am Coll Cardiol* 1988; **11**: 130A (abst).

25 Bom N, Lancée CT, Slager CJ, de Jong N. Ein Weg zur intraluminaren Echoarteriographie. *Ultraschall Med* 1987; **8**: 233–6.

26 Pandian NG, Kreis A, Brockway B et al. Ultrasound angioscopy: real-time, two-dimensional, intraluminal ultrasound imaging of blood vessels. *Am J Cardiol* 1988; **62**: 493–4.

27 Roelandt JR, Bom N, Serruys PW, Gussenhoven WJ, Lancée CT, Sutherland GR. Intravascular high-resolution real-time cross-sectional echocardiography. *Echocardiography* 1989; **1**: 9–16.

28 Lancée CT, Bom N, Roelandt J. Future directions in intravascular ultrasound: from micro-motors to imaging guidewire systems. *Echocardiography* 1995; **12**: 275–81.

29 Stegall HF, Stone HL, Bishop VS, Laenger C. A catheter-tip pressure and velocity sensor. *Proc 20th Ann Conf Eng Med Biol* 1967; **27**: 4 (abst).

30 Reid JM, Davis DL, Ricketts HJ, Spencer MP. A new Doppler flowmeter system and its operation with catheter mounted transducers. In: Reneman RS, ed. *Cardiovascular Applications of Ultrasound* (Amsterdam/London: North Holland Publishing Co., 1974): 183–92.

31 Hartley CJ, Cole JS. A single-crystal ultrasonic catheter-tip velocity probe. *Med Instrum* 1974; **8**: 241–3.

32 Sibley DH, Millar HD, Hartley CJ, Whitlow PL. Subselective measurement of coronary blood flow velocity using a steerable Doppler catheter. *J Am Coll Cardiol* 1986; **8**: 1332–40.

33 Gichard FD, Auth DC. Development of a mechanically scanned Doppler blood flow catheter. *IEEE Ultrasonics Symp Proc* (New York: IEEE, 1975): 306–9.

34 Martin RW, Pollack GH, Philips J. An ultrasonic catheter tip instrument for measuring volume blood flow. *IEEE Ultrasonics Symp Proc* (New York: IEEE, 1975): 301–5.

35 Segal J, Kern MJ, Seolt NA et al. Alterations of phasic coronary artery flow velocity in humans during percutaneous transluminal coronary angioplasty. *J Am Coll Cardiol* 1992; **20**: 276–86.

36 Webster WW. Catheter for removing arteriosclerotic plaque. International patent PCT/US84/00474, 1984.

37 Angelsen BAJ, Linker D. Laser catheter delivery system for controled atheroma ablation combining laser angioplasty and intra-arterial ultrasonic imaging. US Patent 4 887 605, 1989.

38 Crowley RJ, Hamm MA, Joshi SH, Lennox CD, Roberts GT. Ultrasound guided therapeutic catheters: recent developments and clinical results. *Int J Card Imaging* 1991; **6**: 146–56.

39 Yock PG. Catheter apparatus. European Patent no. 0234951, 1987.

40 Slager CJ, Essed CE, Schuurbiers JCH, Bom N, Serruys PW, Meester GT. Vaporization of atherosclerotic plaques by spark erosion. *J Am Coll Cardiol* 1985; **5**: 1382–6.

41 Hodgson JM, Cacchione JG, Berry J, Savakus AD, Eberle M. Combined intracoronary ultrasound imaging and angioplasty catheter: initial in vivo studies. *Circulation* 1990; **82**: III676 (abst).

42 Serrruys PW, Jullière Y, Zijlstra F et al. Coronary blood flow velocity during percutaneous transluminal coronary angioplasty as guide for assessment of the functional result. *Am J Cardiol* 1988; **61**: 253–9.

3 Technical aspects of intravascular ultrasound

Lothar Koch and Thomas Roth

Introduction

The application of ultrasound in medical diagnosis has increased considerably due to the miniaturization of ultrasonic transducers. The use of ultrasound catheters in vessels (intravascular ultrasound, IVUS) produces high-resolution cross-sectional images of the vessel thus providing information on the vascular wall and its pathology. This information is especially important for the application of new interventional devices in cardiology. The knowledge of the basic principles of ultrasound physics and image formation in the IVUS equipment will help in the interpretation of IVUS images. It is hoped that the following brief remarks on the technical aspects of intravascular ultrasound will be of use to physicians. For more detailed information on medical ultrasound the reader is referred to the references.[1-7]

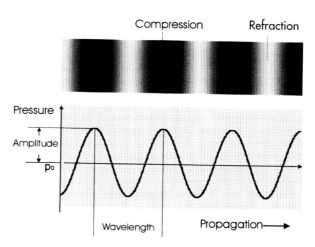

Figure 3.1. Longitudinal wave. Sound travels through a medium in the form of compression waves.

Sound waves

Sound waves are compression waves in gas, liquids, or bulk material. The direction of propagation of the wave coincides with the direction of the vibration of the particles in the medium (longitudinal waves, Fig. 3.1). (In bulk material transversal waves may also be created, where the particles move perpendicular to the direction of the propagation of the wave; in liquids there are also surface waves.) Ultrasound is sound with frequencies above the audible range, that is, above 20 kHz. In medical diagnostics the frequencies are in the range of a few MHz.

The propagation speed c of sound waves in a medium is determined by its bulk modulus E and density ρ:

$$c = \sqrt{\frac{E}{\rho}} \tag{1}$$

The less compressible a material, the higher the speed of sound.

The intensity I of the sound wave at a given point, that is, the flow of energy through the unit area at this point is related to the pressure amplitude p by

$$I = \frac{p^2}{2 \cdot \rho c} \tag{2}$$

The physical property of a medium which determines the reflection of sound waves is its acoustic impedance Z, the product of the propagation velocity c and density ρ:

$$Z = c \cdot \rho \tag{3}$$

Some numerical values for the speed of ultrasound and acoustic impedance are given in Table 3.1.

Table 3.1 **Speed and acoustic impedance in various materials.**[6]		
Material	**Speed (m/s)**	**Acoustic impedance (10^6 kg/m² per second)**
Air	330	0.0004
Water (20 °C)	1 480	1.48
Blood	1 570	1.61
Muscle	1 580	1.70
Fat	1 450	1.38
Bone	3 500	7.80

Table 3.2 **Wavelength in soft tissue at different frequencies.**	
ν (MHz)	λ (mm)
2	0.77
5	0.31
7	0.22
10	0.15
20	0.08
30	0.05

The wavelength λ, the distance of two consecutive points of equal pressure, is related to frequency ν and the propagation speed c as follows:

$$\lambda = \frac{c}{\nu} \qquad (4)$$

For a given medium, the higher the frequency, the smaller the wavelength. Some numerical values for wavelengths of ultrasound in soft tissue (propagation speed $c = 1540$ m/s) are given in Table 3.2.

The propagation of a sound wave in tissue is influenced by physical effects of which the most important are reflection, refraction, scattering, and absorption.

Reflection and refraction

As a sound wave passes from one medium into another with a different acoustic impedance, a part of the incident wave is reflected at the boundary and a part spreads in the second medium, generally with an altered direction of propagation (Fig. 3.2).

The angle α_3 of the reflected part of the wave is equal to the angle α_1 of the incident wave. The angle α_2 of the direction of propagation of the refracted, transmitted part of the wave depends on the velocities of sound c_1 and c_2 in the two media and is given by Snell's Law:

$$\frac{\sin(\alpha_1)}{\sin(\alpha_2)} = \frac{c_1}{c_2} \qquad (5)$$

As the ultrasound speeds in biological soft tissues are very similar there is only a little deviation from the direction of the incident wave which often may be ignored.

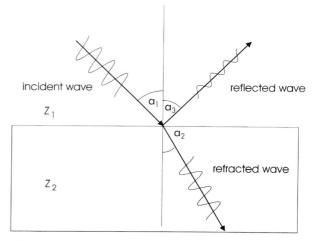

Figure 3.2. Reflection and refraction. Part of the incident wave is reflected at the boundary between medium 1 and medium 2; part of the wave is refracted and propagates in medium 2.

The reflection coefficient R, that is, the ratio of the reflected intensity I_R and the incident intensity I_I, is determined by the acoustic impedances Z_1, Z_2 of the two media, the incident angle α_1 and the angle of refraction α_2:

$$R = \frac{I_R}{I_I} = \frac{(Z_2 \cdot \cos(\alpha_1) - Z_1 \cdot \cos(\alpha_2))^2}{(Z_2 \cdot \cos(\alpha_1) + Z_1 \cdot \cos(\alpha_2))^2} \qquad (6)$$

or

$$R = \frac{\left(Z_2 \cdot \cos(\alpha_1) - \rho_1 \cdot \sqrt{c_1^2 - c_2^2 \cdot \sin^2(\alpha_1)}\right)^2}{\left(Z_2 \cdot \cos(\alpha_1) + \rho_1 \cdot \sqrt{c_1^2 - c_2^2 \cdot \sin^2(\alpha_1)}\right)^2} \qquad (7)$$

In the special case of normal incidence of the sound wave on the boundary ($\alpha_1 = 0°$) the calculation of the reflection coefficient R is simpler:

$$R = \frac{(Z_2 - Z_1)^2}{(Z_2 + Z_1)^2} \qquad (8)$$

The acoustic impedances of different soft tissues are only slightly different, so that the reflection coefficients are very small (typically 1%, Table 3.3.). At boundaries between soft tissue and bone or air a substantial part of the incident energy is reflected. (It should be noted that the value of the reflection coefficient is the same for moving from medium 1 to medium 2 and for moving from medium 2 to medium 1; the only difference is a phaseshift of π in the reflected wave when reflected on a medium of higher acoustic impedance.)

Reflection and refraction describe the phenomena at smooth boundaries with large dimensions compared to the wavelength. If the boundary is not smooth (that is, its roughness is comparable to the dimensions of the wavelength) parts of the incoming wave are reflected in different directions, so in addition to the directed specular reflection there is nondirectional diffuse reflection (Fig. 3.3.).

Scattering

If in a medium the sound wave strikes a discontinuity of dimensions comparable with or smaller than the wavelength, part of the intensity of the wave is scattered in all directions. These discontinuities (scattering centers) are local changes in compressibility, density, or both. The scattered parts of the wave resulting from the randomly distributed different scatterers superimpose. Depending on the phase relations of the contributing scattered waves at a given point there may be enhancement of the intensity or the waves may cancel. Tissue is a grainy medium, because it is composed of cells. The scattering in the grainy medium is the reason that homogeneous regions of tissue show a 'speckle' structure in ultrasound images (Fig. 3.4).

Absorption and attenuation

Besides the loss of energy due to scattering and reflection a sound wave propagating in tissue loses energy mainly by absorption. The mechanical energy of the wave is transformed into heat which is dissipated within the medium. The absorption depends on the medium and strongly increases with frequencies in the frequency range used in medical diagnosis.

Table 3.3 **Coefficients of reflection (%) for perpendicular incidence calculated with values from Table 3.1.**

	Fat	Blood	Muscle	Bone
Air	99.88	99.90	99.90	99.98
Fat		0.59	1.08	48.90
Blood			0.07	43.20
Muscle				41.20

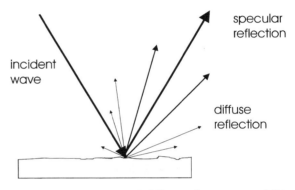

Figure 3.3. Specular and diffuse reflection. In addition to the directed specular reflection there is also nondirectional diffuse reflection at rough surfaces. Parts of the incoming wave are reflected in different directions.

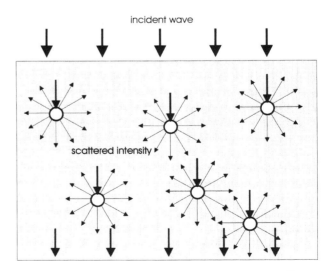

Figure 3.4. Scattering. In a medium containing small discontinuities (indicated by the circles) part of the intensity of the wave is scattered in all directions.

The dependencies of the amplitude A and of the intensity I of the wave on the traveled distance are described by the exponential laws:

$$A = A_0 \cdot e^{-(\gamma s)} \tag{9}$$

$$I = I_0 \cdot e^{-(2 \cdot \gamma s)} \tag{10}$$

The absorption coefficient is designated γ; normally its units are dB/cm. (The notation dB (decibel) is a logarithmic measure for ratios and is defined as follows: $A = 10*\log(I/I_0)$ dB. The value -3 dB means $I/I_0 = 0.7$; -6 dB: $I/I_0 = 0.5$; -20 dB: $I/I_0 = 0.01$; $+6$ dB: $I/I_0 = 2$; $+20$ dB: $I/I_0 = 100$.) There is also a loss of intensity due to the spreading of the ultrasonic beam.

Table 3.4 shows some numerical values for attenuation coefficients.

Table 3.4 **Attenuation coefficients for different tissues at 1 MHz.**[6]	
Tissue	**Attenuation coefficient (dB/cm)**
Blood	0.2
Muscle	1.5
Bone	10.0
Fat	0.6

Generation and detection of ultrasound waves

For the generation of ultrasound waves in medical diagnostics the piezoelectric effect is used. Certain crystals such as PZT (lead zirconate–titanate) have the property of changing their geometric form when a voltage is applied to their surfaces. They transform ('transduce') an electrical signal into mechanical movement. If the crystal (transducer) is excited with a continuous wave voltage signal it will mechanically vibrate. This vibration will create a compression wave in the surrounding medium. The piezoelectric effect is reversible: if a pressure wave strikes the crystal weak electrical signals are induced; the crystal can act as a microphone.

For imaging with the pulse echo method (see below), short ultrasound pulses are needed. In this case a short voltage pulse is applied to the crystal. The crystal will start vibrating and it will continue to ring even after the voltage pulse has already ceased. The length of the ultrasound pulse is determined by the ringing of the crystal. Strong damping is applied to the crystal by bonding some damping material to its back surface. This damping will reduce the length of the ultrasound pulse to a few cycles (Fig. 3.5).

Generally, the same element is used for the generation and detection of ultrasound. To detect the returning echoes one has to wait until the ringing amplitude of the crystal has dropped below the

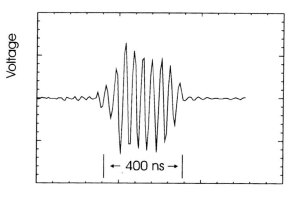

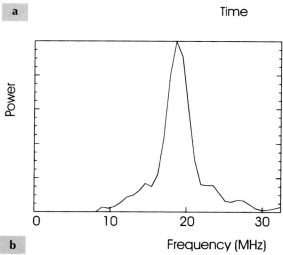

Figure 3.5. (a) Ultrasound pulse of a 20 MHz transducer; (b) power spectrum of the ultrasound pulse.

small amplitudes of the expected echoes. This causes an 'acoustic dead zone' immediately in front of the transducer in which no echoes can be detected.

The pulse echo method

An ultrasonic transducer is excited with a short voltage pulse and creates a short ultrasound pulse which travels as directed through the tissue. If the pulse reaches a boundary between two different tissues a part of the pulse is reflected and travels back towards the transducer. These echoes are then received by the transducer, now acting as a microphone, and create a voltage signal (Fig. 3.6). The delay τ between the transmitted pulse and received echo depends on the ultrasound speed c and the traveled distance of the echo. If the sound velocity is known, the distance between the transducer and the reflecting boundary may be calculated:

$$d = \frac{1}{2} \cdot c \cdot \tau \tag{11}$$

With a velocity of sound in blood and soft tissue of approximately 1500 m/s, an echo delay of 1 µs corresponds to a traveling distance of 1.5 mm and the distance of the reflecting boundary is 0.75 mm.

The largest echo amplitudes in the echo signals result from specular reflections at boundaries between different tissues. These very strong echoes may only be received by the transducer when the ultrasound beam is almost perpendicular to the boundary. If this is not the case the specular echo will miss the transducer, but, because most of the boundaries are rough, weaker echoes resulting from diffuse reflection are detected. Further weak echoes result from scattering of ultrasound waves at inhomogeneities within the tissues.

When moving the transducer different regions are scanned. By transforming the amplitude values of the echo signal into intensity values and combining the scans received during the movement of the transducer a two-dimensional cross-sectional image of the investigated region can be generated (Fig. 3.7).

Ultrasonic fields and beams

The shape of the ultrasonic field depends on the relation of the dimensions of the transducer compared to the wavelength. If the sound source is small compared to wavelength concentric radial waves are radiated. In the case of a large sound source highly directed planar waves are emitted. If the dimensions of the source are comparable to the wavelength the ultrasonic field is determined by diffraction and can show a complex shape. For a disc-shaped transducer element oscillating at a definite frequency the pressure amplitude along the transducer axis is given by:

$$p(z) = p_0 \cdot \sin\left(\frac{\pi}{\lambda} \cdot \left(\sqrt{d^2 + z^2} - z\right)\right) \tag{12}$$

where p_0 is the maximal pressure amplitude, z the distance along the axis, and d the diameter of the disc (Fig. 3.8).

Up to a distance of $d^2/(4\lambda)$ in front of the transducer there are rapid oscillations of the intensity. This region is known as the near field or Fresnel zone. Beyond this region, in the far field, or Frauenhofer zone, the intensity decreases at the inverse square of

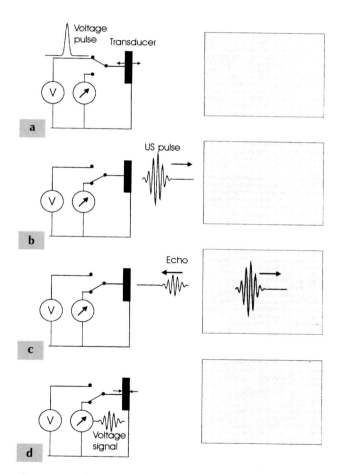

Figure 3.6. The pulse echo method. **(a)** An ultrasonic transducer is excited with a short voltage pulse. A short ultrasound pulse is generated. **(b)** The ultrasound pulse travels as directed through medium 1. **(c)** At the boundary between medium 1 and medium 2 a part of the pulse intensity is reflected and travels back towards the transducer. **(d)** As the echo strikes the transducer a voltage signal is generated. From the delay between the transmitted pulse and the received echo the distance between the transducer and the reflecting boundary may be calculated.

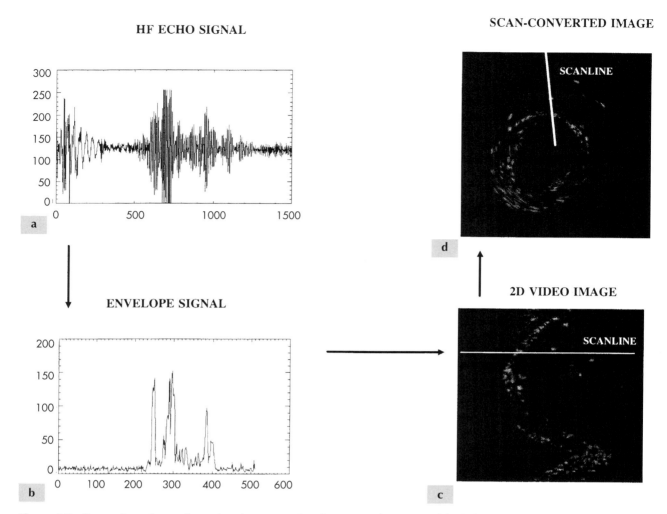

Figure 3.7. Generation of two-dimensional cross-sectional images. The received high-frequency echo signal (**a**) is demodulated to obtain the envelope signal (**b**). This signal is then digitized giving the intensity information of one scanline. The scanlines generated during the movement of the transducer are combined in a two-dimensional image (**c**). For IVUS this image has to be scan-converted to obtain the correct display (**d**).

the distance. In the near field the ultrasonic beam is parallel, its diameter corresponding to the diameter of the crystal. In the far field the beam is diverging with an angle of divergence φ, given by

$$\sin(\varphi) = 1.22 \cdot \frac{\lambda}{d} \tag{13}$$

For a transducer of 0.7 mm diameter and a frequency of 20 MHz in water (wavelength about 0.08 mm) the near field extends to about 1.5 mm and the beam is diverging at about 8° (values for a frequency of 30 MHz are: near field 2.5 mm, divergence 5°).

If the transducer is not used in continuous mode but excited with an electrical pulse it does not emit a single frequency but a frequency band. In this case the resulting ultrasonic field results from a superposition

of the contributions of the single frequency components. The superposition leads to strong reduction of amplitude fluctuations in the near field (Fig. 3.9).

Although the ultrasonic beam shape may be calculated for arbitrary transducer geometry an exact knowledge is achieved only by measurement, since the beam shape is influenced by the mounting of the crystal.

The region from which the transducer receives echoes when it acts as a microphone has the same shape as the ultrasonic beam. The local distribution of the total sensitivity of the transducer in pulse echo mode is calculated by multiplying the local distribution of receiving sensitivity with the beam intensity distribution.

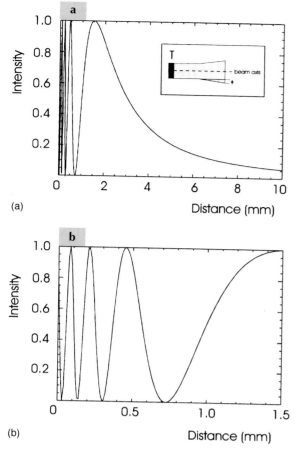

(a)

(b)

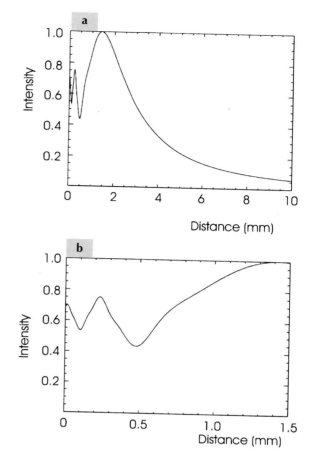

Figure 3.8. Intensity distribution on transducer axis for a circular transducer with a diameter of 0.7 mm and a frequency of 20 MHz. The near field extends to $d^2/(4\lambda)$ = 1.5 mm. The beam shape is sketched in the insert in (a). The angle of divergence φ is 8°. (b) Enlarged display of the intensity distribution in the near field. (T = transducer.)

Figure 3.9. (a) Intensity distribution on transducer axis for a circular transducer with a diameter of 0.7 mm in pulsed mode. The distribution was calculated for the pulse displayed in Fig. 3.5. (b) Enlarged display of the intensity distribution in the near field. The amplitude fluctuations in the near field are reduced.

Resolution

The resolution of an imaging technique measures its ability to display separately objects which are separated by only a small distance. The lateral resolution of IVUS, that is, the resolution perpendicular to the beam axis, is directly related to the beam cross-section. If a point-like scattering object, for example, a small metal sphere, is moved in front of the transducer an echo signal is received as long as the object is within the beam. The signal is largest in the center of the beam and decreases towards the borders. The point-like object is thus smeared out to a longitudinal zone in the imaging.

If a second object is brought close to the first object their reflections start to overlap if their distance is smaller than the beam width. If the objects further approach each other they can no longer be separated into single objects in the image. Usually, the numerical value for the resolution is taken to be the object distance at which the signal decrease in the center of the overlap is still one-half of the maximal amplitude (Fig. 3.10). A typical value for lateral resolution of a 20 MHz catheter is 0.5 mm.

The axial resolution is determined by the length of the ultrasound pulse. A point reflector is smeared out in time. If the reflections of two objects placed in a row overlap in time they cannot be separated in the receiver (Fig. 3.11). The shorter the pulse length, the better the axial resolution. The axial resolution of a transducer is generally better than its lateral resolution: it is approximately 0.2 mm for a

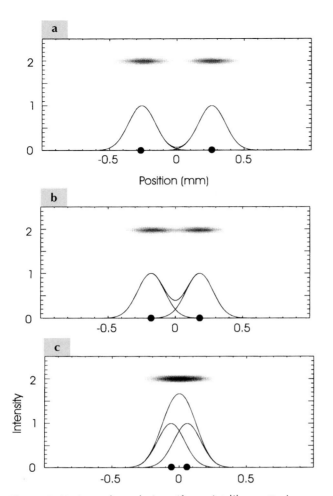

Figure 3.10. Lateral resolution. If a point-like scattering object, for example a small metal sphere, is moved in front of the transducer an echo signal is received as long as the object is within the beam (**a**). If a second object is brought close to the first object their reflections start to overlap if their distance is smaller than the beam width (**b**). If the objects further approach each other they can no longer be separated into single objects in the image (**c**). The appearance of the echoes in the video image is shown schematically in each diagram.

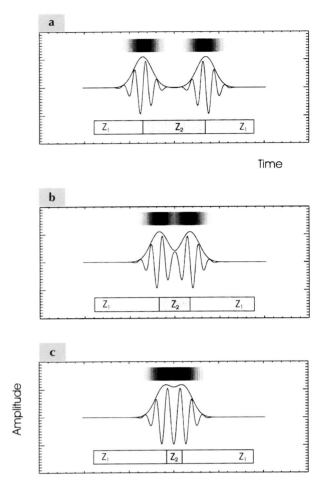

Figure 3.11. Axial resolution. The axial resolution is determined by the length of the ultrasound pulse. The diagrams show schematically the reflection of an ultrasound pulse on two boundaries as indicated at the foot of each diagram. The boundaries are smeared out in time. If the reflections of the two boundaries overlap in time they cannot be separated in the receiver (**c**). The appearance of the boundaries in the video image is also shown schematically in each diagram.

20 MHz IVUS catheter. The lateral resolution in the outer parts of an IVUS image may become worse due to interpolation during the scan conversion process (see below).

IVUS system

Figure 3.12 shows a block schematic diagram of a typical IVUS system. The ultrasound transducer for imaging is integrated in the catheter tip. (The possible transducer configurations are discussed below.)

A clock oscillator controls the pulse repetition frequency and all timing in the machine. For real-time display, about 25 cross-sectional images per second are required. If the vessel is scanned with 250 scan lines for one cross-section the pulse repetition frequency has to be 6250 Hz; that is, the difference in time between two successive transmission pulses is 80 μs.

The transmitter generates a short voltage pulse, which is applied to the piezoelectric crystal in the transducer. Normally the amplitude (transmission power) and the duration (transmission frequency) of

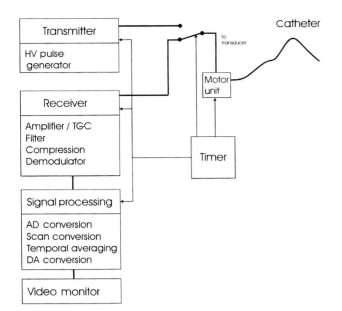

Figure 3.12. IVUS system schematic.

The echo signal is compressed by an adjustable logarithmic amplifier (compression) to avoid a loss of information when it is transformed into the video image. This is necessary because the human eye can only distinguish between about 200 gray levels whereas the dynamic range of the received signal is much larger (about 50 dB).

By demodulation an intensity signal (envelope signal) is derived from the high-frequency echo signal. The intensity signal is digitized, usually by 8-bit AD conversion, corresponding to 255 intensity levels. Further processing is carried out with the digital signal.

During the scanning of the vessel cross-section a series of intensity scan lines are generated, which have to be transformed geometrically for display (scan conversion, Fig. 3.13). Close to the transducer the single scans overlap whereas in large distances the cross-section may not be completely covered. Therefore during the transformation the intensity information of pixels close to the transducer is calculated by averaging over several scans; the brightness values of pixels in large distances for which there is no information available are interpolated from intensity values of adjacent scans.

It is possible to average over several consecutive images to increase image quality by reducing the image noise. (Temporal averaging, postprocessing, has the disadvantage that the display is not then able to follow rapid movements.)

The calculated two-dimensional cross-sectional image is displayed on a video monitor. Also, in this last stage of the processing, the image may be manipulated by changing the grayscale via an adjustable look-up table.

As the image is present in the system in digital form the actual image may be used as a still image (freeze). In the frozen image measurements of areas and distances may be made.

the exciting voltage pulse can be adjusted with the system. Typical values are: amplitude between 50 V and 100 V, duration between 100 ns and 30 ns, corresponding to transmission frequencies between 10 MHz and 30 MHz.

The receiver amplifies the small voltage signals which are generated as the returning echoes strike the transducer. As described earlier, an ultrasound pulse is attenuated as it travels through tissue. To compensate for this loss in echo amplitude for distant structures, a time-dependent amplification may be used (depth compensation, time gain compensation [TGC]). It is customary to have an additional control to adjust the global amplification (master gain, overall gain). Filters are implemented to reduce noise in the signals.

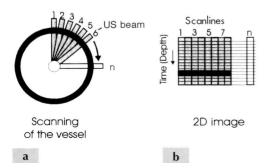

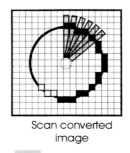

Figure 3.13. Scan conversion. The scanlines generated during the movement of the transducer (a) are combined in a two-dimensional array (b). This array has to be scan-converted to obtain the correct display (c).

IVUS catheter

The developments during recent years have led to flexible imaging catheters with diameters of 1–1.5 mm (3–5 F.) which are advanced into the coronary arteries using guide wires.[8] Transducers using ultrasound frequencies of between 10 MHz and 30 MHz are integrated into the catheter tip.

Different transducer technologies are available for construction of such catheters, each of them having special advantages and drawbacks. Possible configurations are mechanically scanned single-element or electronically scanned multielement transducers assembled in the catheter tip (Fig. 3.14).[9]

In catheters with a single element, either the crystal or a mirror in front of a stationary crystal is mechanically rotated. A real-time display of 25 cross-sectional images per second requires a rotational speed of 1500 revolutions per minute. The rotation is achieved by a flexible shaft which is driven by a motor at the proximal end of the catheter.

If used in highly tortuous vessels the friction of the drive-shaft may lead to nonuniform rotation producing a distortion of the image (rotation angle artifact, see below). A protection circuit switches off the motor if the friction becomes too great. A newly developed catheter with a micro-motor integrated in the catheter tip avoids the problems related to the use of a drive-shaft.[10]

Due to the 'ringdown' of the piezocrystal after excitation, imaging immediately at the surface of the crystal is not possible; there is an acoustic 'dead zone'. In catheters with rotating mirrors this dead zone is reduced due to the longer pathway of the ultrasound inside the catheter. This arrangement has the drawback that the mounting of the crystal and the electric wires connected to the crystal generate the dropout of an image sector by acoustic shadowing.

In catheters with a rotating single crystal or rotating mirror the region between the crystal and the sheath which is traveled by the ultrasound has to be filled with liquid to acquire optimal acoustic coupling. A certain reflection at the catheter sheath is inevitable.

In array systems (suggested as early as 1972 by Bom et al.[11]) single elements or groups of single elements are electronically switched to scan the cross-section of the vessel; their advantage is the lack of any moving parts. To achieve good lateral resolution a large number of single elements (up to 64) have to be assembled in the array cylindrically around the catheter tip. It is then no longer possible to have individual connecting wires for each single element:

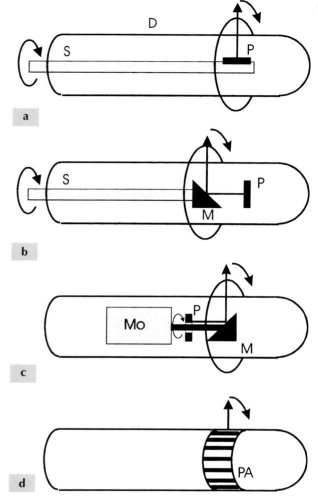

Figure 3.14. Catheter tip configurations: **(a)** rotating transducer, shaft-driven; **(b)** rotating deflecting mirror, shaft-driven; **(c)** rotating deflecting mirror, driven by micro-motor; **(d)** multielement array. (P: piezoelectric element; M: mirror; Mo: micro-motor; S: drive-shaft; PA: array of piezoelectric elements; D: sonolucent dome.)

the addressing of the single elements is done sequentially by a multiplexer integrated in the catheter tip.

It is difficult to obtain high-quality images with multielement arrays because their construction requires the use of PVDF (polvinylidine fluoride) as piezoelectric material. The piezoelectric parameters of this material are not as good as those of PZT (lead zirconate–titanate) used in single-element transducers. Also, the small dimensions of the single elements of the array are not optimal for beam geometry. There is an acoustic dead zone as the piezoelectric elements are just below the catheter sheath. Crosstalk between adjacent elements has to be avoided.

In the selection of frequency two aspects have to be taken into account. With increasing frequency the (axial) resolution increases, but the absorption also increases so that the penetration depth decreases. With frequencies above 30 MHz scattering on erythrocytes becomes important. The resonant frequency of a piezocrystal is determined by its geometry but the broadness of the resonant curve also allows the excitation with other frequencies away from the maximum. So, for example, a 30 MHz catheter can also be used at frequencies of 20 or 10 MHz with decreased performance.

IVUS image artifacts

Ringdown artifact

During the time period of the transmission pulse the receiver is electronically switched off to avoid an overload of its circuitry. When the receiver is opened again to detect returning echoes the trailing edge of the transmission pulse will show up in the image as a bright ring around the blank central region (Fig 3.15). The appearance of this ringdown artifact depends on the amplifier settings for near field gain.

The central black circular region (catheter blank) is generated electronically: it is not an 'image' of the catheter. This has to be taken into account when the diameter of this region is used as a reference for distance measurements: the measured diameter of the black circle may be larger than the geometrical diameter of the catheter.

Guide wire artifact

The guide wire may show up in the image as a bright echo signal if this is not centrally guided as in the array system (Fig. 3.15). Behind the guide wire is acoustic shadowing. New types of rotating crystal catheters allow a pullback of the transducer within the catheter sheath. While imaging with these catheters the guide wire is retracted proximal to the transducer so that the guide wire cannot disturb the image.

Acoustic shadowing

Behind calcified plaque there is acoustic shadowing, that is, no tissue is visible behind the plaque. This is because a great part of sound intensity is reflected at the boundaries between tissue and calcified plaque (Fig. 3.15).

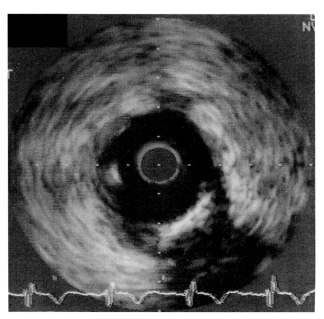

Figure 3.15. Acoustic shadowing: calcium present at five o'clock causes ultrasonic shadowing. Guide wire artifact: the bright spot in the lumen between eight and nine o'clock is the image of the guide wire. Ringdown artifact: the bright ring in the center of the image around the catheter blank is the ringdown artifact. It is caused by the detection of ringing of the crystal after excitation. (3.5 F. catheter; 20 MHz transducer; 1 mm calibration.)

If materials with high acoustic impedance are present multiple reflections may occur if the boundary is perpendicular to the beam. In this case, part of the returning echo is reflected by the catheter, travels back to the boundary, and is reflected again. The multiple echoes are equally spaced.

Echolucent zones

The interpretation of echolucent zones, regions in the image showing no speckle structure, is not always easy. Flowing blood and lipid pools appear to be homogenous for ultrasound frequencies up to about 30 MHz.

Position-related artifacts

For optimal imaging the catheter tip should be placed centrally in the vessel lumen and parallel to the vessel axis, which is not always feasible. In the case of a noncentral position the angle of incidence of the ultrasound on the vessel wall varies. Due to the dependency of reflection on incident angle the

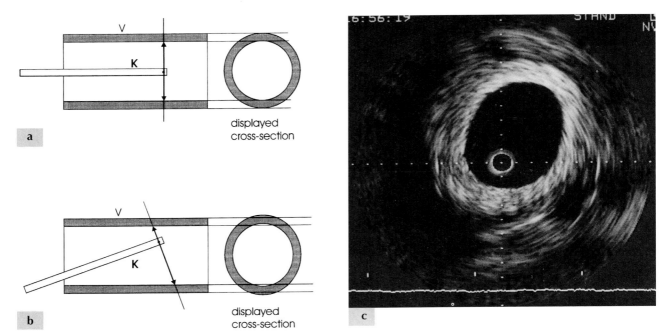

Figure 3.16. Schematic of the influence of the different catheter positions (**a+b**). If the catheter tip is not parallel to the vessel axis the cross-section of a vessel with circular shape will show an elliptical shape in the IVUS image. Figure 3.16(**c**) shows the elliptical shape of a circular-shaped, normal pig vessel ('in vitro'). In addition in the same image there is an intensity variation due to noncentral positioning of the catheter tip. Where the sound beam is almost perpendicular to the wall (around seven o'clock and one o'clock) the reflected intensity is higher. (4.8 F. catheter; 20 MHz transducer; 1 mm calibration.)

brightness of the vessel wall will vary around the cross-section even if the morphology of the vessel wall does not change (Fig. 3.16).

If the catheter tip is not parallel to the vessel axis the cross-section of a vessel with circular shape will show an elliptical shape in the IVUS image. This effect is only important in large vessels; in the coronary arteries the possible deviation is rather limited (Fig. 3.16).

System settings

Besides the position of the catheter tip the system settings (TGC, compression, etc.) have a strong influence on imaging. It is easier to compare different images if they were acquired with similar settings. The various possibilities for adjustment of the system make it difficult to classify tissue using brightness as the only parameter.

Rotation angle artifact

The friction of the drive-shaft used with mechanically rotated transducers may cause nonuniform rotation producing a distortion of the image. This

will lead to incorrect estimation of the angular extent of plaque (Fig. 3.17).

Movement artifacts

The pulsation of the heart often causes lateral movement of the catheter tip. As the complete cross-section is not acquired at once but scanned during one rotation of the ultrasound beam any motion of the catheter tip during this time will lead to a distortion in the display of the cross-section (Fig. 3.18).

Measurements

Distances measured in IVUS images are derived from measurements of the echo travel time. For calculations in the system a constant sound speed (generally the sound speed in blood) is used. The errors due to differences in sound speed may be neglected in soft tissues as the velocities are only slightly different. In calcium the speed of sound is almost twice as high. Calcified plaque is therefore displayed incorrectly with reduced thickness. In invitro studies one has to take into account that the sound velocity in water at 20 °C is about 6% smaller than that of blood at 37 °C.

Vessel cross-section   Displayed cross-section

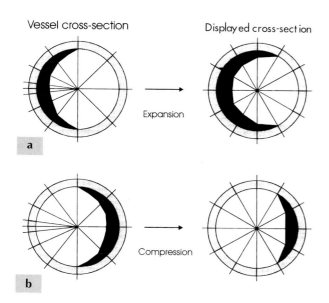

Figure 3.17. Rotation angle artifact. The friction of the drive-shaft used in mechanically rotated catheters may cause nonuniform rotation producing a distortion of the image. The left part of the diagram shows the actual vessel cross-sections; the lines indicate the direction of the ultrasound beam. The right part shows the displayed images; the lines indicate the scanlines used for scan conversion. **(a)** If the plaque (dark area) is in the region of low rotation speed it will be displayed expanded. **(b)** If the plaque is in the region of high rotation speed it will be displayed compressed. (Adapted from ref. 12.)

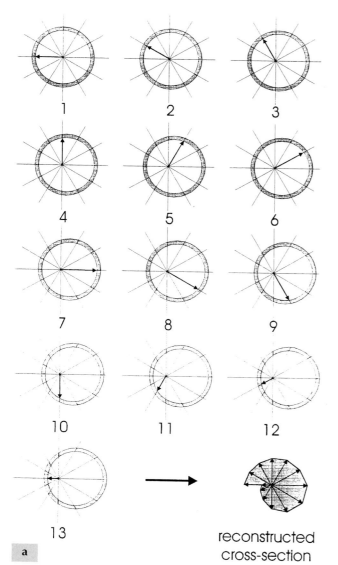

reconstructed cross-section

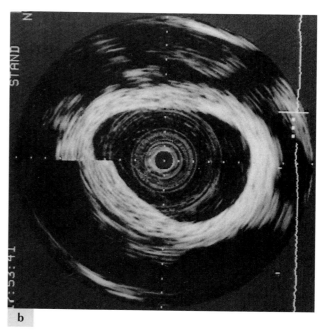

Figure 3.18. Movement artifact. If during one rotation of the ultrasound beam (indicated by the arrows) the catheter tip is moving fast relative to the vessel wall the display of the cross-section will be distorted. In the example shown the catheter, which is centered at the start of the rotation (1), is shifted continuously (2–13). The resulting distorted display of the vessel lumen reconstructed from one revolution is shown at bottom right. The effect is demonstrated in the IVUS image on the right side. (4.8 F. catheter; 20 MHz transducer; 1 mm calibration.)

Future developments

The miniaturization of imaging catheters will continue leading to 'imaging wires'. Several therapeutic techniques, such as atherectomy and laser ablation, will be combined with ultrasound imaging. Further development of signal processing and signal analysis will help in the interpretation of IVUS images.

References

1 Hill CR, ed. *Physical Principles of Medical Ultrasonics* (Chichester: Ellis Horwood, 1986).

2 Kremkau FW. *Diagnostic Ultrasound: Principles, Instrumentation and Exercises*, 2nd edn (New York: Grune and Stratton, 1984).

3 McDicken WN. *Diagnostic Ultrasound: Principles and Use of Instruments*, 2nd edn (New York: Wiley, 1981).

4 Wells PNT. *Biomedical Ultrasonics* (London: Academic Press, 1977).

5 Woodcock JP. *Ultrasonics* (Bristol: Adam Hilger, 1979).

6 Evans DH, McDicken WN, Skidmore R, Woodcock JP. *Doppler Ultrasound: Physics, Instrumentation, and Clinical Applications* (New York: Wiley, 1989).

7 Bom N, Lancée CT, Gussenhoven EJ, Li W, ten Hoff H. Basic principles of intravascular imaging. In: Tobis JM, Yock PG, eds. *Intravascular Ultrasound Imaging* (New York: Churchill Livingstone, 1992): 7–15.

8 Roelandt JRTC, Di Mario C, de Feyter PJ et al. Intravascular ultrasound: instrumentation, image interpretation, promises and pitfalls. In: Hanrath P et al. eds. *Cardiovascular Imaging by Ultrasound* (Dordrecht: Kluwer Academic Publishers, 1993): 325–41.

9 Bom N, ten Hoff H, Lancée CT, Gussenhoven WJ, Bosch JG. Early and recent intraluminal ultrasound devices. *In J Card Imaging* 1989; **4**: 79–88.

10 Lancée CT, Bom N, van Egmond FC, Honkoop J, Roelandt JRTC. A micromotor system for intraluminal ultrasound scanning. *Thoraxcenter J* 1993; **5**: 8–12.

11 Bom N, Lancée CT, van Egmond FC. An ultrasonic intracardiac scanner. *Ultrasonics* 1972; **10**: 72–6.

12 ten Hoff H, Korbijn A, Smit ThH, Klinkhammer JFF, Bom N. Image artefacts in mechanically driven ultrasound catheters. *Int J Card Imaging* 1989; **4**: 195–9.

4 Technical aspects of intracoronary Doppler

Carlo Di Mario, Lucia Di Francesco and Akira Itoh

Introduction

Intracoronary Doppler has several advantages for the assessment of coronary flow. Since there is a direct relationship between velocity and volumetric flow (where blood flow = vessel cross-sectional area × mean flow velocity) the differences or changes in Doppler coronary flow velocities can be used to represent changes in absolute coronary flow provided that the cross-sectional area remains constant. Doppler flowmeters directly measure the red blood cell velocity so that flow markers are not required, allowing a continuous assessment of flow velocity. Since the catheter can be selectively inserted in epicardial vessels, regional flow velocity measurements are possible. Intracoronary Doppler, however, also has several limitations. The most important limitation of intracoronary Doppler is the extreme dependency of the velocity measurements on the position of the Doppler probe within the vessel. If the sampling volume is small, or a large angle is present between ultrasound beam and long axis of the vessel, the measurement of flow velocity can be impossible or misleading, with an underestimation of the peak coronary flow velocity. This limitation has been partially solved by recent technical developments, as will be discussed in this chapter. The different Doppler transducers available for intracoronary blood flow velocity measurements, the technique of assessment of coronary flow reserve and the methods for calculating absolute coronary flow from velocity and area measurements will be described.

Intracoronary Doppler probes

Doppler probes mounted on angiographic catheters

In 1977 Hartley and Cole reported the recording of Doppler tracings at the ostium of the native coronary vessels and of coronary venous bypass grafts using a 20 MHz piezoelectric circular crystal mounted at the tip of a standard 8 F. Sones catheter.[1] In 58 patients the velocity pattern could be recorded in basal conditions and the hyperemic response to contrast media injection was measured.

Recently, Kern et al. described a left Judkins angiographic catheter with a 20 MHz crystal mounted caudally (6 o'clock position) at the tip of the catheter.[2]

With both systems, however, no selective measurements can be made in the vessel(s) of interest and a contamination of the coronary flow due to aortic flow components may be present. Furthermore, the presence of the relatively large catheter in the coronary ostium may, to some extent, obstruct the coronary blood flow, especially during hyperemia.

Intracoronary Doppler catheters

Side-mounted probes

At the University of Iowa, special suction-mounted epicardial Doppler probes were designed for intraoperative and experimental use.[3] In order to apply Doppler velocimetry during selective coronary catheterization, a Doppler crystal was mounted on one side of a 3 F. (1 mm) Rentrop perfusion catheter with a flexible guide wire at the tip.[4] The orientation of the beam at 45° from the long axis of the catheter was designed to avoid flow interference from the catheter. Although this design resulted in a reduction of the maximal recorded velocities due to the nonparallel orientation of the ultrasonic beam with the maximal flow velocity vector, this limitation was accepted because the main goal of the investigators was the evaluation of relative flow changes.[5] Coronary blood flow velocity measured with this catheter correlated well with flow measurement performed with microspheres, timed volume collection of coronary sinus flow, electromagnetic flowmeters and coronary blood flow velocity recorded with epicardial Doppler probes.[4,5]

With this system, for the first time, selective measurements of coronary flow velocity became possible during cardiac catheterization. Further technical development allowed an easier and safer integration of Doppler measurements in the catheterization laboratory during coronary interventions due to the availability of an internal lumen for a movable guide wire in the second-generation catheters.

End-mounted probes

Sibley et al.[6] obtained subselective Doppler recordings using a circular end-mounted crystal on a flexible 3 F. (1 mm) catheter amenable to guide wire insertion. This system was designed to minimize the angle between the ultrasonic beam and the centerline of the intravascular flow profile (subsequently called δ-angle), thus allowing the measurement of maximal intravascular velocity. In the Doppler equation the relationship between Doppler frequency shift and velocity is inversely proportional to the cosine of the δ-angle. Therefore, with an end-mounted crystal and a theoretical δ-angle of 0°, changes of 15° in either direction would induce a negligible reduction (−3.5%) of the measured frequency shift. On the contrary, the side-mounted probes with an angle of 45° with the centerline of flow may have a change of the δ-angle of up to 15%, resulting in a shift of Doppler frequency by as much as 23% from baseline.[7]

The flow stream interference due to the presence of the catheter in the bloodstream is of concern if velocities close to the transducer have to be measured. Tadaoka et al.[8] reported that, in an in-vitro model, a blunt or M-shaped velocity profile, depressed at the centerline, is present several millimeters distal to the catheter tip, resulting in underestimation of flow velocity away from the transducer. A distance of at least 10 catheter diameters was required to have a complete restoration of the flow velocity profile.

Double side-mounted probes

A possible solution to the angle dependency of the Doppler flow velocity measurements is the use of two piezoelectric crystals located on the side of the Doppler catheter in such a way that a right-angle between the transducers is obtained. The true blood flow velocity is then calculated as:

$$\text{True blood flow velocity} = [(\text{Vel. 1st transducer})^2 \times (\text{Vel 2nd transducer})^2]^{-2}$$

A prototype of this still-experimental system was validated in an in-vitro continuous flow model and yielded accurate flow velocity measurements, independent of the catheter position.[9]

Intracoronary Doppler balloon catheters

Custom-designed coronary balloon catheters with an end-mounted 20 MHz Doppler crystal have been successfully used at the Thoraxcenter, Rotterdam, The Netherlands, to record intracoronary velocities during and after successive balloon inflations.[10] The system allowed the recording of high-quality Doppler tracings distal to the stenosis before, during and after balloon inflation. The maximal hyperemic velocity after balloon inflation was found to be a useful guide for the assessment of the result of angioplasty.

Doppler guide wire probes

Although side- and end-mounted Doppler catheters have been extensively used in research cardiac catheterization laboratories, mainly for assessing relative changes of coronary velocities, several limitations have precluded a more widespread clinical application of these devices.

1) Catheters of 1 mm diameter are unlikely to be an obstacle to flow in proximal coronary arteries with a diameter of 3–4 mm, as also confirmed at high flow rates in experiments in calves. If, however, the recording is obtained across or distal to a stenotic segment, the obstruction due to the catheter may induce marked reduction or disappearance of the anterograde flow.
2) The insertion of the Doppler catheter before and after coronary interventions results in repeated and complex exchange procedures and in the inability to monitor coronary blood flow velocities during the most critical phases of the procedure.
3) Optimal position of the sample volume inside the vessel is required to record a high-quality signal, including the highest blood velocities. The lack of steerability and the small sample volume of the Doppler catheters described above result in a high number of unsuccessful procedures.
4) With 20 MHz transducers activated with a pulse repetition frequency of 62.5 kHz, velocities up to 110 cm/s can be recorded, so that the high velocities across a stenosis cannot be accurately measured.
5) Only zero-crossing detectors are commercially available in combination with these Doppler probes.

The Cardiometrics (Mountain View, CA) FloWire is available as a 0.36 mm or 0.46 mm, 175 cm long,

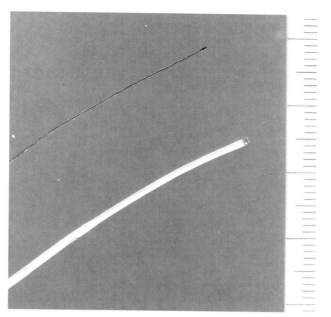

Figure 4.1. End-mounted 3 F. Doppler catheter (Schneider, Zurich, Switzerland) (right side) compared with a 0.46-mm Doppler guide wire (Cardiometrics, Mountain View, CA) (left side).

flexible and steerable guide wire with a tip-mounted 12 or 15 MHz piezoelectric ultrasound transducer (Fig. 4.1). It has handling characteristics similar to traditional angioplasty guide wires, with a distal end which is straight or preshaped in a 30° J-curve but which can be further modified by the operator. An extension wire (Cordis Corporation, Billerica, MA) is also available when an over-the-wire technique is required.

Substituting a Doppler-tipped guide wire for a standard angioplasty guide wire, phasic coronary flow velocity measurements are easily performed in an angioplasty procedure. Recently, support-types of Doppler guide wires were manufactured to help application in procedures where a rigid body of wire is required to facilitate the insertion of stents or directional atherectomy catheters into the coronary vessels. The wire creates less disturbance of the flow profile distal to its tip when placed within a vessel and can be passed into the smaller coronary arteries without creating significant stenoses. The flexibility and steerability of the Doppler FloWire are designed for crossing intracoronary arterial obstructions and maintaining a stable prolonged placement in the distal portion of the coronary artery during coronary angioplasty procedures. The forward-directed ultrasound beam diverges at 30° so that the sampling

volume is approximately 0.65 mm thick by 2.25 mm in diameter when maintained 5.2 mm beyond the transducer, distal to the area of flow velocity profile distortion induced by the Doppler guide wire.[11] This broad ultrasound beam provides a relatively large area of insonification, sampling a large portion of the flow velocity profile. Although this setting and insonification angle is mostly sufficient to obtain high-quality signals in multiple positions in the coronary tree, and especially in smaller coronary vessels (that is, distal to the stenosis), more recently a modified Doppler guide wire ('wide beam') has been introduced further to increase the ability of recording velocity in the proximal segment of the vessel or in other large vessel segments (after stenting) or along curved segments. In this guide wire the larger sample volume is the combined result of a larger angle of insonification and a longer distance between transducer and sample volume.

An adjustable pulse repetition frequency of 16–94 kHz, pulse duration of 0.83 ms and sampling delay of 0.5 ms provide satisfactory parameters for spectral signal analysis. Flow velocities higher than 4 m/s can be accurately measured due to the lower frequency and high repetition frequency of this system (Fig. 4.2). The signal transmitted from the piezoelectric transducer is processed from the quadrature Doppler audio signal by a real-time spectral analyzer using on-line fast Fourier transformer providing a scrolling grayscale spectral display. The frequency response of this system calculates approximately 90 spectra per second. The spectral analysis of the signal and the Doppler audio-signals are video-recorded for later review. Simultaneous electrocardiogram and blood pressure are displayed with the spectral velocity.

The Doppler guide wire has been validated during intravascular measurement of coronary arterial flow velocity by Doucette et al.[11] The Doppler flow velocity signal was recorded in model tubes with pulsatile blood flow. In four straight tubes with internal diameters varying from 0.79 to 4.76 mm, the peak spectral flow velocity was linearly related to absolute flow velocity measured by on-line electromagnetic flowmeters ($r > 0.98$ for each tube). Quantitative volumetric flow was calculated from vessel cross-sectional area and mean flow velocity. The average peak velocity was less accurate in larger tubes (>7.5 mm) and a slightly reduced correlation with absolute flow was observed in tortuous segments. In four canine circumflex coronary arteries, the electro-magnetic flow probe and Doppler flow vessel also demonstrated high correlations in both the proximal and distal segments ($r^2 = 0.93$–0.99 in the proximal vessel and 0.86–0.99 in the distal vessel). Using quantitative angiography to determine arterial diameter, quantitative flow velocity correlations for the two

a

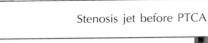

Stenosis jet before PTCA

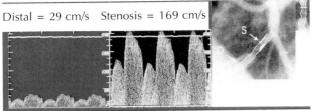

Distal = 29 cm/s   Stenosis = 169 cm/s

Area stenosis doppler = 83%   Angio = 72% ·

b

Stenosis jet after PTCA

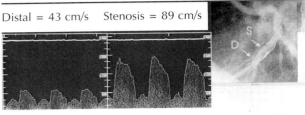

Distal = 43 cm/s   Stenosis = 89 cm/s

Area stenosis doppler = 52%   Angio = 20%

Figure 4.2. (a) Quantative angiography (right panel) and flow velocity measurements distal and within a stenosis of the left anterior descending coronary artery. Note the relatively similar results of the direct measurement of area stenosis with angiography and of its calculation with Doppler based on the continuity equation. **(b)** The same measurements after coronary angiography showing an area stenosis smaller than 20%. The presence of a velocity of the stenotic jet more than double the velocity distal to the stenosis indicates a lumen area reduction greater than 50%.

techniques were $r = 0.95$ in the model cannula and $r = 0.85$ in the proximal coronary artery. These data indicate that the Doppler guide wire accurately measures phasic flow velocity patterns and linearly tracks changes in flow rates in small, predominantly straight coronary arteries.

Motion artifacts, especially when heart rate is high, might influence flow velocity, but this phenomenon did not impair the accuracy of the measurements in the initial validation studies. Changes of pulsatility intensity examined in the in-vitro system demonstrated satisfactory tracking and correlation with electromagnetic flow responses at rapid heart rates. During in-vivo pacing experiments (up to 150 beats/min), an excellent correlation was found between the average peak velocity of the Doppler guide wire system and flowmeter response.

The in-vivo studies with the Doppler guide wire established several important features applicable to patient use. In a recent multicenter study applying intracoronary Doppler during balloon angioplasty,[12] the Doppler guide wire could be used as primary wire to cross the stenosis in 289/297 patients (97%) and basal velocity measurements before balloon angioplasty could be obtained proximal and distal to the stenosis in 74% and 99% of patients, respectively. In most cases (93%), the inability to measure flow velocity proximal to the stenosis was not due to technical failure but to a too-proximal position of the lesion under evaluation. The potential for recording very high velocities can be used to measure the velocity of the stenotic jet and calculate the percentage area stenosis from velocity measurements based

on the continuity equation. This technique, already explored using Doppler catheters for mild stenoses,[13] has been shown to be applicable with the Doppler guide wire and yields a good correlation with independent measurements of stenosis severity with quantitative angiography (Fig. 4.2).[14] Unfortunately, flow velocity tracings suitable for quantitative analysis are difficult to record in the stenotic segment as a result of misalignment of the guide wire with the stenotic jet and reduced intensity of the backscatter from blood in segments with high shear stress leading to a disaggregation of the large red blood cell rouleaux.[15] The low success rate in the recording of flow velocity within the lesion has been confirmed recently in the large multicenter study DEBATE (Doppler Endpoints Balloon Angioplasty Trial Europe) in which high-quality recordings of the stenotic jet were obtained in 12% and 22% of patients before and after balloon angioplasty, respectively.[12] A setting in which the application of the continuity equation appears more feasible is the evaluation of the velocity changes within the stented segment in order to detect segments of residual lumen reduction requiring further stent expansion (Fig. 4.3).

Assessment of coronary flow reserve

Since the original work of Gould, Lipscomb, and Hamilton,[16] the assessment of coronary flow reserve has been viewed as a method of establishing the severity of a stenosis located in one of the major

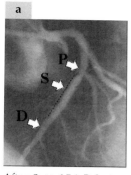

After 2 × 154 P-S stent

Distal	Within stent	Proximal
LA = 6.1 mm²	LA = 8.8 mm²	LA = 6.2 mm²

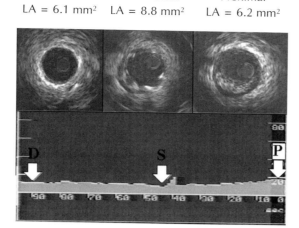

Figure 4.3. (a) Left panel: angiographic result after implantation of two 14 mm Palmaz–Schatz (P–S) stents. Three ultrasonic cross-sections distal, within the stent and proximal to the stent are shown and measured. Note that these three positions are also indicated in the velocity trend recorded during the pullback of the Doppler guide wire. **(b)** Corresponding Doppler measurements. Note that a reduction in flow velocity occurs at the site of the increased lumen area within the stent. Note also the optimal recordings obtained throughout the pullback with the exception of a minor artifact within the stent. APV: time-averaged peak velocity. (LA: luminal area.)

Distal	Within stent	Proximal
APV = 12 cm/s	APV = 8 cm/s	APV = 18 cm/s

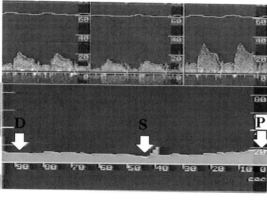

After 2 × 154 P-S stent

epicardial vessels. It is assumed that the reduction in hyperemic flow through the stenotic lesion would be an indicator of stenosis severity. This assumption is derived from the complex hemodynamic principles regulating the coronary circulation. At rest, flow is independent of the driving pressure over a wide range (60–180 mmHg) of physiological pressures, a phenomenon classically described as autoregulation of the coronary circulation. During maximal vasodilatation, flow becomes linearly related to the driving pressure.[17] The presence of a flow-limiting stenosis in a major epicardial vessel generates a pressure drop across the stenotic lesion which is the result of viscous and turbulent resistances, so that the driving pressure distal to the stenosis decreases exponentially in response to the flow increase.[18]

The coronary flow reserve concept is appealing to the clinician because it constitutes a functional surrogate to the anatomic description of the lesions located in the epicardial vessels (Fig. 4.4). Many investigators have shown in animal experiments that a decrease in flow reserve may discriminately detect lesions of increasing severity.[19] Although the concept may be easily and accurately applied in an optimal physiological situation in humans,[20,21] it should be recognized that coronary flow reserve is influenced by several factors independent of the hydrodynamic characteristics of the stenotic lesion. Since flow reserve is a ratio, similar values may be obtained at very different levels of resting and hyperemic flow. Changes in basal resting flow without changes in hyperemic flow will considerably affect the ratio. Furthermore, any factors affecting the hyperemic pressure flow relationship would likewise modify the flow reserve and thereby change the assessment of the severity of the coronary lesion under study. The hyperemic pressure flow relationship is influenced by factors such as heart rate, preload, myocardial hypertrophy or disease of the microvasculature.[22]

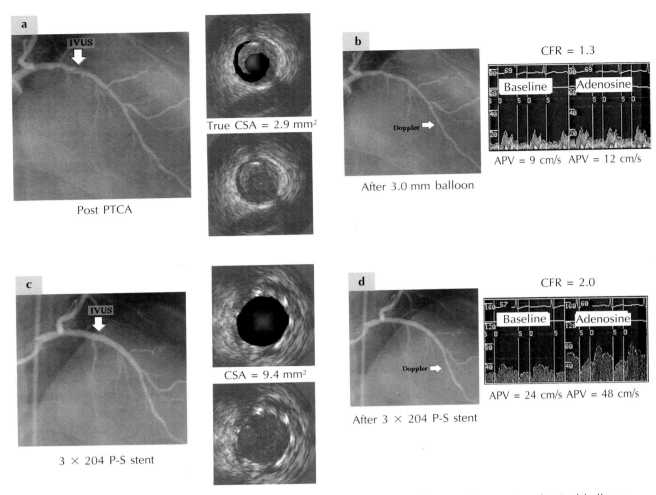

Figure 4.4. (a) Right panel: cineangiogram showing a moderate dissection after percutaneous transluminal balloon angioplasty (PTCA) of the left anterior descending coronary artery. Note that the ultrasonic cross-sections at the site of dilatation show a circumferential dissection with a minimal free lumen around the catheter. **(b)** Corresponding Doppler measurements in baseline conditions and after adenosine 18 μg. **(c)** Angiographic result after implantation of three 18-mm Palmaz–Schatz stents: note the optimal result, confirmed with intracoronary ultrasound. **(d)** Corresponding Doppler measurements after stent implantation. CFR: coronary flow reserve; CSA: cross-sectional area.

Effects of the pharmacologic agents used to induce maximal hyperemia

An increase in coronary blood flow can be observed either during reactive hyperemia induced by transluminal occlusion or by pharmacologically induced hyperemia. Widely used vasodilator agents are dipyridamole, nitroglycerin, papaverine, and adenosine. The hyperosmolar ionic and low osmolar nonionic contrast media cannot be used because they do not produce maximal vasodilatation.[23] Nitrates have a predominant effect on large conductance vessels so that the flow changes due to peripheral vasodilatation are partially masked by the large simultaneous increase in cross-sectional area in the proximal arterial segments. Continuous infusion of an adequate dose of dipyridamole results in

maximal coronary vasodilatation, but it has the disadvantage of a long duration of action, which makes the repeated assessment of the coronary hyperemic response of the coronary vascular bed or the assessment of different coronary vascular bed response during the same procedure impossible.

Bookstein and Higgins[23] have shown in dogs that the hyperemic response after an intracoronary bolus injection of adenosine-triphosphate or papaverine is of the same magnitude as that occurring after a 15-second occlusion of the coronary artery. The dose range of intracoronary papaverine needed to produce maximal coronary vasodilatation has been established in humans by Wilson and White.[24] Selective intracoronary infusion of papaverine produced a maximal hyperemic response in most

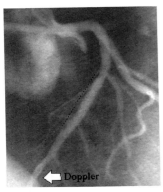

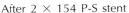

After 2 × 154 P-S stent

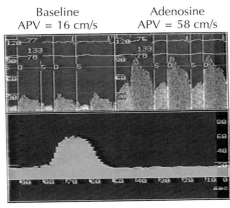

Baseline
APV = 16 cm/s

Adenosine
APV = 58 cm/s

CFR = 3.7

Figure 4.5. Measurement of coronary flow reserve after stenting in the same case as Fig. 4.3. Note that the maximal velocity increase occurs 10–15 s after flushing of 18 µg of adenosine intracoronary, and that the velocity returns to basal values within 30 s from the injection. (CFR: coronary flow reserve; APV: average peak velocity.)

(80%) coronary arteries after 8 mg and in all coronary arteries after 12 mg. Papaverine in this dose range (8–12 mg) produced a response equal to that of an intravenous infusion of dipyridamole in a dose of 0.56–0.84 mg/kg of bodyweight.

The coronary vasodilatation after intravenous or intracoronary adenosine is of a comparable magnitude to that observed after papaverine. The time from intracoronary injection of adenosine to peak hyperemia, as well as the total duration of the hyperemic response, is about four times shorter than that of papaverine (Fig. 4.5).[25] Furthermore, adenosine does not prolong QT-interval and avoids the potentially dangerous ventricular arrhythmias observed after papaverine.[26] Wilson et al.[27] reported that an intracoronary bolus or infusion of adenosine increases coronary velocity to levels similar to those recorded after papaverine without significant systemic effects or symptoms. Adenosine can also be administered intravenously. Kern et al. have shown that a continuous intravenous infusion of 140 mg/kg per minute induces maximal coronary vasodilatation in the vast majority of patients with the presence of mild hypotension and bradycardia.[28] The frequent development of symptoms (flushing, 35%; chest discomfort, 34%; headache, 21%; dyspnea, 19%) and of first- to second-degree atrioventricular block (<10%) rarely requires discontinuation of the infusion.[29] In view of the extremely high safety profile, absence of side-effects to the patient and ease of use, low-dose intracoronary adenosine is the agent and route of administration of choice. The maximum effect is reached after premedication with nitroglycerin.

Intracoronary papaverine has been reported to increase coronary blood flow velocity by between four and six times the resting value in patients with normal coronary arteries.[24,30] In these series, however, a highly selected patient population was studied, with the exclusion of myocardial hypertrophy, previous myocardial infarction or of any other condition known to increase the baseline flow (anemia, hyperthyroidism, etc.).

Using papaverine 8.0–12.5 mg and a Doppler guide wire in an unselected series of patients with coronary artery disease, the present authors observed in 81 arteries without hemodynamically significant coronary artery stenosis a coronary flow reserve of 2.9 ± 0.95, with a large individual variability (range 2.1–4.2).[31]

Effect of the pharmacologic agent used to induce hyperemia on stenosis geometry

The ideal vasodilator should dilate the resistance vessels exclusively without affecting the geometry of the flow-limiting stenosis in the epicardial coronary artery. Unfortunately, as indicated by studies with intracoronary papaverine,[32] the agents used to induce vasodilatation of the resistance vessels also influence the epicardial coronary arteries but only to a level of 5%.

The vasodilatory effect of papaverine on the epicardial arteries has two opposite consequences for the accuracy of the measurements of flow reserve. The vasodilatation of the epicardial vessel in which the Doppler guide wire is positioned will lead to a larger area during hyperemia than at baseline, so that the ratio between hyperemic and basal velocity will underestimate the true flow ratio. On the other hand, a direct vasodilatation after papaverine of the stenotic segment may lead to an opposite result. Because of these factors a predilatation with nitroglycerin 100–200 µg or isosorbide dinitrate 1–3 mg is mandatory in order to overcome this limitation.

Using intracoronary adenosine (12–18 mg) a predilatation with nitrates is not strictly required, since the low dose used has a selective effect on the resistance vessels without inducing changes in the area of the epicardial arteries.[33] Intracoronary nitrates, however, remain highly recommended when reproducible measurements must be obtained in different phases of the same procedure (for example, before and after balloon angioplasty) or in different procedures.

Factors influencing the accuracy of Doppler-based coronary flow reserve as an index of stenosis severity

The basal coronary flow is ultimately determined by the myocardial oxygen demand. Heart rate, preload, mean aortic pressure and inotropic status are the most important determinants of the cardiac workload and, consequently, of the myocardial oxygen consumption and baseline coronary flow. The flow velocity ratio can also be affected by other factors inducing a change in resting flow velocity, both increasing myocardial oxygen consumption (for example, thyrotoxicosis) or producing a resting high flow state (for example, anemia). During maximal hyperemia, coronary flow is linearly positively correlated with aortic pressure and negatively correlated with heart rate. To address this problem, an index of resistance has been proposed by Wilson et al.[5] calculated as the quotient of:

$$\frac{\text{mean aortic pressure and peak flow}}{\text{peak flow velocity}}$$

and

$$\frac{\text{resting aortic pressure}}{\text{resting blood flow velocity}}$$

McGinn et al.[34] have studied the influence of heart rate, arterial pressure and ventricular preload on the long-term variability of serial coronary flow reserve measurements. In 45 patients with normal left ventricular function (38 cardiac allograft recipients, five patients with normal coronary arteries and two patients with minimal coronary artery disease (<50% diameter stenosis), coronary flow reserve measurements were highly reproducible in the absence of conditions known to affect resting or hyperemic coronary blood flow. Increases in heart rate or preload reduced coronary flow reserve because resting coronary blood flow velocity was increased while hyperemic coronary blood flow velocity was unchanged. In contrast, changes in mean arterial pressure did not alter coronary flow reserve. Interpretation of coronary flow reserve measurements should account for the variable hemodynamic conditions at which the flow velocity measurements are obtained.

In 34 patients studied at the Thoraxcenter, Rotterdam, The Netherlands, flow velocity measurements were repeated over a six-month interval, showing a variability which was larger for baseline velocity and coronary flow reserve.[35] This study showed that moderate spontaneous variations in heart rate over time were sufficient to impair the reproducibility of repeated measurements of baseline velocity and, to a lesser extent, of hyperemic velocity. Since opposite changes in baseline and hyperemic velocity occur with an increase in heart rate, coronary flow reserve decreased with an increase in heart rate. Atrial pacing or a normalization of the coronary flow reserve for heart rate should then be considered in order to overcome this limitation. As reported by McGinn et al.,[34] the changes in aortic pressure from the initial study to follow-up had a more limited influence on the changes in flow velocity and coronary flow reserve. When considering long-term changes, as in the Rotterdam study, the effects of risk-factor modifications in regard to smoking, elevated cholesterol, diabetes mellitus, and hypertension should be considered. These factors not only induce progression or regression of the atherosclerotic changes at an epicardial level, with consequent permanent changes in lumen area, but modify the endothelium-dependent and independent coronary vasodilatation of the resistance vessel.

A final technical note concerns the possible induction of flow obstruction due to the large guiding catheter engaged in the ostium. In this case, after selective injection of the vasodilator the catheter should immediately be pulled out from the ostium without moving the Doppler probe. A careful monitoring of the pressure waveform recorded through the guiding catheter can facilitate the detection of damping of velocity. Use of diagnostic or smaller guiding catheters (6–7 F.) is an easier alternative possibility to prevent flow obstruction allowed by the use of the Doppler guide wire.

Calculation of volume flow from flow velocity measurements

Two crucial steps are required to calculate absolute (volume) flow accurately from flow velocity measurements: the calculation of the mean blood flow velocity in a given vascular cross-section and the accurate measurement of the cross-sectional area at the site of measurement.

Assessment of mean blood flow velocity
The measurement of the mean blood flow velocity requires an adequate Doppler sampling of flow velocity within a vessel, including: (a) ultrasound beam parallel to the centerline of flow; (b) flow

profile entirely, or almost entirely, included in the Doppler sample volume; and (c) spectral analysis of the Doppler frequency available in order to identify all the different velocities in the sample volume, including the maximal velocity. Theoretically, mean blood flow velocity can be measured from the weighted average of the velocity spectrum.[36] Several technical shortcomings limit the practical usefulness of the measurement of mean blood flow velocity from the velocity spectrum:

1) the filtering process necessary to remove the high intensity/low velocity signals from vessel wall contact artefacts (wall 'thumps') affects the accuracy of the measurement of mean velocity;
2) measurements derived from the intensity-weighted velocity spectrum mean velocity are more sensitive than the maximal velocity to a variety of noise components of the signal;
3) the mean velocity calculated from the intensity-weighted velocity spectrum is inaccurate if the entire parabolic profile of the artery is not included in the sample volume. Small changes in the position of the tip of the catheter inside the vessel are also more likely to change the mean than the maximal velocity;
4) the weighting factors for the different velocities of the velocity spectrum cannot be reliably determined as signal intensity is modified by several unknown parameters such as rouleaux formation.[37,38]
5) inhomogeneities in the distribution of ultrasonic beam power may cause significant errors in the measurement of mean coronary blood flow velocity.[39]

A different approach is based on the use of the maximal blood flow velocity which is less sensitive to the presence of noise and is more easily included in the sample volume based on the above-described characteristics of the Doppler system. Mean blood flow velocity can be estimated from the maximal blood flow velocity in the presence of a laminar flow field and a fully developed velocity profile (Fig. 4.6).

An important limitation to the applicability of this formula is that the velocity profile is assumed to be parabolic and fully developed. The distance L necessary to allow the full development of a parabolic flow profile is defined by the equation:[40]

$$L = (0.03 \ R_e) \ d$$

where R_e is the Reynolds number and d the diameter of the conduit. Consequently, the velocity measurement should be taken at a distance of four to six times the vessel diameter to allow a complete development of the velocity profile at the Reynolds numbers present in normal epicardial coronary

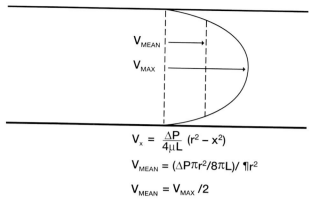

$$V_x = \frac{\Delta P}{4\mu L} \ (r^2 - x^2)$$

$$V_{MEAN} = (\Delta P\pi r^2 / 8\pi L) / \P r^2$$

$$V_{MEAN} = V_{MAX} / 2$$

Figure 4.6. Diagram showing the fixed relation (2:1) between maximal and mean flow velocity in a conduit with a laminar parabolic velocity profile. The fixed relation between maximal and mean velocity in a conduit with a laminar parabolic velocity profile can also be derived from the classical equations describing the velocity of each streamline of flow according to its distance X from the centerline of flow and from the Poiseuille equation. ΔP: pressure gradient; μ: viscosity; r: conduit radius; L: length of the segment.

arteries (150–200 units). The same issues must be considered when sampling velocity distal to major bifurcations of the vessel. Also, in the presence of changes of the vascular diameter, the measurement of mean blood flow velocity from maximal velocity can be misleading if the stenotic segment is too short to allow a full development of the velocity profile. The non-Newtonian characteristics of blood will induce a flatter-than-expected velocity profile so that the mean blood flow velocity may be underestimated by deriving this parameter from the maximal flow velocity.[41] These considerations underline the difficulties in obtaining reliable volumetric flow measurements based on blood flow velocity despite the recent progress in Doppler probe technology and signal analysis.

Assessment of the cross-sectional area at the site of the Doppler sample volume

A high-quality angiogram, suitable for measurement of the cross-section at the site of the Doppler sample volume, can be performed almost simultaneously with the acquisition of the Doppler recording using a Doppler guide wire. It must be noted, however, that more accurate measurements are obtained when the probe is positioned in an arterial segment of uniform caliber, so that a mean cross-sectional area over a short arterial segment immediately distal to the Doppler probe (approximately 5 mm for the Doppler guide wire) can be obtained.

An alternative method is the combination of intra-coronary Doppler and two-dimensional coronary ultrasound imaging. A continuous recording of high-quality echographic cross-sections, suitable for automated quantitative analysis, can be achieved with modern ultrasound imaging catheters. Although prototype systems of combined Doppler-imaging ultrasound catheters have been tested,[42] the introduction of the Doppler guide wire allows a simultaneous assessment with ultrasound catheters compatible with 0.36-mm guide wires. The slightly different position of the Doppler sample volume and of the echographic cross-section and the presence of electrical interference when both transducers are active are minor limitations of this approach. Another advantage of intracoronary ultrasound is the possibility of detecting the area changes through-out the cardiac cycle, so that the phasic changes in flow velocity can be matched with the correspond-ing area changes. Since fairly large area changes (>15%) have been reported with intracoronary ultra-sound in relatively normal vessel segments during the cardiac cycle,[43,44] this method can increase the accuracy of flow measurements in comparison with the standard technique of assessment (time-averaged velocity multiplied for a single cross-sectional area, normally at end-diastole).

Conclusions and future directions

The last few years have seen rapid advances in coronary Doppler probe technology and signal analysis and the development of new approaches to the interpretation of flow velocity measurement. These changes have transformed a complex technique reserved to a few research laboratories into a reliable diagnostic tool which can be used for the assessment of stenosis severity and for the evalu-ation of the results of coronary interventions. Combined Doppler and imaging ultrasound systems can be applied for a continuous measurement of absolute coronary flow as well as for the simultane-ous study of morphological and functional charac-teristics of the coronary system.

References

1   Hartley CJ, Cole JS. An ultrasonic pulsed Doppler system for measuring blood flow in small vessels. *J Appl Physiol* 1974; **37**: 626–32.

2   Kern MJ, Courtois M, Ludbrook P. A simplified method to measure coronary blood flow velocity in patients: validation and application of a new Judkins-style Doppler-tipped angiographic catheter. *Am Heart J* 1990; **120**: 1202–9.

3   Wright CB, Doty DB, Eastham CL. Measurement of coronary reactive hyperemia with a Doppler probe: intraoperative guide to hemodynamically significant lesions. *J Thorac Cardiovasc Surg* 1980; **80**: 888–96.

4   Marcus ML. *The Coronary Circulation in Health and Disease.* (New York: McGraw-Hill, 1983).

5   Wilson RF, Laughlin DE, Ackell PH et al. Transluminal, subselective measurement of coronary artery blood flow velocity and vasodilator reserve in man. *Circulation* 1985; **72**: 82–92.

6   Sibley DH, Millar HD, Hartley CJ, Whitlow PL. Subselective measurement of coronary blood flow velocity using a steerable Doppler catheter. *J Am Coll Cardiol* 1986; **8**: 1332–40.

7   Hatle L, Angelsen B. Physics of blood flow. In: Hatle L, Angelsen B, eds. *Doppler Ultrasound in Cardiology.* (Philadelphia: Lea and Febiger, 1982): 8–31.

8   Tadaoka S, Kagiyama M, Hiramatsu O et al. Accuracy of 20 MHz Doppler catheter coronary artery velocimetry for measurement of coronary blood flow velocity. *Cathet Cardiovasc Diagn* 1990; **19**: 205–13.

9   Akamatsu S, Kondo Y. Velocity measurement with a new Doppler catheter independent of incident angle. *Circulation* 1992; **86**: I869.

10   Serruys, PW, Jullière Y, Zijlstra F et al. Coronary blood flow velocity during PTCA: a guide-line for assessment of functional results. *Am J Cardiol* 1988; **61**: 253–9.

11   Doucette JW, Douglas Corl P, Payne HP et al. Validation of a Doppler guide wire for intravascular measurement of coronary artery flow velocity. *Circulation* 1992; **85**: 1899–1911.

12   Sunamura M, Di Mario C, Piek JJ et al. Intracoronary Doppler guidance during angioplasty. Result of the second interim analysis. In: de Feyter PJ, Di Mario C, Serruys PW, eds. *Quantative Coronary Imaging.* (Delft: Barjesteh, Meeuwes & Co., 1995): 250–67.

13   Nakatani S, Yamagishi M, Tamai J, Takaki H, Haze K, Miyatake K. Quantitative assessment of coronary artery stenosis by intravascular Doppler catheter technique. *Circulation* 1992; **85**: 1786–91.

14   Di Mario C, Meneveau N, Gil R et al. Maximal blood flow velocity in severe coronary stenoses measured with a Doppler guidewire. *Am J Cardiol* 1993; **71**: 54D–61D.

15   Yuan YW, Shung KK. Ultrasonic backscatter from flowing whole blood. *J Acoust Soc Am* 1988; **84**: 52–8.

16   Gould KL, Lipscomb K, Hamilton GW. Physiologic basis for assessing critical coronary stenosis: instantaneous flow response and regional distribution during coronary

hyperemia as measures of coronary flow reserve. *Am J Cardiol* 1974; **33**: 87–94.

17 Klocke FJ. Measurements of coronary flow reserve: defining pathophysiology versus making decisions about patient care. *Circulation* 1987; **76**: 245–53.

18 Sugawara M. Stenosis: theoretical background. In: Sugawara M, Kajiya F, Kitabatake A, Matsuo H, eds. *Blood Flow in the Heart and Large Vessels.* (Berlin: Springer-Verlag, 1989): 91.

19 Gould KL, Kirkeeide RL, Buchi M. Coronary flow reserve as a physiologic measure of stenosis severity. *J Am Coll Cardiol* 1990; **15**: 459–74.

20 Wilson RF, Marcus ML, White CW. Prediction of the physiologic significance of coronary arterial lesions by quantitative lesion geometry in patients with limited coronary artery disease. *Circulation* 1987; **75**: 723–32.

21 Harrison DG, White CW, Hiratzka LF, Eastham CL, Marcus ML. The value of lesional cross-sectional area determined by quantitative coronary angiography in assessing the physiologic significance of proximal left anterior descending coronary. *Circulation* 1984; **69**: 111–19.

22 Klocke FJ. Cognition in the era of technology: 'seeing the shades of gray'. *J Am Coll Cardiol* 1990; **16**: 763–9.

23 Bookstein JJ, Higgins CB. Comparative efficacy of coronary vasodilatory methods. *Invest Radiol* 1977; **12**: 121–8.

24 Wilson RF, White CW. Intracoronary papaverine: an ideal coronary vasodilator for studies of the coronary circulation in conscious humans. *Circulation* 1986; **73**: 444–51.

25 Zijlstra F, Juillière Y, Serruys PW, Roelandt JRTC. Value and limitations of intracoronary adenosine for the assessment of coronary flow reserve. *Cathet Cardiovasc Diagn* 1988; **15**: 76–83.

26 Wilson RF, White CW. Serious ventricular dysrhythmias after intracoronary papaverine. *Am J Cardiol* 1988; **62**: 1301–30.

27 Wilson RF, Wyche K, Christensen BV, Laxson DD. Effects of adenosine on human coronary arterial circulation. *Circulation* 1990; **82**: 1595–603.

28 Kern NJ, Deligonul U, Aguirre F, Hilton TC. Intravenous adenosine: continuous infusion and low dose bolus administration for determination of coronary vasodilator reserve in patients with and without coronary artery disease. *J Am Coll Cardiol* 1991; **18**: 718–26.

29 Abreu A, Mahmarian JJ, Nishimura S, Verani MS. Tolerance and safety of pharmacologic coronary vasodilatation with adenosine in association with thallium 201 scintigraphy in patients with suspected coronary artery disease. *Am J Cardiol* 1991; **18**: 730–6.

30 Zijlstra F, van Ommeren J, Reiber JHC, Serruys PW. Does quantitative assessment of coronary artery dimensions predict the physiologic significance of a coronary stenosis? *Circulation* 1987; **75**: 1154–62.

31 Serruys PW, Di Mario C, Kern MJ. Intracoronary Doppler. In: Topol EJ, ed. *Textbook of Interventional Cardiology* 2nd edn. (Philadelphia: WB Saunders, 1994): 1324–404.

32 Zijlstra F, Reiber JHC, Serruys PW et al. Does intracoronary papaverine dilate epicardial coronary arteries? Implications for assessment of coronary flow reserve. *Cathet Cardiovasc Diagn* 1988; **14**: 1–6.

33 Sudhir K, MacGregor JS, Barbant SD et al. Assessment of coronary conductance and resistance vessel reactivity in response to nitroglycerin, ergonovine and adenosine: in vivo studies with simultaneous intravascular two-dimensional and Doppler ultrasound. *J Am Coll Cardiol* 1993; **21**: 1261–8.

34 McGinn AL, White CW, Wilson RF. Interstudy variability of coronary flow reserve: influence of heart rate, arterial pressure, and ventricular preload. *Circulation* 1990: **81**: 1319–30.

35 Di Mario C, Gil R, Serruys PW. Long-term reproducibility of flow velocity measurements in 34 patients with coronary artery disease *Am J Cardiol* 1995; **22**: 123–7.

36 Evans DH, Schlindwein FS, Levene MI. The relationship between time-averaged intensity-weighted mean velocity and time-averaged maximum velocity in neonatal cerebral arteries. *Ultrasound Med Biol* 1989; **15**: 429–35.

37 De Kroon MGM, Slager CJ, Gussenhoven WJ, Serruys PW, Roelandt JRTC, Bom N. Cyclic changes of blood echogenicity in high-frequency ultrasound. *Ultrasound Med Biol* 1991; **17**: 723–8.

38 Shung KK, Cloutier G, Lim CC. The effects of hematocrit, shear rate and turbulence on ultrasonic blood spectrum from blood. *IEEE Trans Biomed Eng* 1992; **39**: 462–9.

39 Denardo SJ, Talbot L, Hargrave V, Ports TA, Yock PG. Advantage of peak velocity over mean velocity measurements made by Doppler catheters. *Circulation* 1992: **86**: I870.

40 Caro CG, Pedley TJ, Schroter RC, Seed WA. Flow in pipes and around objects. In: Caro CG, Pedley TJ, Schroter RC, Seed WA, eds. *The Mechanics of the Circulation.* (Oxford: Oxford University Press, 1978): 44–73.

41 Ling SC, Atabek HB, Fry DL, Patel DJ, Janicki JS. Application of heated-film velocity and shear probes to hemodynamic studies. *Circ Res* 1968; **23**: 789–801.

42 Linker DT, Torp H, Groenningsaether A et al. Instantaneous arterial flow estimated with an ultrasound imaging and Doppler catheter. *Circulation* 1989; **80**: II580 (abst).

43 McPherson DD, Sirna S, Collins SM et al. Can atherosclerotic coronary arteries vasodilate? An intraoperative high-frequency epicardial echocardiographic study. *Am J Cardiol* 1995; **76**: 21–5.

44 Weissman NJ, Palacios IF, Weyman AE. Dynamic expansion of the coronary arteries: implications for intravascular ultrasound measurements. *Am Heart J* 1995; **130**: 46–51.

5 Normal values: coronary flow

Carlo Di Mario and Morton Kern

Introduction

In patients with coronary artery disease the main goal of intervention is the re-establishment of normal flow to the myocardium. Naturally there is interest in establishing a precise definition of the normal values of coronary flow. Chapter 2 discussed the differences in pattern of flow in the three major coronary arteries and in the left main coronary artery. This chapter reports the results of basal and hyperemic flow velocity measurements obtained in angiographically normal or near-normal arteries in two centers with wide experience of intracoronary Doppler. Since subtle but important differences are present in the methodology used and in the clinical characteristics of the patients studied, no attempts at combination or meta-analysis of data were made.

Systodiastolic changes and reproducibility of measurements: the Rotterdam experience

In order to define the normal range of coronary flow velocity, the time-averaged blood flow velocity was measured in 81 proximal and mid-coronary segments in arteries without hemodynamically significant coronary stenoses. Three patient groups were distinguished: patients with chest pain but without hemodynamically significant coronary stenoses ($n = 5$ (6%)); normal arteries in patients undergoing revascularization of a different artery with greater than 50% diameter stenosis ($n = 41$ (51%)); and arteries of cardiac transplant recipients, studied between 1 year and 7 years after transplan-

tation and without angiographically visible narrowings of epicardial arteries or disease of the distal coronary vessels ($n = 35$ (43%)). Wall irregularities were present in 42% of the arteries but in none of these cases did a computer-assisted automatic quantitative angiographic system detect greater than 30% diameter stenoses.

A 0.018 inch (0.46 mm) or 0.014 inch (0.32 mm) Doppler guide wire was advanced into a straight, smooth and regular proximal or mid segment of the studied artery and the flow velocity signal was recorded. Time-averaged peak blood flow velocity and mean and integrals of diastolic and systolic velocity components were measured using a custom-designed analysis system after digital conversion of the video-signal. After calibration, the contours of the Doppler envelope were traced using an electronic pen. The systolic and diastolic components were defined based on the simultaneously recorded electrocardiogram (QRS complex), aortic pressure (dicrotic notch), and flow velocity pattern (sudden increase in flow velocity at end-diastole). A repeated independent analysis of 10 Doppler tracings from the same observer or from a second observer showed less than 5% intraobserver and interobserver variability for all the analyzed parameters.

The time-averaged peak velocity (mean ± SD of all the coronary measurements) was 23 ± 11 cm/s. A large range of velocity measurements was observed (9–61 cm/s). Maximal blood flow velocity was 42 ± 17 cm/s (range 14–82 cm/s). The time-averaged peak velocity and the diastolic-to-systolic velocity ratio (mean velocities and integrals) are reported for the left anterior descending, left circumflex and right coronary arteries in Fig. 5.1.

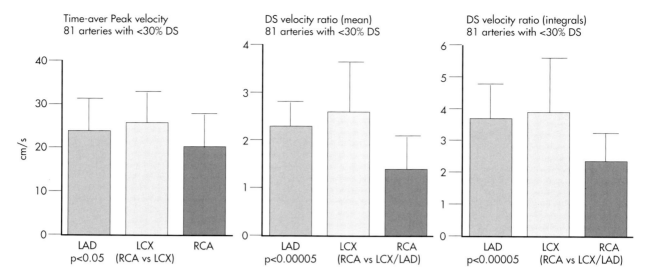

Figure 5.1. Time-averaged peak velocity (left), diastolic-to-systolic ratio of the mean velocity (centre) and diastolic-to-systolic ratio of the velocity integrals (right) in the left anterior descending (LAD), left circumflex (LCX) and right coronary arteries (RCA) in 81 arteries without hemodynamically significant stenoses.

In a smaller series of normal or near-normal arteries in patients with single-vessel coronary artery disease (31 arteries) the long-term reproducibility of flow velocity measurements was tested in both basal and hyperemic conditions.[1] An intracoronary bolus of 8–12 mg of papaverine was used to induce maximal hyperemia. Five minutes after the injection of papaverine, a baseline flow velocity and a cineangiogram were recorded (Fig. 5.2). During measurement of hyperemic and basal velocity, heart rate and aortic blood pressure were simultaneously recorded. After a follow-up period of 4–7 months (mean 5.8 months) hyperemic and baseline coronary flow velocity were recorded in the same position.

No significant differences between initial and follow-up measurements were present for baseline and hyperemic velocity and for coronary flow reserve (Table 5.1). The standard deviation of the difference between initial and follow-up measurements was higher in baseline conditions (± 31%) than during hyperemia (± 23%). The largest dispersion of the data was observed for coronary flow reserve (SD ± 36%). Regression analysis confirmed that a better correlation was present for the hyperemic measurements than for the baseline measurements ($r = 0.59$ and 0.46, respectively) (Fig. 5.3). The correlation between initial and follow-up measurements was very poor for coronary flow reserve ($r = 0.22$). Absolute coronary flow and coronary flow resistance, on the other hand, showed a high correlation between corresponding measurements after a 6-month interval.

Reproducibility of flow reserve

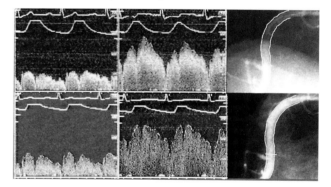

Figure 5.2. Doppler flow velocity measurements in the mid segment of an angiographically normal right coronary artery (magnified and after automated computer-assisted contour detection, right panels) at baseline (basal, left panels) and at the peak effect of papaverine (hyperemic, mid panels) in the initial study and at follow-up. Note the similar velocity pattern and flow reserve. Velocity scale: 120 cm/s.

Minimizing the technical sources of measurement variability in order to detect true changes due to pharmacological or mechanical interventions is a major challenge even for the most recent and sophisticated invasive methods of selective measurement of coronary velocity and diameter. The large sample volume of the Doppler guide wire

Table 5.1 **Hemodynamic, flow velocity and area changes from the initial assessment to follow-up.**

Parameter	Status	Initial evaluation	Follow-up evaluation	P-value
Heart rate (beats/min)	Baseline	67 ± 12	71 ± 11	>0.05
	Papaverine	74 ± 12	74 ± 12	NS
Mean aortic pressure (mmHg)	Baseline	111 ± 11	112 ± 13	NS
	Papaverine	104 ± 11	111 ± 14	>0.05
CSA at site Doppler sample volume (mm²)	Baseline	5.56 ± 2.65	5.66 ± 2.70	NS
Time-averaged peak flow velocity (cm/s)	Baseline	23.5 ± 8.6	22.5 ± 5.5	NS
	Papaverine	64.4 ± 18.8	66.3 ± 16.2	NS
CFR		2.9 ± 0.8	3.0 ± 0.8	NS
Coronary blood flow (ml/min)	Baseline	36.6 ± 16.9	37.2 ± 18.9	NS
	Papaverine	104.8 ± 52.6	112.7 ± 61.5	NS
Coronary resistance (mmHg/ml/min)	Baseline	3.75 ± 1.85	3.99 ± 2.47	NS
	Papaverine	1.29 ± 0.69	1.40 ± 1.01	NS

NS: not significant; CSA: cross-sectional area; CFR: coronary flow reserve.

facilitates the acquisition of reproducible measurements since moderate variations in the orientation of the Doppler crystal inside the vessel do not influence the final measurements.[2] The recording of a high-quality Doppler spectrum, required in all cases, indicates that the centerline of flow is included in the Doppler sample volume. Since the Doppler shift is influenced by the cosine of the angle between ultrasound beam and maximal velocity vector, for a Doppler-tipped transducer negligible changes are produced by relatively large deflections of the probe from the centerline of flow (−6% for a 30° angle). For a given flow, velocity is inversely correlated with the cross-sectional area at the site of the measurement. The better correlation of flow measurements than of velocity measurements confirms the importance of the area changes determined by variations in coronary tone or by minor differences in the position of the guide wire along the vessel. Using intracoronary adenosine (12–18 µg)[3,4] a predilatation with nitrates is not strictly required since the low dose used has a selective effect on the resistance vessels without inducing changes in the area of the epicardial arteries.[5] Intracoronary nitrates, however, remain highly recommended when reproducible measurements must be obtained in different phases of the same procedure (for example, before and after balloon angioplasty) or in different procedures to overcome the spontaneous variations in coronary vasomotor tone.

The basal coronary flow is ultimately determined by the myocardial oxygen demand. Heart rate, preload, mean aortic pressure and inotropic status are the most important determinants of the cardiac workload and, consequently, of the myocardial oxygen consumption and baseline coronary flow. During maximal hyperemia, coronary flow is linearly positively correlated with aortic pressure and negatively correlated with heart rate.[6] Spontaneous variations in heart rate over time are sufficient to impair the reproducibility of repeated measurements of baseline velocity and, to a lesser extent, of hyperemic velocity. Since opposite changes in baseline and hyperemic velocity occur with an increase in heart rate, as reported in previous studies,[7–9] coronary flow reserve decreases with an increase in heart rate. Atrial pacing, or a normalization of the coronary flow reserve for heart rate, can overcome this limitation but is not a practical solution for routine clinical use of this technique. The moderate changes in aortic pressure from the initial study to follow-up had a more limited influence on the changes in flow velocity and coronary flow reserve. Alternatively, the application of correction factors for the basal hemodynamic conditions has been proposed.[9]

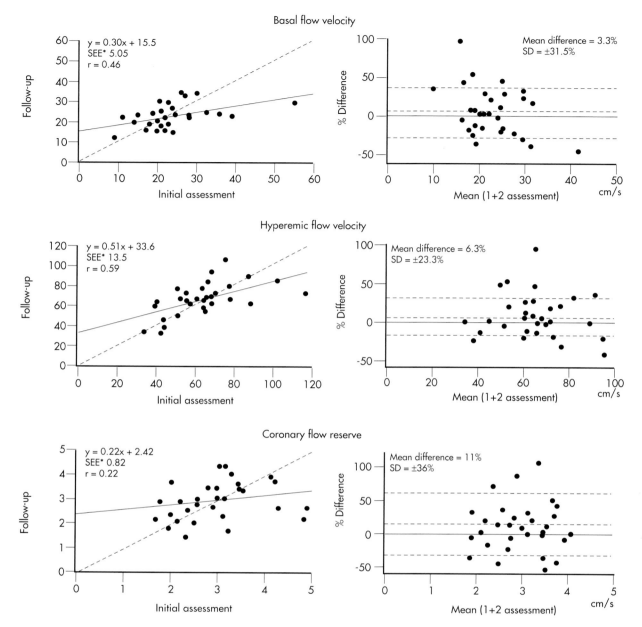

Figure 5.3. Left panels: comparison of follow-up and initial velocity measurements (time-averaged peak velocity) using linear regression. Right panels: the difference between initial and follow-up velocity measurements, expressed as a percentage of the initial velocity, is plotted against the mean of the two measurements. Note that the lowest correlation and the highest standard deviation of the difference, indicating a large dispersion of the repeated measurements, was found for the measurements of coronary flow reserve. (SEE*: standard error of the estimate.) (From Di Mario et al.,[1] with permission.)

Proximal and distal velocity measurements and coronary flow reserve: the St Louis experience[10]

In order to assess the spectrum of coronary vasodilatory reserve in patients with angiographically normal coronary arteries during cardiac catheterization, coronary flow velocity was measured using the Doppler guide wire technique and intracoronary adenosine in 450 coronary arteries of 196 patients. These comprised three groups: (1) atypical chest pain syndromes and angiographically normal coronary arteries; (2) angiographically normal cardiac transplant recipients; and (3) angiographically normal vessels in patients with coronary artery

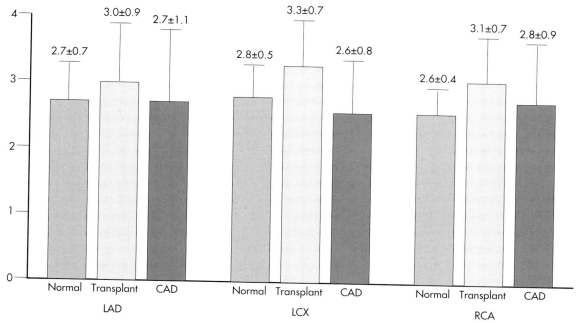

Figure 5.4. Coronary flow reserve in 450 angiographically normal coronary arteries studied between 1991 and 1995. Left anterior descending (LAD), left circumflex (LCX) and right coronary arteries (RCA). CAD: coronary artery disease.

disease (at least one artery with greater than 50% diameter stenosis).[10] Similar measurements of coronary flow reserve were obtained in all three major epicardial coronary arteries (Fig. 5.4). Coronary vasodilatory reserve, on average, was higher in transplant recipients than in the other two groups ($P < 0.05$).

These measurements were obtained in proximal segments of the vessels, but many studies have shown that proximally measured coronary flow reserve in chronically occluded arteries identifies only the contribution of branch flow.[11] Therefore, in a subgroup of 15 patients with 28 angiographically normal arteries, flow velocity measurements were obtained both in the proximal and in the distal epicardial coronary artery segments.[12] The Doppler guide wire was advanced with fluoroscopic guidance 1–2 cm from the origin of each major coronary artery for measurement of proximal velocities and 8–18 μg of intracoronary adenosine was used for computation of coronary flow reserve. Proximal and distal coronary dimensions were measured at the site of flow velocity measurements by quantitative angiography. Two angiographic views which displayed the artery clearly and were approximately 90° orthogonally apart were selected for analysis, and the diameters measured with electronic calipers at the Doppler sampling site;

these measurements were used to calculate the corresponding vessel cross-sectional area assuming a circular shape. Volumetric flow was calculated as the product of the vessel cross-sectional area at the sampling site, the total flow velocity integral, and heart rate. At baseline, the mean velocity was not significantly different either in the proximal or the distal guide wire position (Fig. 5.5a). As expected, all three proximal and distal coronary arteries had proportionally and significantly greater velocity parameters during adenosine-induced hyperemia. Coronary flow reserve did not differ for the left anterior descending, the left circumflex or the right coronary arteries and remained constant between proximal and distal segments (Fig. 5.5b). Chapter 2 explains why minor changes in flow velocity occur despite large differences in cross-sectional area and absolute flow (Figs 5.5a and 5.5b).

What is a normal flow reserve?

The threefold increase in flow velocity from baseline observed after papaverine in these large series of patients is lower than the four- to sixfold increase previously reported in patients with normal coronary arteries.[13,14] In these series, however, a highly selected patient population was studied, with

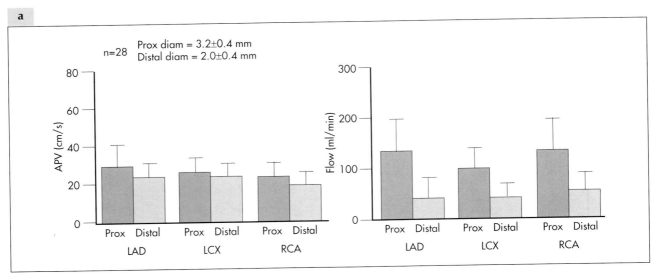

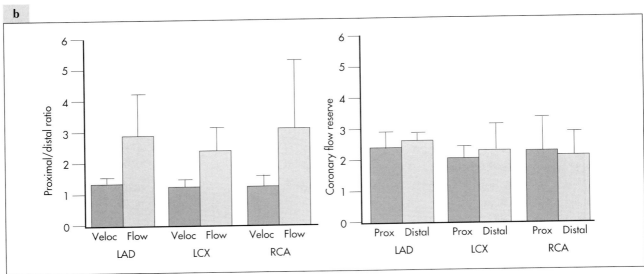

Figure 5.5. (a) Coronary flow velocity and absolute coronary flow proximal and distal to coronary stenoses in the left anterior descending (LAD), left circumflex (LCX) and right coronary artery (RCA). Note that a moderate decrease in flow velocity is observed from proximal to distal despite the almost threefold decrease in flow. Proximal diameter = 3.2 ± 0.4 mm; distal diameter = 2.0 ± 0.4 mm; *n* = 28. **(b)** The proximal-to-distal ratio is close to 1 for flow velocity and greater than 2 for coronary flow. Note that coronary flow reserve is very similar in the proximal and distal segments of the artery. (Redrawn from Ofili et al.,[12] with permission.)

the exclusion of myocardial hypertrophy, previous myocardial infarction or other conditions known to increase the baseline flow (anemia, hyperthyroidism, etc.). These values seem unrealistic when applied to the majority of patients with coronary artery disease. Using the same technique (Doppler catheters and zero-crossing), Zeiher et al. reported a percentage increase in coronary blood flow after papaverine of 361% in normal arteries of patients with coronary artery disease, with a large dispersion of the measurements (standard deviation ± 121%) and a significant reduction in comparison with normal controls.[15] Similar differences were also reported for myocardial flow reserve using positron emission tomography to study the territory of distribution of normal arteries in patients with coronary artery disease.[16] The possible presence of an impaired flow reserve in patients with coronary artery disease independently of the severity of epicardial coronary stenoses is certainly the main limitation to the application of this technique in clinical practice. The definition of a cut-off limit cannot be based on statistical analysis of velocity measurements in normal patients but requires comparison with other techniques used to establish the presence of myocardial ischemia in the territory of distribution of the artery studied. Coronary flow reserve measured with intracoronary Doppler corre- lates well with the results of radioisotopic perfusion tests.[17-20] In particular, lesions with a flow reserve smaller than 2.0 almost invariably show a reduced myocardial perfusion in the territory of distribution of the studied artery. Large clinical studies have reported the safety of deferring angioplasty based on the results of flow velocity measurements and, in particular, using a flow reserve lower than 2.0.[21]

References

1   Di Mario C, Gil R, Serruys PW. Long-term reproducibility of coronary flow velocity measurements in patients with coronary artery disease. *Am J Cardiol* 1995; **73**: 1177–80.

2   Doucette JW, Douglas Corl P, Payne HP et al. Validation of a Doppler guide wire for intravascular measurement of coronary artery flow velocity. *Circulation* 1992; **85**: 1899–911.

3   Wilson RF, Wyche K, Christensen BV, Laxson DD. Effects of adenosine on human coronary arterial circulation. *Circulation* 1990; **82**: 1595–606

4   Kern MJ, Deligonul U, Aguirre F, Hilton TC. Intravenous adenosine: continuous infusion and low dose bolus administration for determination of coronary vasodilator reserve in patients with and without coronary artery disease. *J Am Coll Cardiol* 1991; **18**: 718–29.

5   Sudhir K, MacGregor JS, Barbant SD et al. Assessment of coronary conductance and resistance vessel reactivity in response to nitroglycerin, ergonovine and adenosine: in vivo studies with simultaneous intravascular two-dimensional and Doppler ultrasound. *J Am Coll Cardiol* 1993; **21**: 1261–8.

6   Klocke FJ. Measurements of coronary flow reserve: defining pathophysiology versus making decisions about patient care. *Circulation* 1987; **76**: 245–57.

7   Hongo M, Nakatsuka T, Watanabe N et al. Effects of heart rate on phasic coronary blood flow pattern and flow reserve in patients with normal coronary arteries: a study with an intravascular Doppler catheter and spectral analysis. *Am Heart J* 1994; **127**: 545–51.

8   McGinn AL, White CW, Wilson RF. Interstudy variability of coronary flow reserve: influence of heart rate, arterial pressure, and ventricular preload. *Circulation* 1990; **81**: 1319–30.

9   Rossen JD, Winniford MD. Effect of increases in heart rate and arterial pressure on coronary flow reserve in humans. *J Am Coll Cardiol* 1993; **21**: 343–8.

10   Kern MJ, Aguirre FV, Bach RG et al. Variations in coronary vasodilatory reserve by artery, sex, status post transplantation, and remote coronary disease. *Circulation* 1994; **90**: I154 (abst).

11   Ofili EO, Labovitz AJ, Kern MJ. Coronary flow dynamics in normal and diseased arteries. *Am J Cardiol* 1993; **71**: 3D–9D.

12   Ofili EO, Kern MJ, St Vrain JA et al. Differential characterization of blood flow, velocity, and vascular resistance between proximal and distal epicardial human coronary arteries: analysis by intracoronary Doppler spectral flow analysis. *Am Heart J* 1995; **130**: 37–46.

13   Wilson RF, Marcus ML, White CW. Prediction of the physiologic significance of coronary arterial lesions by quantitative lesion geometry in patients with limited coronary artery disease. *Circulation* 1987; **75**: 723–32.

14   Wilson RF, Johnson MR, Marcus ML et al. The effect of coronary angioplasty on coronary blood flow reserve. *Circulation* 1988; **71**: 873–85.

15   Zeiher AM, Drexler H, Wollschläger H, Just H. Endothelial dysfunction of the coronary microvasculature is associated with impaired coronary blood flow regulation in patients with early atherosclerosis. *Circulation* 1991; **84**: 1984–92.

16   Beanlands RS, Muzik O, Melon P et al. Noninvasive quantification of regional myocardial flow reserve in patients with coronary atherosclerosis using nitrogen-13 ammonia positron emission tomography. *J Am Coll Cardiol* 1995; **26**: 1465–75.

17   Moertl D, Porenta G, Binder T, Sochor H, Probst P. Comparison of stenotic flow reserve by quantitative angiography with intracoronary Doppler flow reserve and myocardial thallium-201 scintigraphy. *Circulation* 1995; **92**: I262.

18   Miller DD, Donouhue TJ, Younis LT et al. Correlation of pharmacological ^{99m}Tc-SestaMIBI myocardial perfusion imaging with post-stenotic coronary flow reserve in patients with angiographically intermediate artery stenoses. *Circulation* 1994; **89**: 2150–60.

19   Joye JD, Schulman DS, Lasorda D et al. Intracoronary Doppler guide wire versus stress single photon emission computed tomographic Thallium-201 imaging in assessment of intermediate coronary stenoses. *J Am Coll Cardiol* 1994; **24**: 940–7.

20   Deychak YA, Segal J, Reiner SR et al. Doppler guide wire flow velocity indexes measured distal to coronary stenoses associated with reversible thallium perfusion defects. *Am Heart J* 1995; **129**: 219–27.

21   Kern MJ, Donouhue TJ, Aguirre FV et al. Clinical outcome of deferring angioplasty in patients with normal translesional pressure-flow velocity measurements. *J Am Coll Cardiol* 1995; **25**: 178–87.

6 Three-dimensional reconstruction of intracoronary ultrasound

Clemens von Birgelen, Pim J de Feyter and Jos R T C Roelandt

Introduction

Two-dimensional intracoronary ultrasound (ICUS) permits the study of the extent, distribution, and therapy of atherosclerotic plaques by unique tomographic visualization of both the vascular lumen and wall.[1–6] Three-dimensional (3D) reconstruction of the ICUS images in vivo has been based on the definition of thresholds in the grayscale intensity.[7-9] Recently, alternative methods and new approaches have been proposed providing new modalities of assessment.[10–13]

Rationale of 3D ICUS

Why three-dimensional reconstruction of the ICUS images? Several clinical and research questions can be better addressed by 3D ICUS than by two-dimensional ICUS or angiography. The therapeutic mechanisms of interventional devices for instance are better studied with ICUS than by angiography[14] since ICUS directly visualizes the vessel wall.[3] The most important limitation of two-dimensional ICUS in pre/post-studies is the matching of the target sites for serial measurement. This problem reflects the lack of the third dimension in the two-dimensional ICUS images. Measurement of the plaque area in an entire coronary segment provides more detailed insight into the complex plaque architecture and avoids the difficult mental conceptualization process.[15-19] Furthermore, measurements of the target lesion and the reference segments are immediately obtained in a reconstructed longitudinal view during on-line 3D reconstruction. This maneuver facilitates the selection of the optimal type and size of interventional device or the evaluation of complications.[8,20] A coronary segment of interest can be examined before and after an interventional procedure,[21-24] thus avoiding incomplete stent deployment with an increased risk of thrombus formation after coronary stenting.[25]

Basic processing steps

The basic processing steps to obtain a 3D reconstruction from the two-dimensional ICUS images are similar for all systems currently available.

Image acquisition

Optimal image quality of the basic ICUS images will result in better 3D reconstructions and therefore machine settings must be optimized before the images are acquired. A zoom function helps to assure the complete visualization of the arterial wall. Starting distal of the stenosis the imaging catheter is withdrawn through the arterial segment which will be reconstructed.

The imaging core of ICUS catheters designed for repeated pullbacks should not have direct contact with the vessel wall. Such catheters are equipped with a 15 cm transparent distal sheath (external diameter ≤ 1 mm) which lodges the guide wire over which the imaging system is introduced and withdrawn. During the ICUS study the common lumen contains the rotating ultrasound cable while the guide wire is pulled back up to a radiopaque marker. The design of this ICUS catheter reduces the risk of nonuniform pullback. The first 5–10 seconds of a continuous pullback are usually required to straighten the imaging core inside the catheter before a constant withdrawal speed is ensured.

Processing steps and utilization of 3D ICUS

Processing steps

- **Acquisition** — continuous or ECG-triggered pullback
- **Digitization** — on-line or off-line
- **Segmentation** — threshold-based, acoustic quantification or contour-detection
- **Reconstruction** — voxel-modeling, shading, rendering techniques

Utilization

- **Visualization** of vascular structures — dynamic or static; transverse, longitudinal, and cylindrical views
- **Measurement** of vessel dimensions — (semi-)automated or manual

Different pullback methods can be used. A continuous-speed pullback which results in an equidistant spacing of adjacent images[26] and a stepwise pullback using an ECG-triggered stepping motor[27] are the most common approaches. Side-branches or spots of calcium are used as topographic landmarks for a reliable comparison of the same arterial segment in serial studies. A modified concept of the continuous-speed pullback is the ECG-triggered video labeling during a uniform pullback of the ICUS catheter. Video frames coinciding with the R-wave of the ECG are automatically labeled and images acquired at the same phase of the cardiac cycle are used for off-line 3D reconstruction. This approach permits the display of the arterial segment and the measurement of the vascular dimensions at any time of the cardiac cycle and minimizes the systolic–diastolic artifacts which can frequently be observed in the uniform-speed pullback approach.

ECG-gating of the image acquisition and pullback is another way to overcome the problem of cyclic motion artifacts. Using a dynamic 3D reconstruction system, initially designed for 3D reconstruction of echocardiographic images (Echoscan, TomTec, Munich, Germany),[28] the arterial segment can be dynamically displayed during the cardiac cycle.[27,29] The upper and lower limits of the R-R interval are defined before the image acquisition starts. During the pullback procedure, a maximum number of 25 ICUS images per cardiac cycle for each scanning plane are sampled in the computer memory, unless the length of the R-R interval fails to meet the preset range.

Image digitization and segmentation

Digitization of the ICUS images can be performed on-line or off-line by sampling the video frames with a framegrabber at a defined digitization frame rate. The segmentation step identifies structures of interest according to a certain grayscale scheme. The segmentation of the grayscale ICUS images can be achieved by the application of dedicated algorithms, discriminating between the blood-pool inside the lumen and structures of the vessel wall.[30] The quality of the final 3D reconstruction and the accuracy of the quantitative analysis are highly influenced by the quality of the segmentation algorithm. Besides the previously mentioned interactive threshold method,[9] segmentation can also be achieved by the application of an acoustic quantification method[10] or a contour detection method.[12,18,31]

The acoustic quantification method (Fig. 6.1) provides the distinction between the blood pool and vessel wall, using an algorithm for statistical pattern recognition (EchoQuant, Indec Systems, Capitola, CA). Comparing the pattern of flowing blood to the pattern of the vessel wall, much more variation in time is found in blood.[32] The algorithm is able to distinguish between these two patterns and thus to detect the interface between blood and vessel wall. Finally, segmentation is performed by removing the blood pool.

The contour detection method which the authors use has been developed at the Thoraxcenter, Rotterdam, The Netherlands, and is based on the application of a minimum cost algorithm for contour detection (Fig. 6.2), which detects the intimal leading edge and the external vascular boundary (lamina externa).[18,31] Another semi-automated contour detection system described by Sonka et al. enables the detection of the plaque borders and the internal and external elastic laminae. First results of an in-vitro study showed good correlation of the lumen and plaque area measurements with observer-defined values.[33,34]

Characteristics of different segmentation methods

	Thresholding	Acoustic quantification	Contour detection
Applicability	• No geometric assumption on lumen shape required • Depends greatly on the image quality • Reliability depends on optimal setting of the thresholds	• No geometric assumptions on the lumen shape necessary • Depends greatly on the image quality	• User interaction is required in irregular lumen shapes • Depends on the image quality
On-line use	• Is possible	• Is feasible	• Is possible
(Semi-) automated detection	• Only detection of the intimal leading edge is possible	• Only detection of the intimal leading edge is possible	• Detection of both the intimal leading edge and the external vessel contour is possible

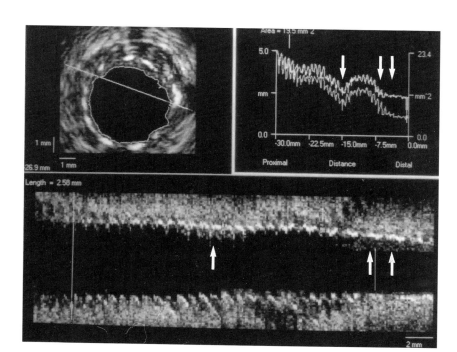

Figure 6.1. In-stent restenosis three months after implantation of a long Wallstent (Schneider, Bülach, Switzerland) in a left anterior descending coronary artery. While the proximal stent shows a good open lumen (left upper panel) focal intimal hyperplasia was found in the mid and distal segments (longitudinal display in lower panel). The diagram (right upper panel), displaying the luminal diameter and area, reflects the luminal encroachment (arrows) by restenotic tissue. The reconstruction was performed using the EchoQuant system (Indec Systems, Capitola, CA).

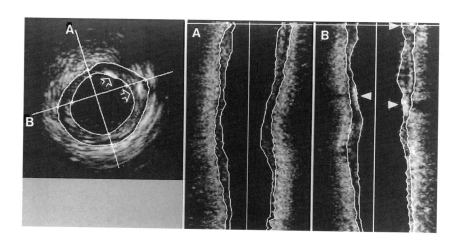

Figure 6.2. Atherosclerotic right coronary artery with spots of calcium. The site of the calcium in the coronary wall, visible in both a longitudinal and a cross-sectional view, is indicated by arrowheads. The detection of the intimal leading edge and the external boundary of the total vessel have been obtained from the contour detection system of the Thoraxcenter.

Advantages of different display formats

Longitudinal	Cylindrical	Lumen cast
• Analysis of luminal patency and vessel wall pathology	• Direct inspection of the intimal surface	• Assessment of the lumen of an entire arterial segment

Image reconstruction and display

Different display formats can be used to show the 3D data set. A longitudinal (Figs. 6.1 and 6.2), a cylindrical (Fig. 6.3), and a lumen cast (Fig. 6.4) format are most commonly generated. General programs for 3D presentation of image data sets allow one to perform oblique and tangential cuts through the reconstructed structures, comparable to the display options available in magnetic resonance imaging systems. A dynamic visualization of the artery after ECG-gated image acquisition is also possible.[27]

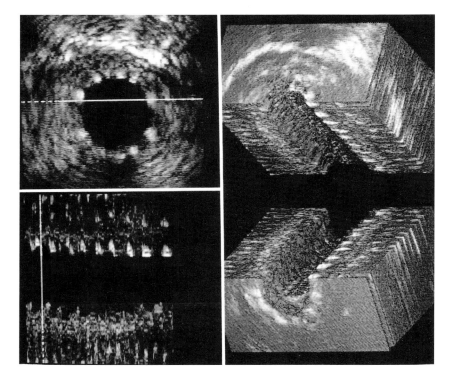

Figure 6.3. Three-dimensional reconstruction of a Wallstent (Schneider, Bülach, Switzerland) in a coronary bypass graft. Using the entire 3D dataset a cylindrical view can be reconstructed (right panel). The cylinder is cut lengthwise and opened like a clam-shell, permitting an insight into the inner surface of the vessel wall. The echogenic metal struts of the well deployed stent are clearly visible in all views. (Reprinted, with permission, from ref. 51.)

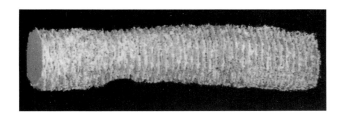

Figure 6.4 Lumen cast. The lumen-cast display of a stented saphenous vein graft permits the rapid assessment of the entire lumen. An inadequate stent expansion was found, suggesting further balloon inflations. (Reprinted, with permission, from ref. 51.)

Systems of 3D reconstruction

Different 3D reconstruction systems are available, providing distinct technical approaches of reconstruction with specific advantages and disadvantages in applicability, imaging, and quantification. The following systems are used at the Thoraxcenter.

The acoustic quantification system

The system (EchoQuant), recently validated in rabbit aortas,[10] requires an Intel Pentium personal computer and the OS/2 operating system. It can be used either on-line or off-line, and sampled ICUS images with a digitization frame-rate of 8.5 frames per second. The length of the reconstructed coronary segment is determined by the pullback speed since the image acquisition and digitization rates are fixed. Using a pullback speed of 1.0 mm/s images of an 8 cm segment can be acquired. Segmentation and reconstruction of a vascular segment of 3 cm length can be performed within 3 minutes. The quality of the automated detection can be checked and manually corrected in individual cross-sectional images.

No geometric assumption on the lumen shape is required and the program may therefore provide accurate segmentation in irregularly shaped lumina, but application of the algorithm may be hampered by the quality of the basic ICUS images.[10,35] Several parameters determining the automated identification process can be adjusted by the user. This is particularly important when the ICUS image quality is not optimal. Since the reconstruction is performed within a few minutes, it can be used in the catheterization laboratory.[35]

A selected cross-sectional image, a longitudinally reconstructed image (Fig. 6.1), and a cylindrical 3D view, presenting the segment opened longitudinally with both halves tilted back (Fig. 6.3), are displayed on the monitor. The results of the automated cross-sectional luminal area measurement are displayed in a diagram. The algorithm is not able to detect the external contour of the total vessel; however, the current version of this program provides an option which allows one to draw manually the external contour of the vessel in selected images. Thus, plaque area can be measured on two-dimensional images as, for instance, the images of the reference or the minimal luminal area.

The Thoraxcenter contour detection system

This system digitizes a user-defined region of interest of a maximum of 200 tomographic images,

requiring a Pentium personal computer (60 MHz) with 16 Mb of internal RAM and a framegrabber. The length of the reconstructed segment is defined by the pullback speed and a user-defined digitization frame-rate. A pullback speed of 1 mm/s and an image processing rate of 10 frames/s (0.1 mm/frame) result, for instance in a reconstructed segment length of 2 cm. The method depends less on the image quality since it operates interactively. Reliable segmentation and 3D reconstruction remain possible even when the image quality is not optimal. However, more user interaction is required in the presence of irregular lumen shapes. On-line application of this system has recently been started.

The contour detection procedure (Fig. 6.5) consists of three steps.[12,31] First, the ICUS images are modeled in a voxel space[36] and two perpendicular cut planes, running parallel to the longitudinal axis of the vessel, are interactively selected. Data located at the interception of these cut planes and the voxel volume are derived to reconstruct two longitudinal images of the vascular segment (Fig. 6.2). The angle and location of the cut planes can be changed interactively by the user in order to optimize the quality of the longitudinal images.

In a second step the contours of the luminal and external vascular boundaries (lamina externa) are semi-automatically defined in the longitudinal images, based on the application of a minimum cost algorithm[37] which has previously been validated[38] and applied in ICUS images.[39] The user is free to add markers, forcing the contours to pass through these sites. The optimal path of the longitudinal contours is updated serially, using dynamic programming techniques. Then, the contours of the longitudinal images are depicted as points in each individual cross-sectional image.

Finally, a contour detection is performed in all the cross-sectional images, using the four edge points derived from the longitudinal contours as landmarks to guide the detection. The accuracy of the final contours can be checked and manual correction may be performed.

The two reconstructed longitudinal images are displayed, and in a third window the user may scroll through the set of cross-sectional ICUS images.

The contour detection system permits the quantitative analysis of lumen and plaque. Each cross-sectional image represents a slice of the reconstructed arterial segment; thus volumetric data can be obtained.[18,19] The cross-sectional image, corresponding to the site of the minimal luminal cross-sectional area, is displayed automatically.

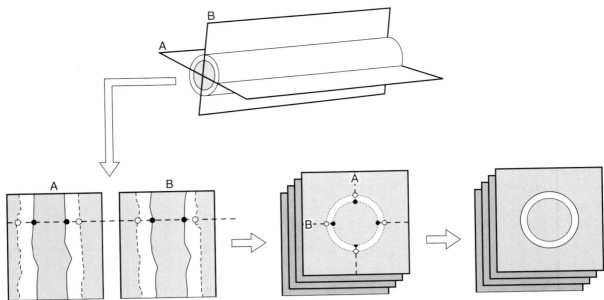

Figure 6.5. Contour detection system. The principle of this method, developed at the Thoraxcenter, Rotterdam, is that the edge information of previously detected longitudinal contours is used to guide the final contour detection on the transverse images. First, two perpendicular cut planes are used to reconstruct two longitudinal sections from the 3D ICUS image data. In a contour detection step the intimal leading edge and the external contour of the vessel are interactively defined, based on the application of a minimum-cost algorithm. Subsequently, contour detection is performed automatically in all the cross-sectional images, using four edge-points, derived from the longitudinal contours, to guide this step. The result of the final contour detection is finally checked and may be corrected by the user.

Area and mean diameter measurements of the total vessel, lumen, and plaque are displayed in diagrams. These diagrams show diameter-obstruction, area-obstruction, and luminal symmetry functions.[12,31]

The dynamic reconstruction system

The 3D reconstruction provided by this system (Echoscan) is based on the definition of thresholds in the scale of gray levels. The applicability of this algorithm depends upon the image quality. However, in instances with optimal basic image quality remarkable reconstructions can be obtained (Fig. 6.6). The ECG-triggered acquisition and the application of filter algorithms are responsible for the smoothness of the vessel contours which do not show cyclic movement artifacts. Since the 3D reconstruction of a coronary artery during the cardiac cycle requires sampling and processing of a large amount of data, the analysis time required for a dynamic assessment is still longer than for a conventional analysis.[40] Using volume rendering techniques the dynamic reconstruction system allows dynamic visualization of the reconstructed segment[27] with a

maximum of 25 frames per cardiac cycle. The reconstruction of various transverse and longitudinal sections is thus possible.

The longitudinal reconstruction of a coronary artery segment is readily available in the cardiac catheterization laboratory.[29] Similar to computer tomography or magnetic resonance imaging, these longitudinal sections can pass through the center of the vessel (Fig. 6.6) or cut the vessel wall tangentially.

Technical challenges

Several factors, including problems related to ICUS[41,42] as well as specific limitations of the 3D reconstruction[43] influence the quality of 3D ICUS. Measurement of both lumen and plaque volumes by 3D ICUS showed minimal short-term biologic variability upon repeated pullbacks of the same coronary artery segment.[44] The quality of the basic ICUS images is crucial. Poor or incomplete visualization of the lumen–plaque and plaque–adventitia

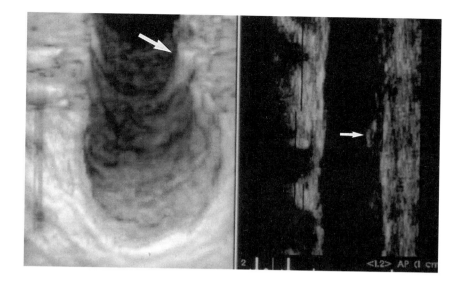

Figure 6.6. ECG-gated reconstruction of a proximal coronary artery with an eccentric plaque (on the right-hand side). A custom-designed pullback device with a stepper motor, developed at the Thoraxcenter, and the Echoscan (TomTec, Munich, Germany) were used to obtain this reconstruction. The plaque is visible on both a longitudinal section through the artery (right panel) and a three-dimensionally reconstructed view (left panel).

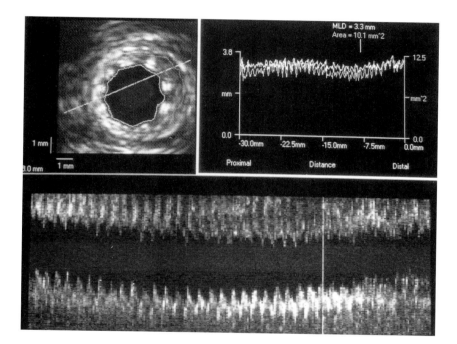

Figure 6.7. Large cyclic movement observed in a coronary vein graft. This longitudinally reconstructed image of a stented bypass graft shows a large saw-shaped artifact resulting from the cyclic movement of the vein graft and the catheter inside the vessel. The artifact is visible in both the longitudinal image display and the graph displaying the measurements of luminal area and minimal luminal diameter (right upper panel). ECG-gated reconstruction systems offer the potential to minimize this limitation. (Reprinted, with permission, from ref. 51.)

boundaries, which is a problem in the presence of calcification, hampers the reconstruction and quantification. Currently available transducers have a limited lateral resolution.[45] Image distortion by nonuniform rotation or a noncoaxial position of the ICUS catheter in the lumen may create complex artifacts in the 3D reconstructions.[43] Although motorized pullback devices or displacement sensors are used, an equal distance between adjacent images cannot always be achieved, as bends of the ultrasound catheter may induce a difference between the movement of the distal transducer and the proximal part of the ICUS catheter.

The movement of the ICUS catheter during the cardiac cycle and systolic-diastolic changes in vessel dimensions originate typical saw-shaped artifacts (Fig. 6.7) of the coronary artery wall.[43,46] These artifacts are more evident in larger arteries with high mobility. The extent of these artifacts in different individuals varies a great deal. ECG-gated image acquisition and pullback have the potential to minimize these cyclic artifacts (Fig. 5.6) and to optimize image acquisition for volumetric measurements.[43,47] However, compared to the continuous pullback, image acquisition by the ECG-gated approach requires a longer acquisition time which may cause problems in patients with very severe coronary stenoses.

Vessel curvatures with a radius of less than 5 cm cause a significant distortion of the three-dimensionally reconstructed image.[48] Overestimation and underestimation of certain portions of the plaque may be caused by vessel curvatures and bending of the ICUS imaging catheter.[43,49] The contour detection system shows artificial curvatures caused by a localized eccentric plaque burden. Other 3D reconstruction systems, as for instance the acoustic quantification system, straighten the display of the coronary segment artificially.

Future directions

Combined use of data obtained from biplane angiography and 3D reconstructed ICUS, provided by the contour detection system,[18,12] may help to overcome many of these limitations and will provide information on the real vessel curvatures and the orientation of the ICUS catheter.[50] Using this technical approach in a geometric vessel phantom of known dimensions, a high accuracy was observed and first applications in humans yielded good results. The use of new forward-locking transducers may also help to overcome some of the current limitations,[13] but the value of this device is still limited by the low image resolution and the large dimensions of the ultrasound transducers. Miniaturization of the imaging catheters and improvement of the computer technology will help to increase future applications of 3D ICUS.

Conclusion

Until recently the application of 3D ICUS appeared to be restricted to research applications, but we feel that 3D ICUS will gain further importance in the future. If the interest, effort, and technical development in this field are sustained, 3D ICUS will become a routine technique supporting both diagnostic and interventional procedures.

References

1 Ge J, Erbel R, Gerber T et al. Intravascular ultrasound imaging in angiographically normal coronary arteries: a prospective study in vivo. Br Heart J 1994; **71**: 572–8.

2 Gerber TC, Erbel R, Görge G, Ge J, Rupprecht H-J, Meyer J. Extent of atherosclerosis and remodeling of the left main coronary artery determined by intravascular ultrasound. Am J Cardiol 1994; **73**: 666–71.

3 von Birgelen C, Di Mario C, Serruys PW. Structural and functional characterization of an intermediate stenosis with intracoronary ultrasound and Doppler: 'case of reverse Glagovian modeling.' Am Heart J 1996; **132**: 694–6.

4 Yock PJ, Linker DT. Intravascular ultrasound: looking below the surface of vascular disease. Circulation 1990; **81**: 1715–18.

5 Ge J, Erbel R, Rupprecht H-J et al. Comparison of intravascular ultrasound and angiography in the assessment of myocardial bridging. Circulation 1994; **89**: 1725–32.

6 Yamagishi M, Miyatake K, Tamai J, Nakatani S, Kojama J, Nissen SE. Intravascular ultrasound detection of atherosclerosis at the site of focal vasospasm in angiographically normal or minimally narrowed coronary segments. J Am Coll Cardiol 1994; **23**: 352–7.

7 Matar FA, Mintz GS, Douek P et al. Coronary artery lumen volume measurement using three-dimensional intravascular ultrasound: validation of a new technique. Cathet Cardiovasc Diagn 1994; **33**: 214–20.

8 Rosenfield K, Kaufman J, Pieczek A, Langevin RE, Razvi S, Ilsner JM. Real-time three-dimensional reconstruction of intravascular ultrasound images of iliac arteries. Am J Cardiol 1992; **70**: 412–15.

9 Rosenfield K, Losordo DW, Ramaswamy K et al. Three-dimensional reconstruction of human coronary and peripheral arteries from images recorded during two-dimensional intravascular ultrasound examination. Circulation 1991; **84**: 1938–56.

10 Hausmann D, Friedrich G, Sudhir K et al. 3D intravascular ultrasound imaging with automated border detection using 2.9 F. catheters. J Am Coll Cardiol 1994; **23**: 174A.

11 Koch L, Kearney P, Erbel R et al. Three dimensional reconstruction of intracoronary ultrasound images: roadmapping with simultaneously digitized coronary angiograms. In: Computers in Cardiology 1993 (Los Alamitos: IEEE Computer Society Press, 1993): 89–91.

12 Li W, von Birgelen C, Di Mario C et al. Semi-automatic contour detection for volumetric quantification of intracoronary ultrasound. In: Computers in Cardiology 1994, (Los Alamitos: IEEE Computer Society Press, 1994): 277–80.

13 Ng K-H, Evans JL Vonesh MJ et al. Arterial imaging with a new forward-viewing intravascular ultrasound catheter, II: three-dimensional reconstruction and display of data. Circulation 1994; **89**: 718–23.

14 von Birgelen C, Umans V, Di Mario C et al. Mechanism of high-speed rotational atherectomy and adjunctive

balloon angioplasty revisited by quantitative coronary angiography: edge detection versus videodensitometry. *Am Heart J* 1995; **130**: 4055–12.

15 Losordo DW, Rosenfield K, Pieczek A, Baker K, Harding M, Isner JM. How does angioplasty work? Serial analysis of human iliac arteries using intravascular ultrasound. *Circulation* 1992; **86**: 1845–58.

16 Dhawale PJ, Rasheed Q, Mecca W, Nair R, Hodgson J McB. Analysis of plaque volume during DCA using a volumetrically accurate three-dimensional ultrasound technique. *Circulation* 1993; **88**: I550.

17 Galli FC, Sudhir K, Kao AK, Fitzgerald PJ, Yock PG. Direct measurement of plaque volume by three-dimensional ultrasound: potentials and pitfalls. *J Am Coll Cardiol* 1992; **19**: 115A.

18 von Birgelen C, Di Mario C, Li W et al. Morphometric analysis in three-dimensional intracoronary ultrasound: an in-vitro and in-vivo study using a novel system for the contour detection of lumen and plaque. *Am Heart J* 1996; **132**: 516–17.

19 von Birgelen C, Slager CJ, Di Mario C, de Feyter PJ, Serruys PW. Volumetric intracoronary ultrasound: a new maximum confidence approach for the quantitative assessment of progression/regression of atherosclerosis? *Atherosclerosis* 1995; **118(Suppl)**: S103–S113.

20 Coy KM, Park JC, Fishbein MC et al. In vitro validation of three-dimensional intravascular ultrasound for the evaluation of arterial injury after balloon angioplasty. *J Am Coll Cardiol* 1992; **20**: 692–700.

21 Rosenfield K, Kaufman J, Pieczek AM et al. Human coronary and peripheral arteries: on-line three-dimensional reconstruction from two-dimensional intravascular US scans. *Radiology* 1992; **184**: 823–32.

22 Mintz GS, Leon MB, Satler LF et al. Clinical experience using a new three-dimensional intravascular ultrasound system before and after transcatheter coronary therapies. *J Am Coll Cardiol* 1992; **19**: 292A.

23 Schryver TE, Popma JJ, Kent KM, Leon MB, Eldredge S, Mintz GS. Use of intracoronary ultrasound to identify the true coronary lumen in chronic coronary dissection treated with intracoronary stenting. *Am J Cardiol* 1992; **69**: 1107–8.

24 Mintz GS, Pichard AD, Satler LF, Popma JJ, Kent KM, Leon MB. Three-dimensional intravascular ultrasonography: reconstruction of endovascular stents in vitro and in vivo. *J Clin Ultrasound* 1993; **21**: 609–15.

25 von Birgelen C, Gil R, Ruygrok P et al. Optimized expansion of the Wallstent compared to the Palmaz-Schatz stent: online observations with two- and three-dimensional intracoronary ultrasound after angiographic guidance. *Am Heart J* 1996; **131**: 1067–75.

26 Mintz GS, Keller MB, Fay FG et al. Motorized ICUS transducer pullback permits accurate quantitative axial measurements. *Circulation* 1992; **86**: I323.

27 Bruining N, von Birgelen C, Di Mario C et al. Dynamic three-dimensional reconstruction of ICUS images based on an ECG gated pullback device. In: *Computers in Cardiology* 1995 (Los Alamitos: IEEE Computer Society Press, 1995): 633–71.

28 Roelandt JRTC, ten Cate FJ, Vletter WB, Taams MA. Ultrasonic dynamic three-dimensional visualization of the heart with a multiplane transesophageal imaging transducer. *J Am Soc Echocardiogr* 1994; **7**: 217–29.

29 Fehske W, Pizzulli L, Hagendorff A, Lüderitz B. Real-time three-dimensional intracoronary ultrasonography: high resolution dynamic images of coronary artery lesions. *J Am Coll Cardiol* 1995; **25**: 180A.

30 Chandrasekaran K, D'Adamo AJ, Sehgal CM. Three-dimensional reconstruction of intravascular ultrasound images. In: Yock PG, Tobis JM, eds. *Intravascular Ultrasound Imaging* (New York: Churchill Livingstone, 1992): 141–7.

31 von Birgelen C, van der Lugt A, Nicosia A, Metz GF et al. Computerized assessment of coronary lumen and atherosclerotic plaque dimensions in three-dimensional intravascular ultrasound correlated with histomorphometry. *Am J Cardiol* 1996 (in press).

32 Li W, Gussenhoven EJ, Zhong Y et al. Temporal averaging for quantification of lumen dimensions in intravascular ultrasound images. *Ultrasound Med Biol* 1994; **20**: 117–22.

33 Sonka M, Zhang X, Siebes M, DeJong S, McKay CR, Collins SM. Automated segmentation of coronary wall and plaque from intravascular ultrasound image sequences. In: *Computers in Cardiology 1994* (Los Alamitos: IEEE Computer Society Press, 1994): 281–4.

34 Sonka M, Zhang X, Siebes M et al. Semi-automated detection of coronary arterial wall and plaque borders in intravascular ultrasound images. *Circulation* 1994; **90**: I550.

35 von Birgelen C, Kutryk MJB, Gil R et al. Quantification of the minimal luminal cross-sectional area after coronary stenting: two- and three-dimensional intravascular ultrasound versus edge detection and videodensitometry. *Am J Cardiol* 1996; **78**: 520–5.

36 Kitney R, Moura L, Straughan K. 3-D visualization of arterial structures using ultrasound and voxel modeling. *Int J Card Imaging* 1989; **4**: 135–43.

37 Li W, Bosch JG, Zhong Y et al. Image segmentation and 3D reconstruction of intravascular ultrasound images. In: Wei Y, Gu B, eds. *Acoustical Imaging*, Vol. 20. (New York: Plenum Press 1993): 489–96.

38 Li W, Gussenhoven EJ, Zhong Y et al. Validation of quantitative analysis of intravascular ultrasound images. *Int J Card Imaging* 1991; **6**: 247–54.

39 Di Mario C, The SHK, Madretsma S et al. Detection and characterization of vascular lesions by intravascular ultrasound: an in-vitro study correlated with histology. *J Am Soc Echocardiogr* 1992; **5**: 135–46.

40 Masotti L, Pini R. Three-dimensional imaging. In: Wells PNT, ed. *Advances in Ultrasound Techniques and Instrumentation* (New York: Churchill Livingstone, 1993): 69–77.

41 Ge J, Erbel R, Seidel I et al. Experimentelle Überprüfung der Genauigkeit und Sicherheit des intraluminalen Ultraschalls. *Z Kardiol* 1991; **80**: 595–601.

42 Di Mario C, Madretsma S, Linker D et al. The angle of incidence of the ultrasonic beam: a critical factor for the image quality in intravascular ultrasonography. *Am Heart J* 1993; **125**: 442–8.

43 Roelandt, JRTC, Di Mario C, Pandian NG et al. Three-dimensional reconstruction of intracoronary ultrasound images: rationale, approaches, problems and directions. *Circulation* 1994; **90**: 1044–55.

44 Dhawale P, Rasheed Q, Berry J, Hodgson J McB. Quantification of lumen and plaque volume with ultrasound: accuracy and short-term variability in patients. *Circulation* 1994; **90**: I164.

45 Benkeser PJ, Churchwell AL, Lee C, Abouelnasr DM. Resolution limitations in intravascular ultrasound imaging. *J Am Soc Echocardiogr* 1993; **6**: 158–65.

46 Di Mario C, von Birgelen C, Prati F et al. Three-dimensional reconstruction of two-dimensional intracoronary ultrasound: clinical or research tool? *Br Heart J* 1995; **73(Suppl 2)**: 26–32.

47 Dhawale PJ, Wilson DL, Hodgson J McB. Optimal data acquisition for volumetric intracoronary ultrasound. *Cathet Cardiovasc Diagn* 1994; **32**: 288–99.

48 Waligora MJ, Vonesh MJ, Wiet SP, McPherson DD. Effect of vascular curvature on three-dimensional reconstruction of intravascular ultrasound images. *Circulation* 1994; **90**: I227.

49 Klein HM, Günther RW, Verlande M et al. 3D-surface reconstruction of intravascular ultrasound images using personal computer hardware and a motorized catheter control. *Cardiovasc Intervent Radiol* 1992; **15**: 97–101.

50 Slager CJ, Laban M, von Birgelen C et al. ANGUS: A new approach to three-dimensional reconstruction of geometry and orientation of coronary lumen and plaque by combined use of coronary angiography and ICUS. *J Am Coll Cardiol* 1995; **25**: 144A.

51 von Birgelen C, Di Mario C, Reimers B et al. Three-dimensional intracoronary ultrasound imaging: methodology and clinical relevance for the assessment of coronary arteries and bypass grafts. *J Cardiovasc Surg* 1996; **37**: 129–39.

7 Tissue characterization

Paulina Ramo and Timothy Spencer

Introduction

Since intravascular ultrasound (IVUS) imaging was first performed eight years ago it has emerged as a promising new imaging modality for the study of vascular disease. In the context of IVUS in coronary artery disease, tissue characterization seeks to define the structure and content of atherosclerotic plaque based on the changes that occur in sound waves during their physical interaction.[1] IVUS imaging has several advantages over transthoracic ultrasound which affect the feasibility and diagnostic utility of clinical tissue characterization of the heart. These include the short distance of the interrogated tissue from the transducer, relatively homogeneous fluid path, relatively limited pathology of the tissues of interest, and high resolution of the data acquisition system.

The sensitivity and specificity of current IVUS imaging in identifying calcium is about 90% and the presence of calcium has been shown to be associated with greater frequency of deep medial leaks and with greater lumen gain.[2] Accurate identification of other lesion morphology could also be potentially useful in the diagnosis and treatment of coronary disease at many levels. These include: (a) to help decision-making as regards to therapeutic strategy (for example, fibrinolytic treatment versus mechanical recanalization); (b) when choosing between different interventional strategies (such as percutaneous transluminal coronary angioplasty (PTCA) versus stent implantation versus rotablator versus directional coronary atherectomy and laser treatment); (c) detection of plaques prone to rupture; and (d) identification of lesions requiring intensive lipid-lowering therapy.

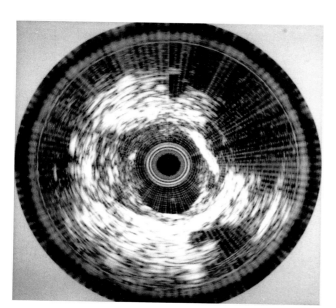

Figure 7.1. Intravascular ultrasound image of a calcified atherosclerotic plaque at 2 o'clock with an acoustic shadow and reverberations behind the plaque.

Methods of ultrasound signal analysis

Qualitative assessment of ultrasound images

The simplest way to achieve tissue characterization and the current interpretation of plaque morphology are based on the visual assessment of the IVUS video images. According to the first videodensitometric classification of an atherosclerotic plaque,[3] (a) hypoechoic regions represent lipid depositions, (b) 'soft' echoes arise from fibromuscular tissue, (c) bright echoes are reflected from collagen and fibrous tissue and (d) bright echoes with acoustic shadowing represent the presence of calcium.

In current clinical practice, calcium is identified by a bright ultrasound echo with an acoustic shadow and reverberations behind the plaque (Figs 7.1 and 7.2). Dense fibrosis appears as regions in which echodensity is higher than that of adventitia (Figs 7.3, 7.4 and 7.5). Videodensitometric sensitivity in

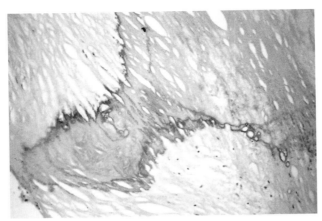

Figure 7.2. Calcified plaque; area of heavy calcification identified with standard H and E staining.

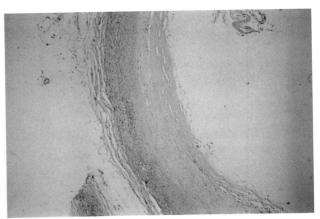

Figure 7.4. H and E staining of a dense fibrotic plaque; the plaque consists of dense, hyaline collagen with small numbers of cells.

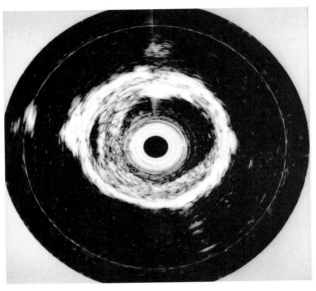

Figure 7.3. IVUS image of a fibrotic plaque at 12 o'clock.

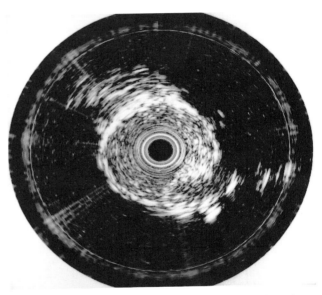

Figure 7.5. IVUS image of a restenosed veingraft with moderately fibrotic tissue (increased cellularity and collagen content in comparison with loose fibrotic plaque).

identifying dense fibrosis (fibrous connective tissue with dense extracellular collagen) is about 63–77%.[4–6] Although the term 'soft' has not been shown to be associated with the compressibility of the plaque, it is still widely used to describe sonolucent plaques composed possibly of thrombus, lipid, and/or loose fibrotic tissue (Figs 7.6, 7.7 and 7.8). The videodensitometric sensitivity in identifying lipid has been shown to be about 23–46%[6] and for thrombus about 57%. Because of the low sensitivity of IVUS video images in identifying thrombus and because of its clinical importance,[7] other ultrasonic features of thrombotic material have been used to discriminate thrombus from lipid and loose fibrotic tissue. These include (a) sonolucent material with slight synchronic pulsation, (b) imprint of the intravascular ultrasound catheter, (c) irregular borders, (d) intensity about half the adventitia, (e) microchannels (older thrombus) and (f) scintillation appearance of the video image.

The main reasons for the low sensitivity of IVUS video images in discriminating different plaque types are the postprocessing of the ultrasound

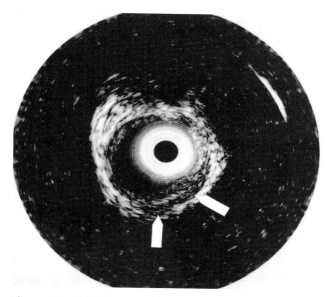

Figure 7.6. IVUS image of intimal thickening consisting of loose fibrotic tissue and lipid-filled foam cells (arrowed region).

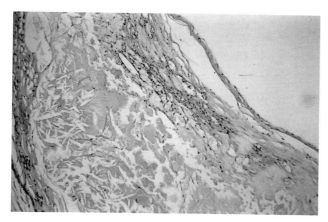

Figure 7.7. Histological section of a loose fibrotic plaque (loose, edematous connective tissue with few cells and small amounts of collagen).

Figure 7.8. Histological section of an atheromatous plaque with foam cells, free lipid and cholesterol crystals.

signal, the low spatial and dynamic resolution of the video signals and the vulnerability of video images to adjustments in gain settings on the machine.

Quantitative assessment of reflected ultrasound signals

The quantitative assessment of reflected ultrasound signals has the potential to quantify the extent of change. Depending on the site of data collection, it can be less vulnerable to the inherent problems of videodensitometry due to the postprocessing of the ultrasound signal and adjustments in gain settings. Data collection for quantitative analysis can be carried out (a) from the video image; (b) after some of the postprocessing of the ultrasound signal has been done by the IVUS machine itself; or (c) from the so-called 'raw', unprocessed radiofrequency (RF) signal (Fig. 7.9). By collecting the RF data, all postprocessing of the ultrasound signal can be avoided and thus the frequency and phase information of the data preserved. The frequency information, for example, is needed in order to carry out frequency analysis of the reflected signal or attenuation calculations from the ultrasound signal which are shown to be potentially successful approaches for accurate tissue characterization.

Other approaches to analyzing specific characteristics of the sound waves include the analysis of the reflected signal or attenuation of the sound waves in the time domain or the analysis of the pattern of the backscattered ultrasound energy. Time domain analysis of the ultrasound signals is based on the amplitude of the echo signals. It can be potentially available in real time and be applied to the output of commercial ultrasound machines. The collected and processed signal can be integrated to calculate the mean backscattered energy over the bandwidth of the transducer. In real time, the data can be integrated over time to determine the time-averaged integrated backscatter. The frequency information is, however, lost in time-domain-based analysis.

Absolute backscatter
Backscattered power refers to the total reflected ultrasound energy per unit of time. Power reflected from particles smaller than the wavelength of the applied ultrasound or from structures with rough or uneven surfaces will increase as the fourth power of the frequency increases (Fig. 7.10). This so-called Rayleigh scattering is omnidirectional, but most of the tissues, like arterial walls, emit both scattering and specular reflections. Specular reflections are angle-dependent and rise from particles larger than the wavelength. As the size of the scattering particle increases, the backscattered energy will increase

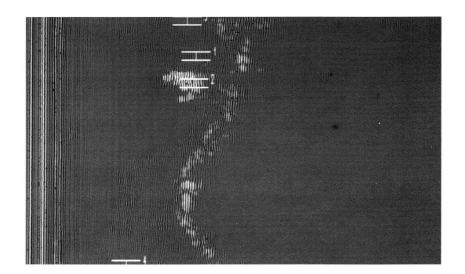

Figure 7.9. Unprocessed radiofrequency signal of an IVUS scanner.

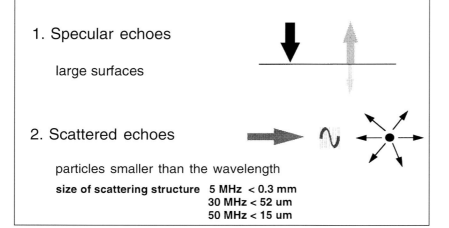

Figure 7.10. Specular and scattered ultrasound reflections.

Table 7.1. **Integrated backscatter (IB, mean ± SD) and mean pixel gray levels (MPGL, mean and range) in different plaque subtypes and intraluminal thrombus.**

Histology	IB (dB) Barzilai et al.[9]	IB (dB) Urbani et al.[11]	MPGL Peters et al.[12]
Normal	−43.2 ± 2.4		
Fibrofatty	−43.9 ± 3.4		
Fibrous	−40.7 ± 3.8	−23.8 ± 5.0	126 (88–169)
Calcified	−30.0 ± 6.4	−11.5 ± 5.2	183 (166–198)
Thrombus		−42.0 ± 5.1	
Fatty		−40.3 ± 5.4	82 (75–94)

roughly as the second power of the increase in the frequency.[8] With 30 MHz central frequency, the size of a Rayleigh scattering structure will be < 52 μm. Backscattered power is a function of frequency and is affected, in addition to the size of the particles, also by their spatial orientation and density, and by the acoustic properties of the tissue components.

For absolute backscatter measurements, the recorded value has to be corrected with a power recorded from a perfect reflector (for example, a ground glass or steel surface) which also excludes the frequency-dependent properties of the transducer.

Calcified plaques have been shown to have higher backscatter when compared to other tissue[9] and are usually larger in size (Table 7.1). Backscattering coefficient from lipid is lower than that measured from fibrotic tissue,[10] but, so far, none of the applied

backscatter analysis has been able to discriminate microcalcification from other types of tissue.

Frequency-dependent analysis of backscatter

Backscattered power is also a function of the frequency of the applied ultrasound signal. Spectral analysis can be applied to the power spectrum of the reflected ultrasound from a region of interest, where the backscattered amplitude (y-axis) is presented as a function of frequency (x-axis) (Fig. 7.11). Spectral slope can be calculated by executing a least-squares linear regression over a given bandwidth. An intercept of this straight line with y-axis provides an additional measure of frequency-dependent attenuation. Both spectral slope and its y-axis intercept have been shown to discriminate loose fibrotic, dense fibrotic and calcified coronary plaques from each other in vitro.[13] These preliminary results show that

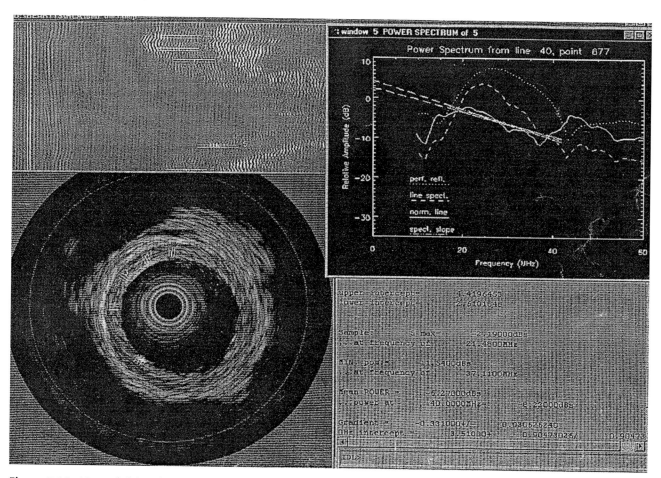

Figure 7.11. Upper left-hand corner: spectral analysis of unprocessed radiofrequency (RF) signal; lower left-hand corner: raw ultrasound signal; upper right-hand corner: scan-converted image of the RF signal; power spectrum of the chosen region of interest, perfect reflector and normalized line (x-axis = frequency, y-axis = amplitude).

the *y*-axis intercept is highest and the spectral slope steepest from calcified plaques, and as the density of extracellular collagen decreases, the slope of the power spectrum becomes flatter and the *y*-axis intercept decreases. These preliminary in-vitro results seem very promising and may offer in the future an additional tool for accurate tissue characterization.

Analysis of attenuation

Many previously published articles concerning ultrasonic tissue characterization deal with measurement of ultrasonic attenuation. Attenuation is the signal loss due to transmission through a given thickness of tissue. Frequency-domain measurement of attenuation slope can be based on spectral slope calculations and processed in two ways: (1) by measuring the rate of attenuation (*y*-axis) versus frequency (dBcm^{-1} MHz^{-1}) or (2) by measuring the rate of change of spectral slope (*y*-axis) with depth (dBMHz^{-1}cm^{-1}).[14] Although attenuation is an important quantitative description and reflects ultrasonic behavior of underlying tissue structure and composition, it is difficult to adapt to an in-vivo situation. The inherent technical problems associated with attenuation measurements are mainly due to the lack of spatial resolution, which makes it difficult to adapt to small sudden changes typical for coronary pathology and the lack of the specificity of observed changes.

Preliminary results from in-vitro attenuation studies have shown that pathological changes, such as lipid pools, cholesterol clefts, necrosis, microcalcification and gross calcification can all lead to abnormally high attenuation slopes and that the resolution of attenuation slope imaging is poor both in spatial and attenuation slope terms.[14] Also, differences in attenuation slope between fibrous plaque and normal tissue are not measurable. This technique seems promising in identifying plaque degeneration, but the specificity of this method needs further improvement before it can be applied to clinical practice.

Backscatter texture analysis

Since the backscattered ultrasound is dependent on both the size and number of scatterers per volume and the degree of their biological variability, one possible way to discriminate different plaque types is to analyze the pattern, that is, the textural information of the composition of the imaged structure in the form of quantitative numerical measures. One of the main advantages of such measurements is that they are not dependent on the absolute backscatter values.

So-called first-order gray-level attributes, such as average gray level, variance, skewness (the asymmetry of the shape of the distribution) and kurtosis (the peakedness of the distribution) of gray levels assess the regional echo amplitude. Such analysis is based on a histogram of echo amplitude distribution (gray-level amplitude on the abscissa and the frequency of occurrence on the ordinate) and data can be derived either from unprocessed RF signal, partially processed data or video data.[15] Videodensitometric analysis of pixel gray level (PGL) distribution of homogeneous coronary atherosclerotic plaques have shown that mean PGL is highest for calcific plaques, and lowest for lipid plaques. PGL is significantly different from calcium, lipid and fibromuscular plaques but the ranges of different plaque types overlap. Also, skewness and kurtosis were able to discriminate lipid, calcific and fibromuscular plaques.[16] Of the first-order statistics, uniformity has been shown to be significantly higher for an older ventricular thrombus than for a fresh one,[18] and gray-scale intensity of IVUS images from whole

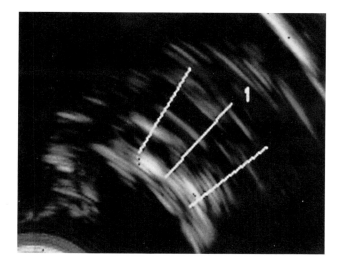 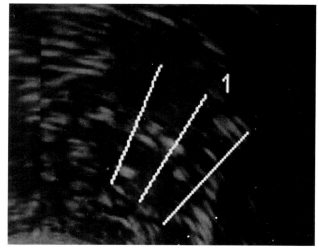

Figure 7.12. Echocardiographic features of a platelet-rich white thrombus (left) and a red thrombus (right).

blood is higher when compared with the mean echogenicity of platelet-rich thrombi.[18]

Quantitative analysis of echo amplitudes can also be assessed by a number of measures involving calculation of features of the two-dimensional spatial pattern of regional gray levels. These measurements give information concerning the heterogeneity of the gray levels and the relative size of the individual echo reflections and thus characterize the image texture.[15] Data derived from unprocessed RF signal have been shown to be more sensitive than standard video images in discriminating platelet-rich thrombus from red clot (Fig. 7.12),[19,20] and may in the future prove to be a reproducible quantitative means of accurate tissue characterization among different laboratories.

Summary and future directions

Standard intravascular ultrasound imaging has already led to semi-quantitative and qualitative assessment of vessel wall morphology. Better understanding and a knowledge of underlying coronary pathology may help in choosing the appropriate strategy for the treatment of coronary disease and acute coronary syndromes and result in improved outcome of the treatment of choice. The improvement of image quality is therefore one of the highest priorities of future IVUS development. High-frequency imaging (up to 60 MHz), which has already been shown to be feasible in vitro (Fig. 7.13)[21] and which would lead to better resolution of IVUS images, together with more advanced signal processing, has the potential to improve significantly our current image quality and interpretation of plaque morphology. Current clinical experience, knowledge from previous studies concerning IVUS-based tissue characterization with improved accuracy of image interpretation may lead to IVUS becoming the reference imaging modality for assessing vessel morphology before and after pharmacological and interventional procedures.

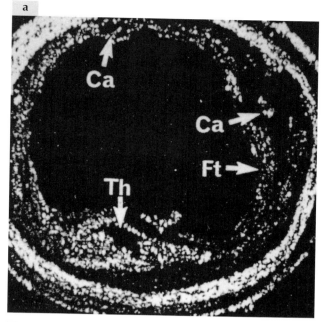

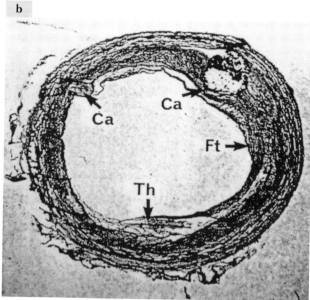

Figure 7.13. (a) Ultrasound backscatter microscopic image (with a 50 MHz central frequency transducer) and (b) histological section of a diseased femoral artery. (Reproduced with permission from Lockwood et al.[21])

References

1 Pearlman JO, Weyman AE. Tissue characterization. In: Weyman AE, ed. *Principles and Practice of Echocardiography*, 2nd edn (London: Lea & Febiger, 1994):1264–85.

2 Fitzgerald PJ, Pohts TA, Yock PG. Contribution of localized calcium deposits to dissection after angioplasty. *Circulation* (1992) **86**:64–70.

3 Gussenhoven WJ, Essed CE, Frielman P et al. Intravascular echographic assessment of vessel wall characteristics: a correlation with histology. *J Card Imaging* (1989) **4**:105–16.

4 Rasheed Q, Phawale PJ, Anderson J, Hodgson JMcB. Intracoronary ultrasound-defined plaque composition: computer-aided plaque characterization and correlation

with histologic samples obtained during directional coronary atherectomy. *Am Heart J* (1995) **129**:631–7.

5   DiMario C, Salem HK, Madretsma S et al. Detection and characterization of vascular lesions by intravascular ultrasound: an in vitro study correlated with histology. *J Am Soc Echocardiogr* (1992) **5**:135–46.

6   Yock PG, Linker DT. Intravascular ultrasound. Looking beyond the surface of vascular disease. *Circulation* (1990) **81**:1715–18.

7   Siegel RJ, Ariani M, Fignbein MC et al. Histopathologic validation of angiography and intravascular ultrasound. *Circulation* (1991) **84**:109–17.

8   Linker OT, Yock PG, Grammingsather A, Johansen E, Angelsen BAJ. Analysis of backscattered ultrasound from normal and diseased arterial wall. *J Card Imaging* (1989) **4**:177–85.

9   Barzilai B, Saffitz JE, Miller JG, Sobel BE. Quantitative ultrasonic characterization of the nature of atherosclerotic plaques in human aorta. *Circ Res* (1987) **60**:459–64.

10   Picano E, Landini L, Distante A, Sarnelli R, Benassi A, L'Abbate A. Different degrees of atherosclerosis detected by backscattered ultrasound: an in vitro study of fixed human aortic walls. *J Clin Ultrasound* (1983) **11**:375–9.

11   Urbani MP, Picano E, Parenti G et al. In vivo radiofrequency-based ultrasonic tissue characterization of the atherosclerotic plaque. *Stroke* (1993) **24**:1507–12.

12   Peters RJG, Kok WEM, Havenith MG, Rijsterborgh H, Wal van der AC, Visser CA. Histopathologic validation of intracoronary ultrasound imaging. *J Am Soc Echocardiogr* (1994) **7**:230–41.

13   Spencer T, Ramo MP, Salter DM et al. Characterization of atherosclerotic plaque by spectral analysis of

intravascular ultrasound: an in vitro methodology. *Ultrasound Med Biol* 1997 (in press).

14   Wilson LS, Neale ML, Talhami HE, Appleberg M. Preliminary results from attenuation-slope mapping of plaque using intravascular ultrasound. *Ultrasound Med Biol* (1994) **20**:529–42.

15   Haralick RM. Statistical and structural approaches to texture. *Proceedings of the IEEE* (1979) **67**:786–803.

16   Peters RJG, Kok WEM, Bot H, Visser CA. Characterization of plaque components with intracoronary ultrasound imaging: an in vitro quantitative study with videodensitometry. *J Am Soc Echocardiogr* (1994) **7**:616–23.

17   Belloti P, Ferdeghini EM, Picano E et al. Echocardiographic quantitative texture analysis of tissue acoustic properties of fresh versus organized ventricular thrombi. *Coron Artery Dis* (1991) **2**:673–7.

18   Frimerman A, Miller KJ, Hallman M, Laniado S, Keren G. Intravascular ultrasound characterization of thrombi of different composition. *Am J Cardiol* (1994) **73**:1053–7.

19   Nailon WH, McLaughlin S, Spencer T, Ramo MP. Comparative study of textural analysis techniques to characterize tissue from intravascular ultrasound. In: *Proceedings of the IEEE International Conference on Image Processing (ICIP '96)*, Lausanne, Switzerland, September 1996. IEEE Signal Processing Society.

20   Nailon WH, McLaughlin S, Spencer T, Ramo MP. Intravascular ultrasound image interpretation. In: *Proceedings of the International Conference on Pattern Recognition (ICPR '96)*, Vienna, Austria, August 1996. IEEE Computer Society Press.

21   Lockwood GR, Ryan LK, Hunt JW, Foster FS. Measurement of the ultrasonic properties of vascular tissues and blood from 35–65 MHz. *Ultrasound Med Biol* (1991) **17**:653–66.

8 Intracardiac ultrasound imaging

Junbo Ge, Günter Görge and Raimund Erbel

Intravascular ultrasound originated from intracardiac ultrasound (ICUS) imaging. In as early as 1956, Cieszynski[1] built a catheter for intracardiac investigation and was able to obtain ultrasonic reflections of soft tissues during model experiments. Using his catheter he was even able to image the inner wall of both ventricles and the pulmonary artery in dogs. He

concluded that diagnosis of heart failure might become possible using intracardiac imaging. Since this technique is invasive, and owing to the technical limitations on image quality as well as the size of the ultrasound catheter, this method has not been implemented during clinical cardiology. Transesophageal echocardiography (TEE), a semi-invasive

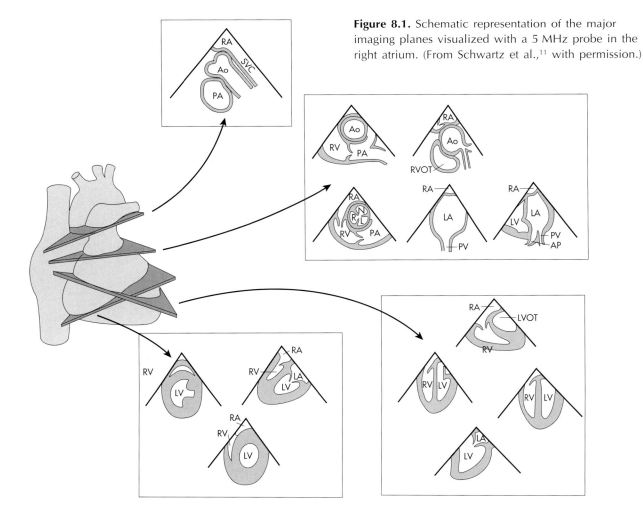

Figure 8.1. Schematic representation of the major imaging planes visualized with a 5 MHz probe in the right atrium. (From Schwartz et al.,[11] with permission.)

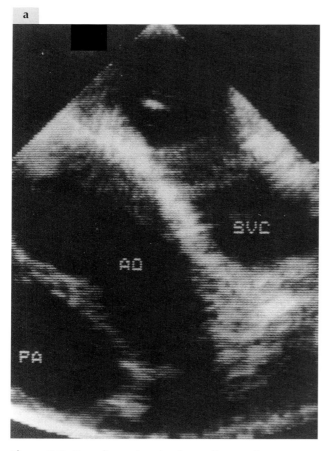

Figure 8.2. Two-dimensional echocardiogram image recorded with a 5 MHz probe placed in the high-right atrium. Image orientation is such that the lower right corner of the image is superior and the right atrium is to the left sector. The superior vena cava (SVC) as it drains into the right atrium, the ascending aorta (AO) and pulmonary artery (PA) are seen. (From Schwartz et al.,[11] with permission.)

technique, and an approach known as intraluminal ultrasound, have been intensively used in recent years; however, in cases of monitoring the cardiac function as well as in cases of complications during interventional therapeutic procedures, patients can be lacking in tolerance if TEE is needed during the entire length of the procedure. As the precursor to high-frequency intravascular ultrasound, ICUS imaging has aroused great interest for evaluating cardiac structures and function.[2–10] It has been noted that the advantage of ICUS imaging is its ability to monitor continuously cardiac structures and function without the risk of contrast-related adverse effects.

Intracardiac ultrasound device

The commonly used intracardiac imaging catheters include 10 MHz, 10 F. or 20 MHz, 8 F. CVIS rotating mirror catheters and 12.5 MHz rotating crystal catheters (Scimed, Boston Scientific Co., Natick, MA, USA). They are mechanically rotated at 600–1800 rpm to provide 360° cross-sectional images via an ultrasound console. Electronic catheters are seldom used in intracardiac imaging because of their technical limitations. In experimental studies, Schwartz et al.[11] and Seward et al.[12] used a small, 5 MHz TEE transducer which was advanced into the right atrium to obtain images of the heart, namely transvascular ultrasound.[11,12]

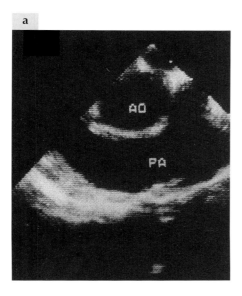
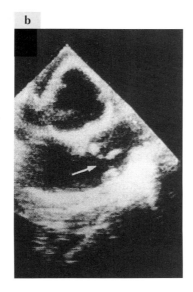

Figure 8.3. From the mid-right atrium, the ascending aorta and pulmonary artery are visualized. **(a)** Ascending aorta (AO) in short axis, main pulmonary artery (PA) in long axis. **(b)** Same image orientation, illustrating the pulmonic valve cusps (arrow). **(c)** Pulmonary trunk (PT) bifurcation into the right pulmonary artery (RPA) and left pulmonary artery (LPA). (From Schwartz et al.,[11] with permission.)

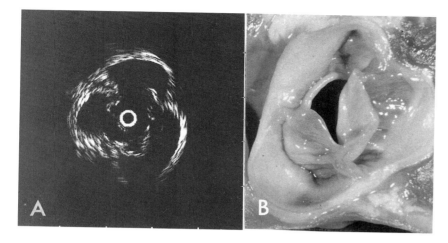

Figure 8.4. Cross-sectional scanning of the aortic valve by use of a 6.2 F 20 MHz catheter (**a**) in comparison with pathology (**b**). The aortic valve is clearly seen.

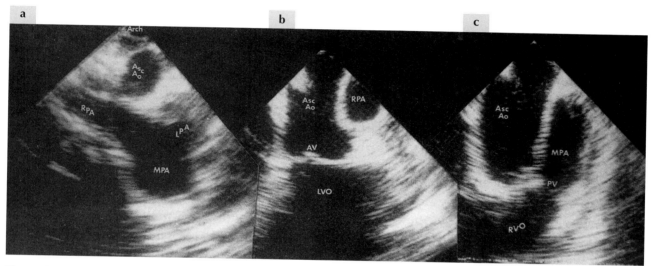

Figure 8.5. Transvascular via aorta: a sequential series of scans (left to right) obtained from a transducer in the aortic arch and upper descending thoracic aorta. (**a**) The plane of section is along the long axis of the right pulmonary artery (RPA), which runs posterior to the ascending aorta. MPA = distal main pulmonary artery; LPA = left pulmonary artery. (**b**) Ascending aorta (AscAO), aortic valve (AV), and left ventricular outflow (LVO) are obtained with slight anteflexion of the scan plane. The right pulmonary artery (RPA) is visualized in short axis. (**c**) Further anteflexion images show the proximal main pulmonary artery (MPA), pulmonary valve (PV), and right ventricular outflow (RVO). (From Seward et al.,[12] with permission.)

Visualization of cardiac structures

By introducing the ultrasound catheter into a cardiac cavity, cross-sectional images of the heart can be obtained. Fig. 8.1 shows the schematic representation of the major imaging planes when placing a TEE transducer in the right atrium. The cardiac chambers and valves can be scanned (Figs 8.2–8.4).

The TEE transducer can also be advanced through the aorta to scan the aorta and periaortic structures (Figs 8.5 and 8.6). In addition, blood flow can be examined when switching to Doppler flow mode.

By advancing a high-frequency ultrasound catheter into the great vessels or ventricular cavity, the structures of the ventricles and surrounding structures are visualized with high resolution in 360°, namely lighthouse echocardiography. Fig. 8.7 shows the

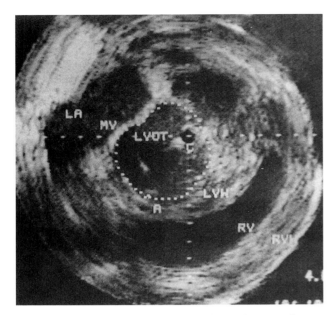

Figure 8.6. Intracardiac image with the catheter in the left ventricular outflow tract (LVOT) obtained using a 10 F., 10 MHz ultrasound catheter. Periaortic structures can also be visualized. (From Chen et al.,[2] with permission.)

Assessment of the cardiac function

Assessment of the cardiac function is very important during operations and in the intensive care unit. Using transthoracic echocardiography it is sometimes very difficult to obtain optimal images because of obesity, pulmonary emphysema, etc. In addition, it can affect sterilization during an operation. Transesophageal echocardiography may avoid some of these drawbacks; nevertheless, it is not accepted for long-term monitoring of the cardiac function. The ideal method of monitoring heart function is via high-resolution images, continuously monitoring without affecting the operation procedure, and without increasing the risk of infection and the patient's discomfort. Intracardiac or transvascular echocardiography have these advantages and therefore can be used to monitor cardiac function. As shown in Fig. 8.7, the left ventricle can be imaged at different levels. Therefore the left ventricular volume can be assessed using Simpson's rule. Figure 8.9 shows the schematic display of the calculation of the left ventricular volume.[2] Close correlation was found in vitro for left ventricular volume between ultrasonic and anatomic measurement.[2] In an experimental study, Chen et al. also found close correlations for heart volume between the measurements derived by ultrasound and the true volume.[2] They also found that there are no significant differences in the ventricular volume between 5 mm and 10 mm intervals (Fig. 8.10). Similarly, close correlation for the left ventricular

cross-sectional images of the left ventricle at different levels obtained by advancing an ultrasound catheter through the aorta into the left ventricle. Abnormalities such as thrombus formation (Fig. 8.8) and septal defects can also be clearly visualized.

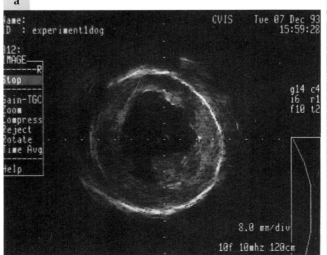

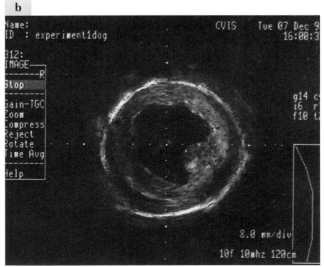

Figure 8.7. Cross-sectional images of the left ventricle in a dog model at different levels obtained by use of a 10 MHz intracardiac ultrasound catheter. The thickness of the myocardium as well as the endocardium are clearly detected.

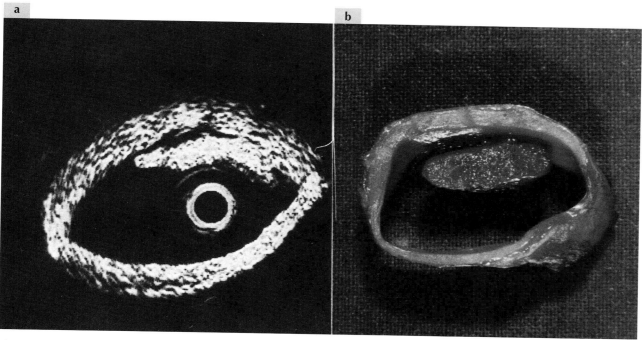

Figure 8.8. In-vitro examination of a mural thrombus in the pulmonary artery with a 20 MHz ultrasound catheter. A dense reflection can be seen.

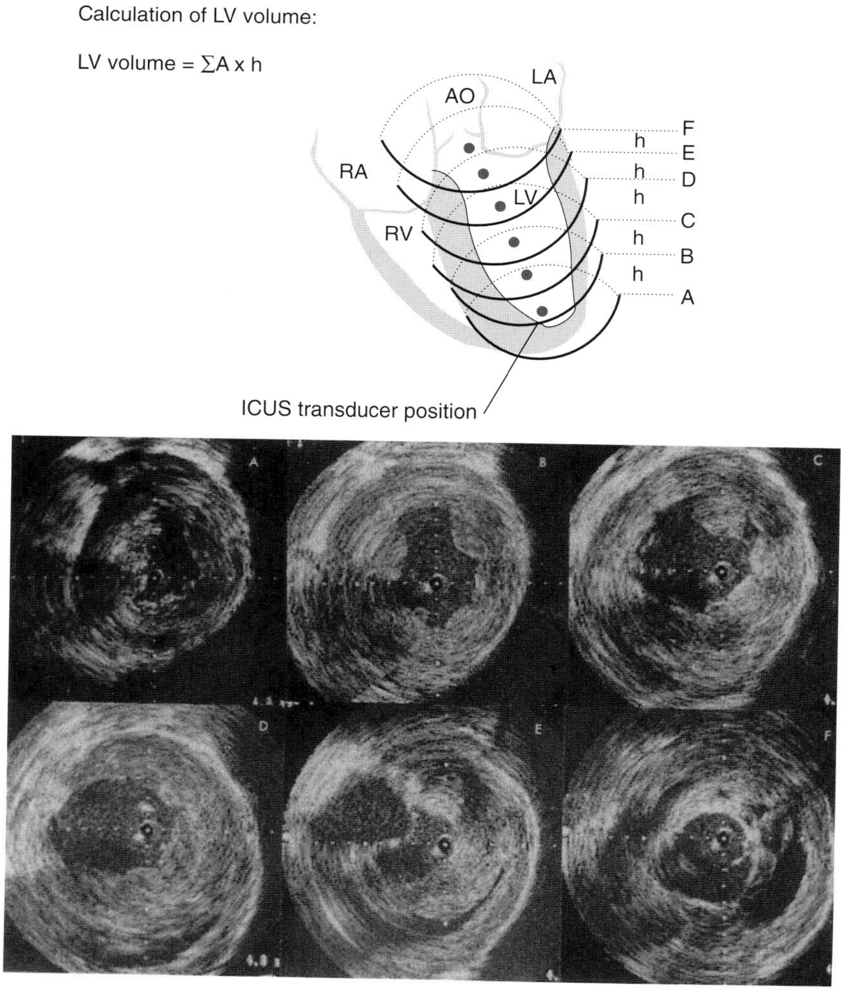

Calculation of LV volume:

LV volume = $\sum A \times h$

Figure 8.9. Cross-sectional images of the left ventricle by advancing the ultrasound catheter into the left ventricle through the aortic valve and the calculation of the left ventricular volume. (From Chen et al.,[2] with permission.)

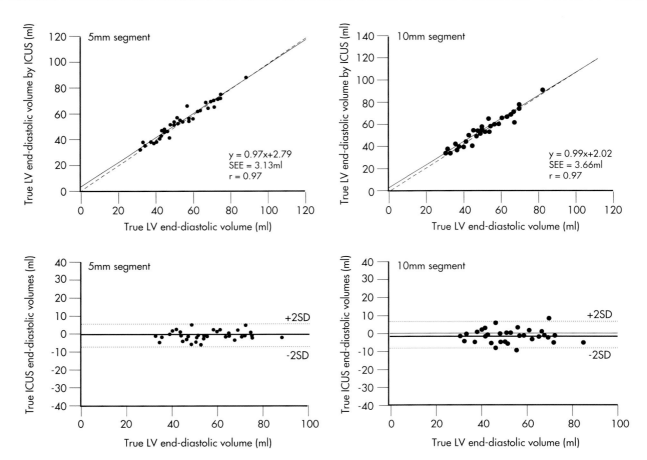

Figure 8.10. Correlation between true left ventricular end-diastolic volume and left ventricular end-diastolic volume by intracardiac ultrasound. No significant differences in the left ventricular volume between 5 mm and 10 mm intervals were found. (From Chen et al.,[2] with permission.)

ejection fraction was obtained between the measurements derived by ultrasound and biplane ventriculography. In an in-vitro study, Ge et al. found that intracardiac ultrasound can accurately assess the left ventricular mass in comparison with anatomic study.[10]

Wall motion analysis

Regional wall motion abnormalities as detected by echo are accurate indices for evaluating regional myocardial ischemia. As intracardiac echocardiography is able to provide high-resolution images of the heart it can be used for wall motion analysis. Ricou et al. found that a 12.5 MHz ultrasound transducer is able to portray the left ventricle when they compared 12.5 MHz and 20 MHz catheters in an experimental study.[13] They also noticed that regional wall motion abnormality is correlated with the coronary perfusion defects. Prada et al reported that regional wall motion abnormality correlates closely with the extent of myocardial infarction ($r = 0.98$). Nevertheless, a significant overestimation exists using ICUS.[14] Chen et al. evaluated left ventricular thickening with a 10 MHz ultrasound catheter in comparison with the measurement derived using a sonomicrometer and found a close relationship between the two methods.[2] In addition, myocardial contrast defects can also be detected in the corresponding area after coronary ligation using a 12.5 MHz ultrasound catheter. McKay et al. reported a good relationship between ICUS and single photon emission computed tomography (SPECT) in the assessment of myocardium viability.[15] In an in-vitro heart model, Prada et al found that right ventricular function can be assessed using the same method as used by Chen et al. in the evaluation of left ventricular function.[16]

ICUS and interventional cardiology

Atrial septum puncture has been successfully guided by transthoracic and transesophageal echocardiography.[17,18] Kyo et al. compared TEE and ICUS in the guidance of atrial septum puncture and found that both imaging methods permitted the imaging of the fossa ovalis.[19] TEE is able to visualize the whole septum while ICUS is not. However, ICUS is more helpful in adjusting the site of puncture and is safer and more comfortable than TEE. Another important role for ICUS in interventional cardiology is the guidance of radiofrequency ablation of arrythmia. Berns et al. and Goli et al. found that ICUS allows the imaging of the position of the ablation catheter in the sinus.[20,21] Tardif et al. reported that ICUS could clearly monitor the ablation procedure and morphologic changes in the ablated area thereafter.[22]

Limitations and future directions

As ICUS is able to assess the whole heart, it provides potential for the assessment of global as well as segmental cardiac function. It offers a new modality for observing valvular morphology, pericardial disease, aortic disease, and atrial septum disorders. In intracoronary interventional procedures, it may allow a new approach to the monitoring of hemodynamic abnormalities and myocardial ischemia, as well as detecting complications. It provides detailed information about ablation procedures. However, as the present ICUS catheters are 10–20 MHz in frequency, the imaging depth is limited. Thus it is necessary to develop a low-frequency catheter or multiple-frequency catheters. The miniaturized TEE catheter provides a greater depth, yet is still too large for intracardiac or transvascular imaging. Moreover, ICUS imaging is now performed in the catheterization laboratory under X-ray guidance. The future ICUS catheter should also be steerable so that it can be used in the intensive care unit to monitor hemodynamics. The combination of ICUS transducers with interventional devices such as ablation catheters, as well as valvuloplasty balloon catheters, presages the intensive use of ICUS in cardiology.

References

1 Cieszynski T. Intracardiac method for the investigation of structure of the heart with the aid of ultrasonics. *Arch Immunol Ther Dow* 1960; **8**: 551–7.

2 Chen CG, Guerrero L, de Prada JAV et al. Intracardiac ultrasound measurement of volumes and ejection fraction in normal, infarcted, and aneurysmal left ventricles using a 10 MHz ultrasound catheter. *Circulation* 1994; **90**: 1481–91.

3 Kiomoto S, Omoto R, Tsunemoto M. Ultrasonic tomography of the liver and detection of heart atrial septal defect with the aid of ultrasonic intravenous probes. *Ultrasonics* 1964; **2**: 82–6.

4 Conetta DA, Christie LG, Pepine CJ, Nichols WW, Conti CR. Intracardiac M-mode echocardiography for continuous left ventricular monitoring: method and potential application. *Cathet Cardiovasc Diagn* 1979; **5**: 135–43.

5 Glassman E, Bronzon I. Transvenous intracardiac echocardiography. *Am J Cardiol* 1981; **47**: 1255–9.

6 Stephen DD, Palacios I, Block P, Weyman AE. Intracardiac echocardiographic evaluation of phasic right atrial free wall dynamics. *Circulation* 1981; **64** (suppl IV): 128.

7 Pandian NG, Kumar R, Katz SE et al. Real-time, intracardiac, two-dimensional echocardiography. *Echocardiography* 1991; **8**: 407–22.

8 Schwartz SL, Gillam LD, Weintraun AR et al. Intracardiac echocardiography in humans using a small-sized (6 F), low-frequency (12.5 MHz) ultrasound catheter: method, imaging plane and clinical experience. *J Am Coll Cardiol* 1993; **21**: 189–98.

9 McKay CR, Spencer K, Hanson P, Dejong S, Smith R, Kerber RE. Intracardiac ultrasound and dobutamine can identify stunned myocardium in a canine model. *J Am Coll Cardiol* 1993; **21**: 75A.

10 Ge J, Liu F, Görge G, Haude M, Baumgart D, Erbel R. In vitro validation of the accuracy of intracardiac ultrasound in the assessment of the left ventricular mass. *Eur Heart J* 1994; **15**: 608.

11 Schwartz SL, Pandian NG, Kusay BS et al. Real-time intracardiac two-dimensional echocardiography: an experimental study of in vivo feasibility, imaging planes, and echocardiographic anatomy. *Echocardiography* 1990; **7**: 443–55.

12 Seward JS, Khandheria BK, Mcgregor CGA, Locke TJ,

Tajik AJ. Transvascular and intracardiac two-dimensional echocardiography. *Echocardiography* 1990; **7**: 457–64.

13 Ricou F, Sahn DJ, Weintraub A et al. Improved visualization of the left ventricle during cardiac catherization by intracardiac scanning with a new 12.5 MHz ultrasound imaging catheter: a study in pigs. *J Am Coll Cardiol* 1992; **19**: 95A.

14 Prada JAV, Chen MH, Padial L et al. Intracardiac ultrasound measurement of normal akinetic endocardial surfaces by reconstructing sequential left ventricular cross-sections. *Circulation* 1994; **90**: I495.

15 McKay CR, Grover-McKay MM, Dejong S et al. Diagnosis of viable myocardium in patients by intracardiac ultrasound: comparison with rest thallium and psotron emission tomography. *Circulation* 1993; **88**: I–112.

16 Prada JAV, Padial L, Chen MH et al. Assessment of the right ventricular volume using a new 10 MHz intracardiac ultrasound catheter: an in vitro validation study. *Circulation* 1994; **90**: I495.

17 Vilacosta I, Iturralde E, Alberto J et al. Transesophageal echocardiographic monitoring of percutaneous mitral balloon valvulotomy. *Am J Cardiol* 1992; **70**: 1040–4.

18 Ballal RS, Mahan EF III, Nanda NC et al. Utility of transesophageal echocardiography in interatrial septal puncture during percutaneous mitral balloon commisurotomy. *Am J Cardiol* 1990; **66**: 230–3.

19 Kyo S, Miyamoto N, Mitsumury M. Brockenbrough transsepta puncture and left atrial cannulation with guidance of transesophageal and/or intracardiac echocardiography. *Circulation* 1994; **90**: I596.

20 Berns E, Mitchel J, Mehran R et al. Ablating catheter placement under direct visualization with the intravascular ultrasound probe: a potential aid to ablative therapy of arrhythmia. *J Am Coll Cardiol* 1990; **15**: 19A.

21 Goli VD, Prasad R, Jackman WM et al. Intracardiac echocardiography from the coronary sinus using 12.5 MHz ultrasound catheter in patients undergoing accessory pathway ablation. *Circulation* 1992; **86**: II439.

22 Tardif JC, Groeneveld PW, Haugh CJ et al. Intracardiac echocardiography can guide microwave ablation of arrhythmic foci: an in vitro study. *Circulation* 1994; **90**: I595.

9 Characteristic plaque morphology

Junbo Ge and Raimund Erbel

Coronary artery atherosclerosis is a long-term, slowly progressing disease. Ischemic coronary heart disease occurs only when the atherosclerotic disease results in severe coronary lumen reduction which affects coronary perfusion and which cannot be compensated for. Contrast coronary angiography is unable to detect the early stage of atherosclerosis (see chapter 11). Based on the early works of pathological observation by Stary,[1,2] the committee on vascular lesions of the Council on Atherosclerosis (American Heart Association) recently classified the atherosclerotic process into six stages (Table 9.1).[3]

Table 9.1 **Classification of atherosclerotic lesions based on pathological observation (modified from refs 1–3).**

Types	Description
Type I (initial lesions)	Lipoprotein accumulation in intima; lipid in macrophages. These changes discernible only microscopically or chemically; no tissue damage is visible.
Type II (fatty streak) IIa (progression-prone; co-localized with adaptive thickening) IIb (progression-resistant)	Lipoprotein accumulation in intima; lipid in macrophages and smooth muscles cells; quantities large enough to be visible to the unaided eye but still no tissue damage.
Type III (preatheroma)	All Type IIa changes plus mutiple deposits of pooled extracellular lipid; macroscopic evidence of tissue damage or disorder.
Type IV (atheroma)	All Type IIa changes plus confluent mass of extracellular lipid (lipid core) with massive structural damage to intima.
Type Va (fibroatheroma)	All Type IV changes plus development of marked collagen layers and smooth muscle cell increase above lipid core.
Vb (calcific lesion)	Any advanced lesion type composed predominantly of calcium; substantial structural deformity
Vc (fibrotic lesion)	Any advanced lesion type composed predominantly of collagen; lipid may be absent.
Type VI (complicated lesion) VIa (fissure, erosion) VIb (hematoma, hemorrhage) VIc (thrombus)	All Type IV and V changes plus a thrombotic deposit and/or hematoma and/or erosion or fissure.

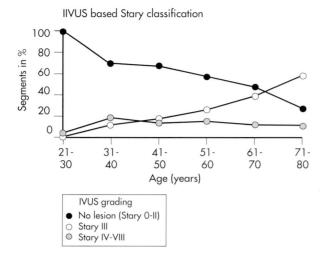

Figure 9.1. Distribution of atherosclerotic lesions in 812 segments of 49 patients with angiographically normal angiograms. As age increases, advanced lesions also increase. Accordingly, normal segments and early lesions decrease.

Intravascular ultrasound (IVUS) is able to provide high-resolution images of the vessel lumen and wall by imaging the vessel from within. It is therefore possible to stage the atherosclerotic process. Erbel et al. evaluated 812 segments in 49 patients who had normal angiograms with IVUS and found 440/812 segments (54%) with plaque formation.[4] Early signs of atherosclerosis are mainly seen in young people. The percentage of advanced lesions increases as the patient's age increases. Even in angiographically normal coronary arteries, advanced atherosclerotic lesions are found, thus explaining the potential risk of acute coronary syndromes in this group of patients (Fig. 9.1).[4,5]

Type I lesions cannot be differentiated by IVUS in normal coronary arteries. Type II lesions present with a circular lumen with smooth wall or slight intimal thickening with the so-called 'three-layer appearance' (Fig. 9.2). Type III lesions present with eccentric intimal thickening but no echolucent areas in the thickened intima (Fig. 9.3). Type IV lesions present with concentric or eccentric plaque formation with a lipid core which show an echolucent area within the plaque (Fig. 9.4(a)). Angiographically, Type I–IV lesions do not cause lumen reduction (75%) because of vessel compensation.

Type Va lesions show a lipid core with a thin fibrous cap covering it (Fig. 9.4(b)). Sometimes focal calcium deposits exist in different types of lesion but can also be present in Type III and IV lesions. Type IV and V lesions are known as 'plaques-at-risk'

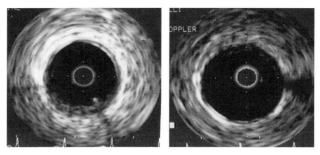

Figure 9.2. IVUS images of normal artery or early stage of atherosclerosis. Left panel: a mild intimal thickening exists between 12 and 3 o'clock which presents a three-layer appearance. An obvious intimal thickening is seen between 4 and 9 o'clock. Right panel: a mild intimal thickening is seen between 5 and 7 o'clock.

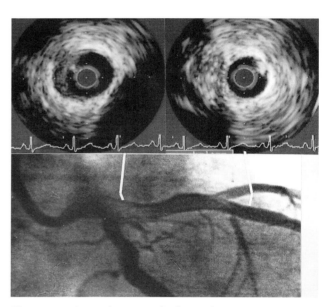

Figure 9.3. An early stage of atherosclerosis (preatheroma) is seen in the IVUS image (upper left) without lumen reduction angiographically.

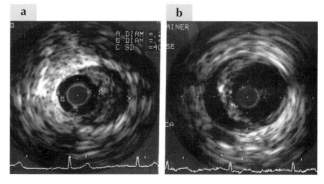

Figure 9.4. (a) Advanced stage of atherosclerosis (Stage IV) which is characterized by a large lipid core (echolucent zone on IVUS). (b) Stage V, which is characterized by a large lipid core and a thin fibrous cap. Both lesions are rather unstable and are known as 'plaque-at-risk' as they can rupture under high-wall shear stress or inflammation of the cap.

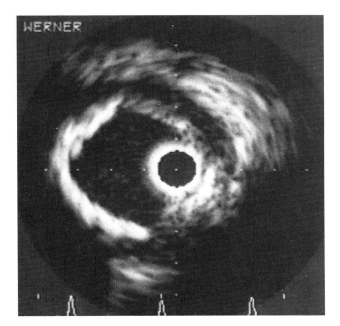

Figure 9.5. Stage Vb (previously Stary VII) lesion (plaque with severe calcification) which is characterized by bright echoes with acoustic shadowing behind (from 6 to12 o'clock).

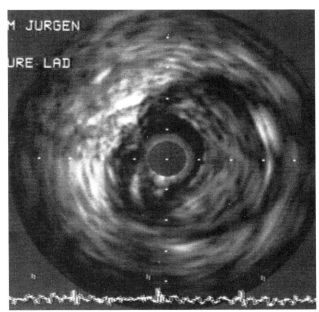

Figure 9.6. Stage Vc (previously Stary VIII) lesion (fibrotic plaque) which presents on IVUS as bright echoes without acoustic shadowing. It is considered to be the result of several episodes of plaque reorganization.

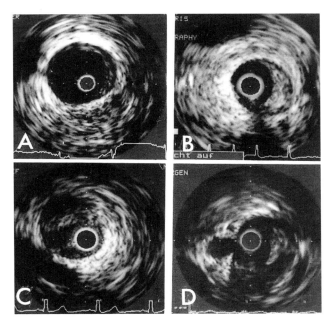

Figure 9.7. Atherosclerotic process at different stages. A and B indicate early stages of atherosclerosis (Stages II and III); C indicates plaque-at-risk with a lipid core and a thin cap (Stage Va); D presents rupture (Stage VIa).

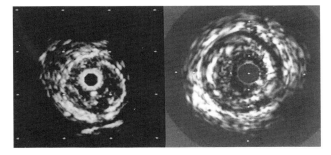

Figure 9.8. Stage VIc (mural thrombus) which is characterized by a speckled reflection and undulation (rain worm movement) mass in the lumen.

show plaque with echodense reflection but without acoustic shadowing (Fig. 9.6). Focal calcium deposits may exist.

Type VI includes three subgroups: VIa presents as a plaque fissure or rupture. With IVUS it shows an emptied plaque with a thin fibrous cap (Fig. 9.7(d)). The emptied plaque cavity is filled when injecting contrast agent. With coronary angiography it is sometimes misdiagnosed as a coronary aneurysm, because the emptied cavity is filled with contrast agent. IVUS is able to differentiate coronary aneurysms from plaque rupture.[6] Ruptured plaques may result in unstable angina, acute myocardial infarction, and sudden death. They may also heal subsequently, with thrombus formation followed by

but can also be present in Type III and IV lesions.[5] Type Vb lesions present mainly with calcium deposits which are characterized by bright echoes and acoustic shadowing (Fig. 9.5). Type Vc lesions

plaque reorganization[7] showing a 'layering effect'.[8] This may explain the layering effect in plaques previously observed in pathological studies. Type VIb is a hematoma or hemorrhage pathologically. It is normally difficult to identify this subtype using IVUS because hematoma or hemorrhage show an echolucent area within the plaque; the lipid core also shows an echolucent area within the plaque. The difference between hematoma or hemorrhage and lipid core may be that the former occurs more frequently in the wall while the latter occurs more frequently in the plaque. Up to now it has been difficult to differentiate these two situations when hematoma exists in plaque. However, it is simple to identify plaque hemorrhage when a communication exists between the lumen and the hemorrhage by injecting contrast agent during IVUS. Type VIc is a thrombus formation. Fresh thrombus can be fairly easily identified by IVUS because it usually presents as a speckled undulating mass in the lumen (Fig. 9.8). Old thrombus is, however, usually differentiated from plaque when it is covered with fibrotic tissue (plaque reorganization). It normally presents with the layering appearance as described above.[6] The underlying lesion leading to plaque rupture is included in classification Type III and VIa, which means that the ruptured plaque (Type VIa) is based on the Stary Type III lesion classification.

References

1   Stary HC. Evolution and progression of atherosclerotic lesions in coronary arteries of children and young adults. *Arterioscler Thromb* 1989; **9 (suppl I)**: 19–32.

2   Stary HC. The sequence of cell and matrix changes in atherosclerotic lesions of coronary arteries in the first forty years of life. *Eur Heart J* 1990; **11 (suppl E)**: 3–19.

3   Stary HC, Chandler AB, Dinsmore RE et al. A definition of advanced types of atherosclerotic lesions and histological classification of atherosclerosis. *Circulation* 1995; **92**: 1355–74.

4   Erbel R, Ge J, Jollet N, Görge G, Haude M. Intravascular-ultrasound-based Stary classification of coronary plaque formation. *J Am Coll Cardiol* 1996; **27**: 40A.

5   Erbel R, Ge J, Görge G et al. Intravaskuläre Sonographie bei koronarer Herzkrankheit, Neu Aspekte zur Pathogenese. *Dtsch Med Wschr* 1995; **120**: 847–54.

6   Kearney P, Erbel R, Rupprecht HJ et al. Difference in the morphology of unstable and stable coronary lesions and their impact on the mechanisms of angioplasty. An in vivo study with intravascular ultrasound. *Eur Heart J* 1996; **17**: 721–30.

7   Ge J, Haude M, Görge G, Liu F, Erbel R. Silent healing of spontaneous plaque disruption demonstrated by intracoronary ultrasound. *Eur Heart J* 1995; **16**: 1149–51.

8   Kearney P, Erbel R, Rupprecht HJ et al. Differences in the morphology of unstable and stable coronary lesions and their impact on mechanisms of angioplasty. *Eur Heart J* 1996; **17**: 721–30.

10 Distribution of atherosclerosis

Vijay T Shah, Junbo Ge, Mahmoud Ashry and Raimund Erbel

Introduction

The location of atherosclerotic lesions in the coronary artery tree is of considerable importance in assessing the myocardial mass at risk as well as the patient prognosis. Severe proximal coronary artery disease jeopardizes a large mass of myocardium, in contrast to distal lesions, which are of minor significance.[1]

Therapeutically it is of the utmost importance to know the location, distribution, and quantification of atherosclerotic plaques in the coronary arteries. This information helps in planning coronary interventions, bypass surgery, progression/regression studies, and, occasionally, intracoronary delivery of drugs.[2]

Since its inception, coronary angiography has been the 'gold-standard' for the in-vivo diagnosis of coronary artery disease. The extent of disease as assessed by coronary angiography also correlates with the clinical picture and short- and long-term prognosis of the patient.[3]

However, comparison between angiography and post-mortem studies has revealed significant discrepancies, particularly in detecting disease of the left main coronary artery (LMCA), reference segment and side branches.[4] This is particularly important when diffuse coronary artery disease is present, or when the plaque is eccentric, or if there is culprit vessel remodeling, or vessel foreshortening due to inappropriate projections.[5]

Intravascular ultrasound (IVUS) has been recognized as the most accurate method available for measuring vessel wall thickness, lumen area, plaque area, and for characterization of plaque morphology in the coronary tree.[6] Even tissue characterization should be possible in the near future.

In-vitro studies: histologic correlation to intracoronary ultrasound

Minimal lipid accumulations occur at a young age in almost everyone and in many locations of the coronary arteries. The locations at which advanced atherosclerotic critical lesions or occlusions are most often found at autopsy are also the same locations where early stages of the disease are found.[7] Intravascular ultrasound imaging has helped

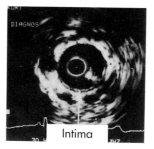

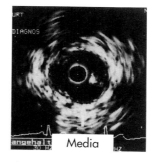
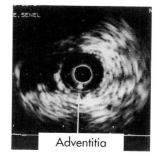

Figure 10.1. Normal three-layered appearance of coronary artery on IVUS (20 MHz transducer). The innermost thin echogenic layer is the intima. The outer thick echogenic layer corresponds to the adventitia. The sonolucent layer in between the two echogenic layers represents the media.

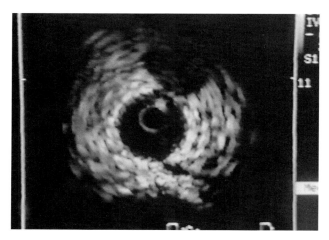

Figure 10.2. Two-layer appearance of coronary artery on IVUS (20 MHz transducer) due to absence of internal elastic membrane and high collagen content of media. At 12 o'clock a guidewire artefact is present.

to obtain high-resolution images of the arterial wall via the use of ultrasound catheters placed within the coronary artery. Initial in-vitro studies by various authors[8] have established the excellent correlation between the ultrasound images and the layers of the arterial wall on histopathological segments. These studies describe normal muscular arteries as having a three-layer appearance with two echogenic zones separated by an echolucent layer which correlates well with the media. Although the width and position of these zones matched the histologic sections, a three-layer ultrasound appearance was not observed until the intimal thickness was greater than 178 μm (Fig. 10.1). Normally this is seen in elderly populations where the intima is thickened. In young patients a monolayer appearance may be seen (Fig. 10.3). With increasing resolution of the transducers the detection of intimal thickness should be possible at an earlier age. However, a two-layer appearance was observed when there was an absence of signals of internal elastic membrane as well as high collagen content of media (Fig. 10.2). Various studies have shown excellent correlation between the morphology of the plaque observed on IVUS and their histologic sections. These observations are useful in interpreting IVUS images in clinical studies.[9]

Single versus multiple vessel distribution

The number of major epicardial coronary vessels severely diseased by atherosclerotic plaques varies with the necropsy studies. In general, severe single vessel disease is more common in patients aged 40 years or younger and in patients aged around 90 years or older. Triple vessel disease is most frequently found in patients aged 41–89 years. The left anterior descending artery (LAD) is the most frequently diseased major vessel (58%), followed by the right (33%) and circumflex (LCX) (25%). The LMCA is least frequently (16%) involved in atherosclerotic plaque formation. Severe LMCA disease is associated with significant disease of the remaining three coronary arteries. Isolated severe LMCA atherosclerosis is a rare finding at necropsy.[10] There are no detailed studies of IVUS imaging in all three major epicardial vessels in patients with single vessel or multivessel disease. However, data from various case-studies in different reports confirm the findings that advanced atherosclerosis is indeed a multivessel disease.[11]

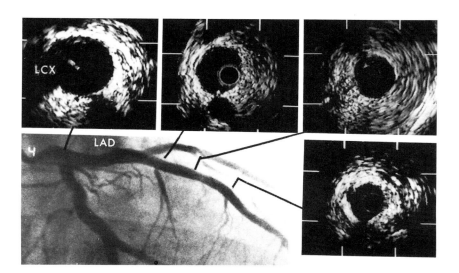

Figure 10.3. Monolayer appearance seen in the ultrasound image of the mid-LAD. This is observed as the intima and media are thin enough to escape ultrasound catheter detection. (4.8 Fr; 20 MHz transducer).

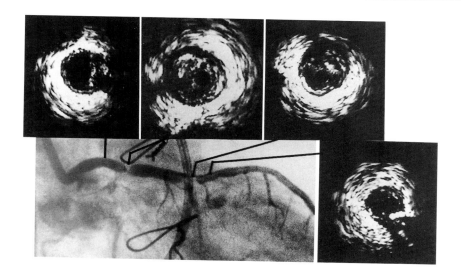

Figure 10.4. Atherosclerotic lesions in the proximal segment of the LAD. Also note the presence of atherosclerotic plaque in angiographically normal reference segments and the left main artery (30 MHz transducer).

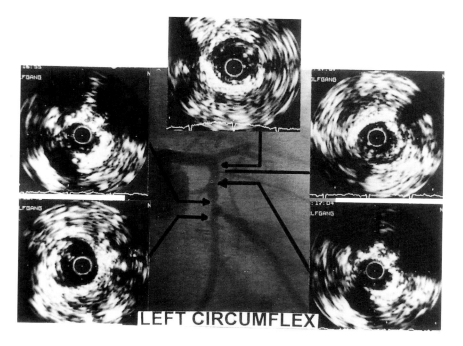

LEFT CIRCUMFLEX

Figure 10.5. Atherosclerotic lesions in the proximal segment of the left circumflex artery with severe superficial calcium (upper right) and deep calcium (lower left) and extensive calcification with shadowing (180°) (upper left, lower right) (30 MHz transducer).

Axial distribution

In-vitro observations have shown that:

(a) in the left coronary artery (LCA) the prevalence of lesions of all types was greatest near the bifurcation. A marked decrease in the prevalence of lesions occurred as one moves distally from the bifurcation along both the LCX and the anterior descending branches;

(b) the LAD is the artery most vulnerable to developing atherosclerosis and the plaques are more frequent in the first 2 cm followed by a rapid decrease in frequency to the seventh-to-eighth centimeter with slight increase in frequency after the eighth (Fig. 10.4);

(c) the first 2 cm in the LCX is the most frequently affected (Fig. 10.5);

(d) lesions in the right coronary artery (RCA) have maximal prevalence at the second-to-third centimeter (Fig. 10.6) and a lower peak prevalence at the eighth-to-tenth (Fig. 10.7).

This pattern of distribution is similar in all age groups and both sexes.[12] Some angiographic studies[13] have shown similar distribution of lesions although significant discrepancies were revealed when compared with post-mortem studies.[14] However, IVUS studies in diseased vessels also show the preponderance of lesions in the proximal segments compared with the distal segments. Lesions were more frequent at or within 5 mm proximal or distal to the origin of side branches.[15,16]

Circumferential distribution

The variation in the distribution of atherosclerotic plaque along the circumference of the coronary arteries results in two different types of cross-sectional luminal shapes: (1) concentric (Fig. 10.8), if the atherosclerotic plaque is distributed evenly along the entire vessel wall circumference; (2) eccentric and focal if the plaque fails to involve the entire circumference (Fig. 10.9) or eccentric and circumferential if the plaque predominantly involves one arc of the circumference (Fig. 10.10). It has been shown that over 70% of all significantly narrowed segments on post mortem have eccentrically placed plaques giving rise to an eccentric lumen.[17] IVUS studies of coronary artery disease segments have confirmed this finding that the majority of the plaques are eccentrically situated and that at the level of bifurcation they are situated typically opposite the flow divider wall (Fig. 10.8).[16,18]

Diffuse versus focal distribution

The atherosclerotic process is diffused, involving all three epicardial coronary arteries.[19] However, it does

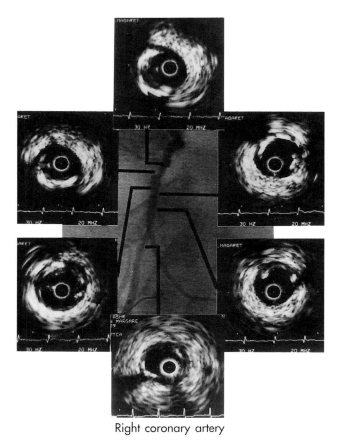

Right coronary artery

Figure 10.6. Atherosclerotic lesions in the proximal segment of the right coronary artery (30 MHz transducer).

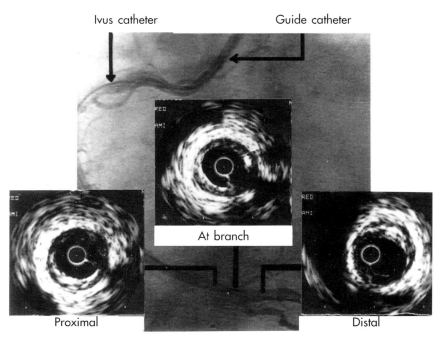

Right coronary artery

Figure 10.7. Atherosclerotic lesions in the RCA at the level of origin of the posterior descending artery (30 MHz transducer).

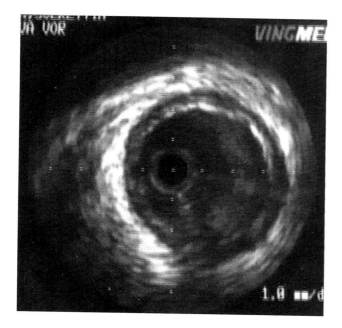

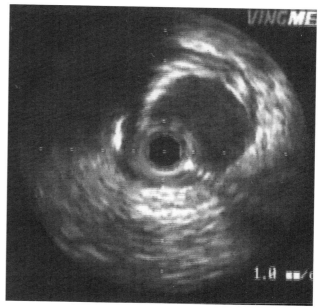

Figure 10.8. Concentric plaque of atherosclerosis on IVUS in coronary artery (30 MHz transducer).

Figure 10.9. Eccentric plaque of atherosclerosis: focal type; not involving the entire circumference of the artery (30 MHz transducer).

not involve every segment of the coronary tree as patches of normal segment are present in between the disease segments (Fig. 10.9).[20] In addition, the focal nature of atherosclerotic process is amplified on IVUS as on histology, since one arc of segment is commonly involved rather than the other normal segment, as in eccentric stenosis.

In angiographically normal or mildly diseased coronary arteries

New cardiac transplant recipients present a unique group in which it is possible to image coronary arteries of young donor hearts. Therefore, studies in these patients are overcoming the ethical problems involved in imaging coronary arteries in normal young people. IVUS studies in these subjects have shown that young (less than 25 years) angiographically normal hearts had a broad range of ultrasound-measured intimal thickness and, in a few, evidence of focal early atheromatous changes.[21] In a recent study it was shown that only 22% had no atherosclerosis on IVUS, 54% had less than 300 μm intimal thickness and 26% had more than 300 μm intimal thickness in the LAD.[22] Even regression of plaque in these patients has been documented.[22]

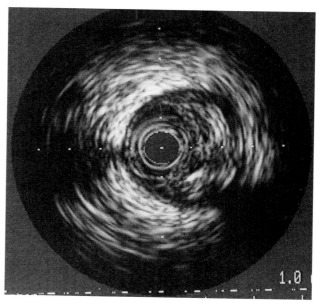

Figure 10.10. Eccentric plaque of atherosclerosis: circumferential type predominantly involving one arc of the segment (30 MHz transducer).

Ultrasound imaging of symptomatic patients with normal angiographic coronary arteries shows identifiable plaques in the range of 17–50% of the examined sites in the LAD. Most (84%) of these

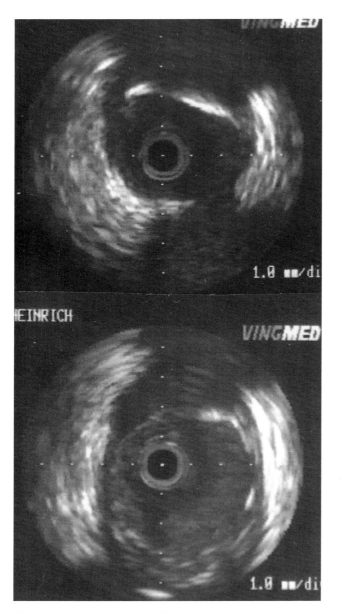

Figure 10.11. At the level of bifurcation: no evidence of atherosclerosis on the flow divider wall (top picture) but present opposite to the divider wall (bottom picture) (30 MHz transducer).

plaques are eccentric in distribution.[24,25] Some studies have shown diffuse atherosclerotic plaques on ultrasound in vessels with normal angiography[26] (Fig. 10.12). A very high percentage of angiographically normal left main coronary arteries have plaques detected on ultrasound, most in the range of 34–89%. Some (4–21%) of these have a significant percentage area stenosis of more than 40%.[27,28]

In reference segments used in quantitative coronary angiography (QCA)

Atherosclerotic plaques in angiographically normal reference segments were analyzed using epicardial echocardiography during cardiac surgery.[29] Subsequently other studies have recently suggested that IVUS is a very sensitive tool for detection of plaques in the reference segments.[30] The reference segments in these studies were defined as those within 10 mm proximal to the target lesion but distal to any major side-branch. These data suggest that most of the plaques detected have a characteristic semilunar appearance and do not protrude significantly into the lumen. In these cases, the smooth coronary lumen contour was preserved, maintaining a circular or midly elliptical configuration that may partially explain the absence of luminal irregularities on contrast angiography (Fig. 10.4). A few plaques, small and confined to one quadrant, clearly protruded into the lumen and disrupt the luminal contour on IVUS. In addition, plaque characteristics ranged from hypoechogenic to calcified, although no calcification was seen on fluoroscopy. However, reference segment plaque distribution was less eccentric than target lesion plaque distribution (Fig. 10.12). Qualitative analysis shows that reference segments contain relatively less calcium and fibrosis and more soft elements. These studies have reported the prevalence of plaques at around 80% in the angiographic normal reference segments although the cross-sectional vessel area was similar to the target vessel area. The plaque area, percentage cross-sectional narrowing, arc of calcium, and eccentricity index of the reference segments were smaller than those of the target lesions.[31]

In relation to myocardial bridges

Previous studies have reported the protective role of intramural coronary arteries and the high incidence of atherosclerosis in the segment proximal to it. IVUS imaging has made it possible to study them in vivo and to confirm this finding.[32]

In relation to coronary aneurysms

IVUS tomographic imaging of coronary aneurysms has not only shown severe atherosclerosis within the aneurysms but also in the segments proximal

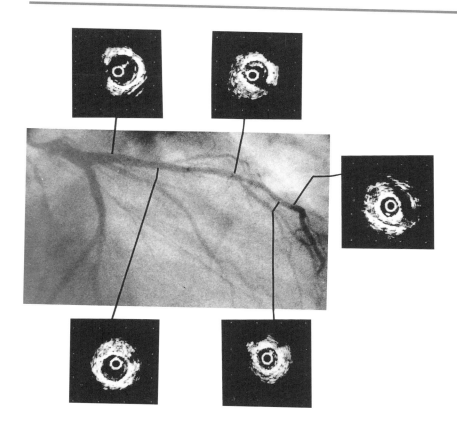

Figure 10.12. Normal angiography of left descending artery showing atherosclerotic plaques on IVUS examination at different sites (30 MHz transducer).

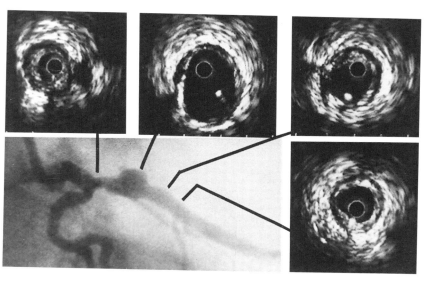

Figure 10.13. IVUS images of angiographic coronary aneurysm showing atherosclerotic plaque in the segment proximal and distal to the aneurysm (30 MHz transducer).

and distal to the true aneurysms (Fig. 10.13). Atherosclerotic pseudo-aneurysms show evidence of plaque rupture at the site of aneurysm or proximal to it.

Limitations

The main limitation of IVUS is the size of the catheter. The smallest size is 2.9 F. (1 mm). This does not allow assessment of tight lesions of coronary arteries with minimal lumen diameter (MLD) less than 1 mm in size. Occasionally it can cause ischemia or produce the Dotter effect. In addition, it requires the insertion of a guide wire through the artery which in itself is an invasive procedure with known risks and complications. Therefore, IVUS cannot be used as a routine diagnostic tool for the detection of distribution of atherosclerosis.

Summary

In conclusion it can be said that the road map provided by contrast angiography can be used to direct the IVUS catheter for a detailed tomographic assessment of the arterial segment, especially when intervention is planned. IVUS imaging has several advantages for the study of the distribution of in-vivo atherosclerosis of coronary arteries. The cross-sectional perspective of the lumen, the tomographic visualization of bifurcation sites, objective assessment of angiographic disease and reference segments: all can now be possible with a high degree of accuracy. However, due to the limitations of the catheter size and the invasive nature of the procedure, it cannot be used routinely in the detection of atherosclerosis in all patients with suspected coronary artery disease.

References

1 Halon DA, Sapoznikov D, Lewis BS et al. Localization of lesions in the coronary circulation. *Am J Cardiol* 1983; **52**: 921–6.

2 Waller BF. Topography of atherosclerotic coronary artery disease. *Clin Cardiol* 1990; **13**: 435–42.

3 Guidelines for Coronary Angiography. A report of the American College of Cardiology/American Heart Association Task Force on assessment of diagnostic and therapeutic cardiovascular procedures. *Circulation* 1987; **76**: 963A–77A.

4 Erbel R, Ge J, Görge P et al. Sonographie bei koronare Herzkrankheit *Dtsch Med Wschr* 1995; 847–54.

5 Hermiller J, Tenaglia A, Kisslo K. In vivo validation of compensatory enlargement of atherosclerotic coronary arteries. *Am J Cardiol* 1993; **71**: 665–8.

6 Nissen SE, Gurley JC, Grines CL et al. Intravascular ultrasound assessment of lumen size and wall morphology in normal subjects and patients with coronary artery disease. *Circulation* 1991; **84**: 1087–9.

7 Stary HC. Evolution and progression of atherosclerotic lesions in coronary arteries of children and young adults. *Arteriosclerosis* 1989; **9**(supplt): 9–32.

8 Fitzgerald PJ, St Goar FG, Conolly AJ et al. Intravascular imaging of coronary arteries. Is three layers the norm? *Circulation* 1992; **86**(1): 154–8.

9 Maheswaran B, Leung CY, Gutfinger DE et al. Intravascular ultrasound appearance of normal and mildly diseased coronary arteries: correlation with histologic specimens. *Am Heart J* 1995; **130**: 976–86.

10 Richard Conti C, Selby JH, Pepine CJ et al. Left main coronary artery stenosis: clinical spectrum, pathophysiology and management. *Progress in Cardiovascular Diseases* 1979; **12**: 73–99.

11 Tobis JM, Mallery J, Mahon D et al. Intravascular ultrasound imaging of human coronary arteries in vivo. *Circulation* 1991; **83**: 913–26.

12 Montegro MR and Eggen DA. Topography of atherosclerosis in the coronary arteries. *Lab Invest* 1968; **18**: 126–33.

13 Schwartz JN, Kong Y, Hackel DB et al. Comparison of angiographic and postmortem findings in patients with coronary artery disease. *Am J Cardiol* 1975; **36**: 174–8.

14 DiMario C, Madresma S. Detection and characterization of vascular lesions by intravascular ultrasound. An in-vitro study correlated with histology. *J Am Soc Echo* 1992; **5**: 135–46.

15 Rasheed Q, Nair R, Sheehan H et al. Correlation of intracoronary ultrasound plaque characteristics in atherosclerotic coronary artery disease patients with clinical variables. *Am J Cardiol* 1994; **73**: 753–8.

16 Ge J, Erbel R, Görge G et al. Atherosclerotic lesions in relation to the origin of side branches in human coronary arteries: evaluation with intravascular ultrasound and angiography. *J Am Soc Echo* 1992; **5**: 320.

17 Freudenberg H, Lichtien PR, Engel HJ. The normal wall segment in coronary stenosis – a postmortem study. *Z Kardio* 1981; **70**: 39.

18 Stary HC et al. Report from the committee on vascular lesions of the council on arteriosclerosis, AHA. *Circulation* 1995; **92**: 1355–74.

19 Arnett EN, Isner JM, Redwood DR et al. Coronary artery narrowing in coronary heart disease: comparison of necropsy and angiographic findings. *Ann Int Med* 1979; **79**: 350–6.

20 Vlodaver Z, Frech R, Van Tassel RA et al. Correlation of the antemortem coronary angiogram and the postmortem specimen. *Circulation* 1973; **47**: 162–9.

21 Ge J, Liu F, Kearney P et al. Intravascular ultrasound approach to the diagnosis of coronary artery aneurysms. *Am Heart J* 1995; **130**: 765–71.

22 Frederick G St. Goar, Fausto J P et al. Detection of coronary atherosclerosis in young adult hearts using intravascular ultrasound. *Circulation* 1992; **86**: 756–63.

23 Haude M, Ge J, Machraoui A et al. Regression of pre-existing coronary artery disease in a donor heart after cardiac transplantation. *Eur J Cardiothorac Surg* 1995; **9**: 399–402.

24 Ge J, Erbel R, Gerber T et al. Intravascular ultrasound imaging of angiographically normal coronary arteries: A prospective study in vitro. *Br Heart J* 1994; **71**: 572–4.

25 Erbel R, Ge J, Rupprecht HJ et al. Intravascular ultrasound and Doppler in angiographically normal coronary arteries. *Circulation* 1986; **4**: 122.

26 Porter TR, Sears T, Feng Xie et al. Intravascular ultrasound study of angiographically mildly diseased coronary arteries. *J Am Coll Cardiol* 1993; **7**: 1858–65.

27 Hermiller JB, Buller CB, Tenaglia AN et al. Unrecognized left main coronary artery disease in patients undergoing interventional procedures. *Am J Cardiol* 1993; **71**: 173–6.

28 Ge J, Liu F, Görge G et al. Angiographically silent plaque in the left main coronary artery detected by intravascular ultrasound. *Coron Artery Dis* 1995; **6**: 805–10.

29 McPherson DD, Hiratzka F, Lamberth WC et al. Delineation of the extent of coronary atherosclerosis by high frequency epicardial echocardiography. *N Engl J Med* 1984; **316**: 304–8.

30 De Franco AC, Tuzcu EM, Eaton G et al. Detection of unrecognized LMCA disease by intravascular ultrasound in patients undergoing interventions. Prevalence and severity. *Circulation* 1993; **88**: 1411.

31 Waller BF. The eccentric coronary atherosclerotic plaques, morphological observations and clinical relevance. *Clin Cardio* 1989; **12**: 14.

32 Ge J, Erbel R, Rupprecht HJ et al. Comparison of intravascular ultrasound and angiography in the assessment of myocardial bridging. *Circulation* 1994; **89**: 1725–32.

11 Coronary artery remodeling in atherosclerotic disease

Junbo Ge and Raimund Erbel

Introduction

An early compensatory mechanism that preserves coronary perfusion in arteries affected by atherosclerosis is the enlargement of the diseased vascular segment. This compensatory enlargement of atherosclerotic coronary arteries has been demonstrated in animal models[1-3] and in histopathologic studies in human beings.[4] It is not apparent on angiography; nevertheless, no in-vivo studies have been performed to assess the remodeling of coronary arteries affected by atherosclerosis apart from an epicardial echocardiographic study performed during open chest surgery.[5]

In order to study the remodeling process, a total of 92 atherosclerotic segments from 46 patients were analyzed.[6] The percentage stenosis, estimated as the ratio between plaque area and vessel area, ranged from 9.2% to 92.8% (mean 34.1 ± 16.9%). The plaque area ranged from 2.0 to 19.6 mm^2 (mean 6.3 ± 3.6 mm^2).

Of the 46 patients studied, no plaque formation was noted in the proximal segment in 37 patients. The vessel area and lumen area of atherosclerotic segments, as well as the area of proximal and distal plaque-free segments were measured. The vessel area is given in Fig. 11.1. The vessel area of the atherosclerotic segment was larger than that of the proximal plaque-free segment (20.4 ± 7.34 mm^2 for the atherosclerotic segment versus 18.66 ± 7.33 mm^2 for the proximal segment; $P = 0.018$). However, the area of the distal plaque-free segment was smaller than that of the proximal plaque-free segment ($P < 0.01$). Figure 11.2 illustrates an example of this IVUS finding. The vessel area of the diseased segment was larger than that of the proximal plaque-free segment. The differences between the areas of

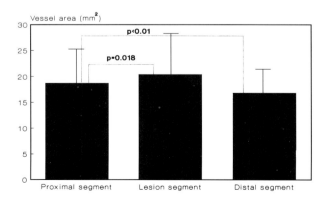

Figure 11.1. Diagram of the measurement of the vessel area of the proximal segment, plaque segment, and distal segment. The vessel area of the plaque segment is larger than that of the proximal segment ($P = 0.018$).

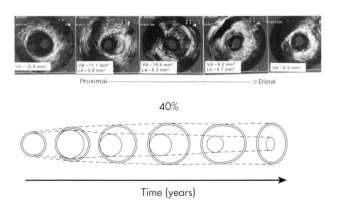

Figure 11.2. Intravascular ultrasound images of the left anterior descending coronary artery proximally to distally. The values of vessel cross-sectional areas of the coronary artery are shown beside every picture. The vessel area of the stenotic segment (19.4 mm^2) is even larger than that of the proximal normal segment (15.9 mm^2). (Glagov et al.[4])

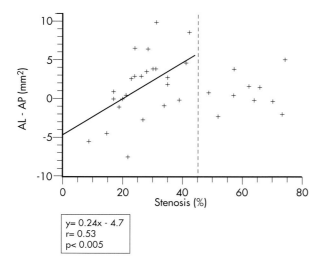

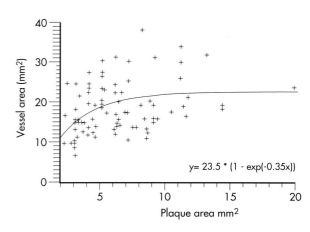

Figure 11.3. Percentage stenosis plotted against the difference between the vessel area of the plaque segment and the vessel area of the proximal segment (AL–AP(approximate)). Stepwise regression analysis showed that good correlation could be obtained between the percentage stenosis and AL–AP if the stenosis is below 45% ($r = 0.53$, $P <0.005$).

Figure 11.4. Correlation between vessel area and plaque area. Exponential correlation is obtained. Vessel area does not increase in relation to the increase in plaque area when the plaque is larger than 7–8 mm².

the atherosclerotic segment and the proximal plaque-free segment were calculated and plotted against the percentage stenosis, a good correlation being found on linear regression analysis up to 45% stenosis (Fig. 11.3). At higher percentage stenoses, no reliable correlation could be found.

The vessel area increased with increasing plaque area. The relation between vessel area and plaque

area can be described as $Y = 23.5*(1-\exp(-0.35\psi))$ (Fig. 11.4). No statistically significant correlation was found when the percentage stenosis and the vessel area were compared.

These data demonstrate that in atherosclerotic arteries the cross-sectional vessel area of the diseased segment is larger than that of the proximal nondiseased segment. This remodeling of the coronary

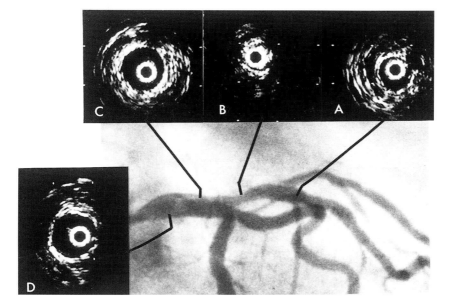

Figure 11.5. Paradoxical remodeling of a coronary arterial segment (B). The vessel area is even smaller than that of the distal reference segment.

Calcified plaque

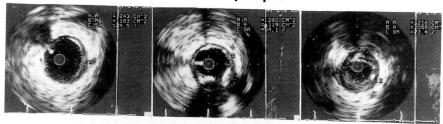

Proximal------------------------------------> Distal

Figure 11.6. IVUS images of a moderately calcified plaque; no effect of the calcium deposit on the vessel remodeling was found.

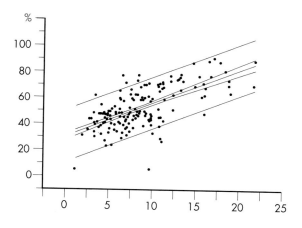

$$Y = -22{,}2543 + -0{,}98377*X^2 + 1{,}84793e\text{-}02*X^3$$

Figure 11.7. Relation between plaque size (X) and percentage stenosis (Y) in eccentric plaques. Percentage stenosis increased slowly in accordance with the plaque size, which indicates that the remodeling process starts at a very early stage of atherosclerosis and continues thereafter.

Figure 11.8. Relation between plaque size (X) and percentage stenosis (Y) in concentric plaques. It shows that the remodeling process in concentric plaques starts at a late stage of atherosclerosis.

arteries affected by atheroma seems to be an intrinsic compensatory mechanism which preserves coronary blood flow, and it begins at an early stage of the atherosclerotic process. The stage of the disease at which this compensatory mechanism becomes insufficient remains to be determined. However, not all atherosclerotic plaques undergo compensatory remodeling. In a recent observation, the authors noticed that some of the lesions undergo a negative remodeling, namely vessel shrinkage (Fig. 11.5). This may address the reason for luminal narrowing in some patients. The vessel area in the lesion segment is even smaller than that of the normal segment. The mechanism of this 'negative remodeling' is still unknown. Medial and adventitial damage, for different reasons, might contribute to

this process because this phenomenon is frequently found in patients who have undergone directional atherectomy, which often damages the media and adventitia during intervention. Although unable to measure the vessel area in cases of severe calcification, the authors did not find any effects of mild to moderate calcification in the process of remodeling (Fig. 11.6). In IVUS studies on peripheral arteries, Pasterkamp et al. also found that paradoxical arterial wall shrinkage contributes to luminal narrowing.[6]

Plaque morphology seems to play an important role in the process of remodeling. The remodeling process in eccentric plaques begins at a very early stage of atherosclerosis (Fig. 11.7) while it begins only at a late stage for concentric plaques (Fig. 11.8).

In segments with plaque areas greater than 8–10 mm² no correlation with increasing vessel size could be found. It appears that the compensatory potential of vessel enlargement is exhausted at this point. The loss of normal vessel tapering, expressed as the difference between plaque and proximal vessel areas, correlated with percentage stenosis until the stenosis exceeded 45% (Fig. 11.4). This suggests that, potentially, more rapid stenosis development will occur if 45% of the vessel's cross-sectional area is occupied by atherosclerotic plaque. Prospective longitudinal studies of patient groups such as the authors' are required to confirm this finding.

This result also explains the considerable discrepancies between coronary angiography and postmortem examinations. It also confirms the result of a post-mortem coronary angiographic/pathohistological study.[7–12]

Limitations of IVUS in the evaluation of artery remodeling

Because ultrasound cannot penetrate heavily calcified tissue, peripheral echo dropout is seen behind calcified plaque. As a result, vessel area cannot be determined in such segments. An IVUS-based study is thus restricted to evaluating atherosclerotic plaque without severely calcified deposits. Since the axial resolution of the 20 MHz transducer used in this study was approximately 150 μm and the lateral resolution approximately 300 μm, accurate definition of the media is not possible. Thus any compensatory thinning of the media which may contribute to luminal enlargement could not be detected. Because tissue characterization, in the absence of validated techniques, remains subjective, the particular remodeling behavior of vessels with different plaque types (calcified, fibrous, or lipid-laden) cannot be reliably assessed.

References

1 Bond MG, Adams MR, Bullock BC. Complicating factors in evaluating coronary arterial atherosclerosis. *Artery* 1981; **51**: 434–9.

2 Marcus ML, Armstrong ML, Heistad DD, Eastham CL, Mark AL. A comparison of three methods of evaluating coronary obstructive lesions: postmortem angiography, pathological examination and measurement of regional myocardial perfusion during maximal vasodilation. *Am J Cardiol* 1982; **49**: 1699–706.

3 Armstrong ML, Heistad DD, Marcus ML, Megan MB, Piegors DJ. Structural and hemodynamic response of peripheral arteries of macaque monkeys to atherogenic diet. *Atherosclerosis* 1985; **5**: 336–46.

4 Glagov S, Weisenberg E, Zarins CK, Stankunavicius R, Kolettis GJ. Compensatory enlargement of human atherosclerotic coronary arteries. *New Engl J Med* 1987; **316**: 1371–5.

5 McPherson DD, Serna AJ, Hiratzka LF et al. Coronary arterial remodeling studied by high-frequency epicardial echocardiography: an early compensatory mechanism in patients with obstructive coronary atherosclerosis. *J Am Coll Cardiol* 1991; **17**: 79–86.

6 Ge J, Erbel R, Zamorano J et al. Coronary artery remodeling in atherosclerotic disease: an intravascular ultrasonic study in vivo. *Coron Artery Dis* 1993; **4**: 981–6.

7 Pasterkamp G, Wensing PJW, Post MJ, Hillen ZB, Mali WPTM, Borst C. Paradoxical arterial shrinkage may contribute to luminal narrowing of human atherosclerotic femoral arteries. *Circulation* 1995; **91**: 1444–9.

8 Vlodaver Z, Frech R, VanTassel RA, Edwards JE. Correlation of the antemortem coronary angiogram and the postmortem specimen. *Circulation* 1973; **47**: 162–9.

9 Grodin CM, Dyrda I, Pasternac A, Campeau L, Bourassa MG. Discrepancies between cineangiographic and postmortem findings in patients with coronary artery disease and recent myocardial revascularization. *Circulation* 1974; **49**: 703–56.

10 Arnett EN, Isner JM, Redwood CR et al. Coronary artery narrowing in coronary heart disease: comparison of cineangiographic and necropsy findings. *Ann Intern Med* 1979; **91**: 350–5.

11 Harrison DG, White CW, Hiratzka LF et al. The value of quantitative coronary angiography in determining the physiologic significance of coronary stenosis in man. *Circulation* 1984; **69**: 1111–19.

12 Stiel GM, Stiel LSG, Schofer J, Donath K, Mathey DG. Impact of compensatory enlargement of atherosclerotic coronary arteries on angiographic assessment of coronary artery disease. *Circulation* 1989; **80**: 1603–9.

12 The acute coronary syndromes

Peter Kearney

Introduction

The underlying mechanisms of unstable angina and acute myocardial infarction have been the subject of intensive investigation over the last two decades. It has become apparent that the acute presentations of coronary ischemia, including unstable angina, non-q-wave myocardial infarction, full-thickness myocardial infarction, and a proportion of cardiac sudden deaths share the common precipitants of variable degrees of intimal disruption, thrombus formation, and acute luminal compromise. Many unresolved issues concerning both the pathophysiology and therapy of acute coronary disease remain, however. The anatomical and functional features that underlie the differing presentations of acute coronary disease, the true prevalence and prognostic significance of so-called 'vulnerable' lipid-rich plaques, and the paradoxically detrimental or neutral effects of fibrinolytic treatment for unstable angina are unexplained or unknown. The mechanism of plaque growth following an acute coronary episode (intimal hemorrhage by way of plaque fissuring as opposed to laminated thrombus formation) and the contribution of such episodes to the natural history of atherosclerosis are also the basis of ongoing debate.

Until recently, the investigation of acute coronary disease has relied upon histopathological case-studies and in living patients has been confined to the angiographic findings during an acute coronary event. The selective nature of cases coming to autopsy precludes a comprehensive study of the full range and severity of acute coronary disease. Angiography too is subject to significant limitations as a means of studying such lesions. Certain angiographic patterns are held to be indicators of intracoronary thrombus. These include smooth central intracoronary filling defects surrounded by contrast, the absence of calcification within the filling defect, contrast staining, and irregular or overhanging margins to the lesion.[1] Such features were shown to

be sensitive indicators of thrombus in a post-mortem angiogram model.[2] A classification of the angiographic appearances associated with unstable angina has been proposed by Ambrose et al.[3] and amended by Braunwald and colleagues.[4]

However, the reported incidence of angiographically recognized coronary thrombi in patients with unstable angina varies very considerably in different studies from 1.3%[1] to over 80%,[5] and an attempt has been made to overcome the limited reproducibility of subjective evaluation by quantifying the 'complexity' of a given lesion in an automated manner.[6] Using angioscopy, the most accurate method of identifying intracoronary thrombus, it has become apparent that contrast angiography is both an insensitive and nonspecific method for thrombus detection.[7–9] The inability to image the vessel wall, the site of many of the events of interest in acute coronary disease, is a further serious drawback.

A number of these shortcomings are overcome by intracoronary ultrasound with which direct visualization of the vessel wall and evaluation of its tissue components can be achieved. The identification of lipid and thrombus, both key factors in acute coronary syndromes, is generally thought not to be reliable using videodensitometric parameters alone.[10,11] The development of more accurate methods based on analyses of radiofrequency data to identify tissue types, discussed later, is the most promising means of addressing these limitations. Nonetheless, existing technology has already provided a number of interesting observations in patients with acute coronary disease.

Unstable angina

The first report of a comparison of ultrasound findings in a series of patients with stable and unstable angina undergoing percutaneous transluminal

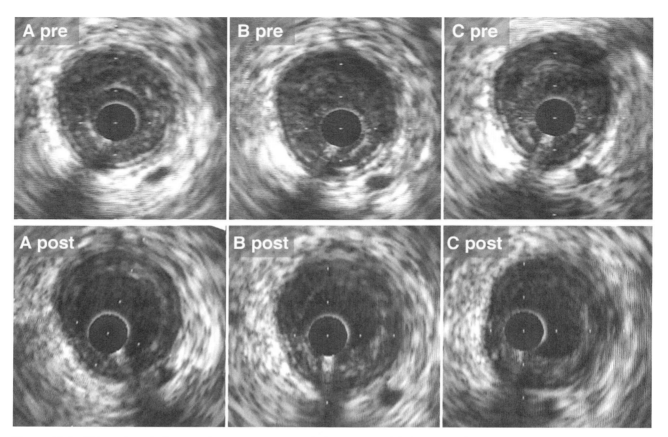

Figure 12.1. This series of ultrasound images was recorded in an unstable lesion in the right coronary artery of a 56-year-old woman before (upper panels) and after (lower panels) balloon angioplasty. In the left upper panel the transducer is positioned in the proximal, less stenotic portion of the lesion, and in the mid and right-hand panels at points more distally. In all the pre-interventional images, a fine circumferential line demarcates an outer from an inner layer. The endoluminal border, and differentiation between the blood-filled lumen and the demarcated inner layer, is most evident in the left-hand panel, but a small rim of free lumen is also seen around the catheter blank in the mid and right-hand images. After percutaneous transluminal coronary angioplasty (PTCA) (lower panels), although an increase in the overall vessel area is evident (vessel stretch), particularly in the proximal, left-hand panel, the neolumen conforms closely in shape with that of the inner layer prior to intervention. Lumen area increase, particularly in the mid and right-hand sites, appears to be predominantly the result of remodeling or 'compression' of the inner layer. Some residual material (possibly mural thrombus) is seen at 6 o'clock in the lower mid and right-hand panels. Calibration 1 mm, 30 MHz transducer.

coronary angioplasty (PTCA) noted a higher incidence of echolucent zones, possibly corresponding with lipid accumulation, in unstable lesions than in stable lesions. Plaque echolucency was a more sensitive indicator of an acute coronary syndrome than were angiographic criteria.[12]

In a more recent study,[13] in which pre-interventional ultrasound was performed in 33 patients with unstable and stable angina, no significant difference in plaque echodensity in each group was found, although there was a trend to more echolucent zones in unstable lesions. The principal finding was the observation that unstable coronary lesions are frequently characterized by a 'layered' pattern within the lesion (Fig. 12.1). The inner part of the lesion was separated from the outer segment in most cases by a fine, circumferential echodense line. The echodensity of the inner layer was frequently no different from the surrounding layer, but in a proportion of cases was relatively echolucent (Fig. 12.2). The distinction between inner and outer layers was further aided in a small proportion of cases by an abrupt difference in texture (Fig. 12.3).

Echographic lesion layering was thought most probably to represent mural thrombus apposed to underlying atheromatous plaque. The reasons put

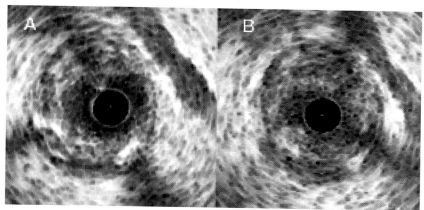

Figure 12.2. This pair of ultrasound images was acquired before (right) and after (left) angioplasty of a stenosis in a patient presenting with postinfarction angina. In this case, a prominent inner layer was identified as a result of a marked difference in the echodensity of inner (hypoechoic) and outer (echogenic) layers. Following angioplasty, a lumen area increase appeared to result almost completely from displacement or remodeling of the echolucent inner layer. The somewhat ragged lumen seen in the right-hand panel was filled with dynamic speckles that were slightly more echogenic (as a result of red-cell-generated backscatter) than the static material occupying the same space prior to angioplasty. Calibration 1 mm, 30 MHz transducer.

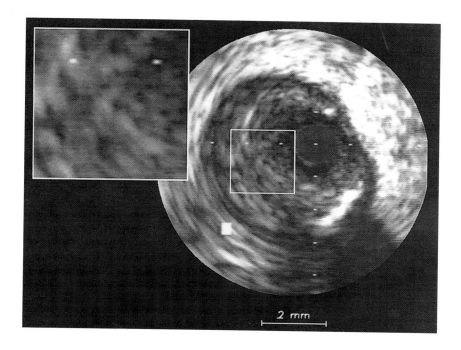

Figure 12.3. This image was acquired within a thrombotic, acute, infarct-related total occlusion of a right coronary artery. Although inner and outer layers are quite readily distinguished within the lesion, this results not from differences in echodensity, but from the presence of a subtle circumferential line, and in this case more obviously because of an abrupt difference in the texture of the material in the inner (granular) and outer (flatter speckled) layers. 30 MHz transducer.

forward for this conclusion were (a) this pattern was highly specific for unstable lesions, in which thrombus is usually found;[14,15] (b) features recognized as characteristic (if not specific) of thrombus were frequently present in the inner layer on the ultrasound images (fine, scintillating speckle or 'granular' pattern);[16,17] and (c) the line demarcating the inner from outer layers may readily be explained as a spectral echo generated at an interface of two tissues offering differing levels of acoustic impedance, such as plaque and thrombus. Further support for a thrombotic basis for this appearance derives

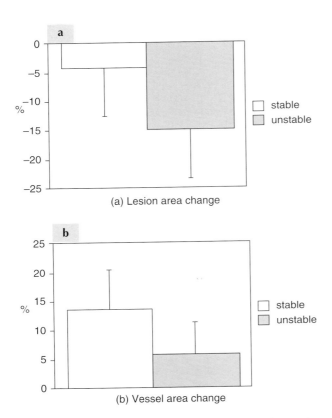

Figure 12.4. Bar graphs depicting the relative change in vessel dimensions following balloon angioplasty in stable and unstable lesions. Error bars indicate one standard deviation. **(a)** The relative reduction in lesion cross-sectional area in stable lesions, −4.1 ± 8.4%, was significantly less than the reduction that occurred in unstable lesions, −14.8 ± 8.3%. **(b)** The relative increase in vessel cross-sectional area, indicative of vessel wall stretch, was +13.5 ± 6.8% in stable lesions, significantly greater than the +5.5 ± 5.6% in unstable lesions.

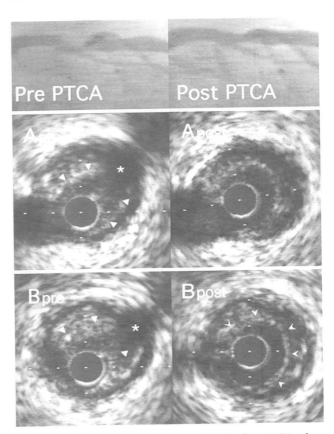

Figure 12.5. The angiograms before and after PTCA of a proximal left anterior descending (LAD) stenosis causing unstable angina are seen in the upper panels. The lower panels show matched IVUS images of the lesion before and after PTCA. A pre: The catheter blank, situated at the origin of the first diagonal branch, is wedged in an eccentric lesion (9 to 7 o'clock), that is divided into outer and inner layers, separated by an echodense line (arrowheads). A post: After PTCA the neolumen corresponds in area and shape with the demarcated inner layer prior to dilatation. Little stretch and no significant change in dimensions of the underlying plaque have occurred. B pre: At a point proximal to the diagonal origin, a layer is again evident (arrowheads) obscured by the guide wire artifact at 2 o'clock (asterisk). B post: The neolumen corresponds in dimensions and shape with the layer evident prior to intervention, but a thin remnant of the layer is evident from 9 to 6 o'clock (hollow arrowheads). Calibration 1 mm; 30 MHz transducer.

from the difference in the mechanisms of angioplasty noted in the same study. Whereas vessel stretch, with or without a wall tear, was the predominant contributor to lumen gain in stable lesions, a significant reduction in lesion cross-sectional area was found only in unstable lesions (Fig. 12.4). This appeared to arise from displacement or remodeling of the circumferentially distributed inner layer, as its shape and size were seen to correspond closely with that of the neolumen following balloon dilatation (Fig. 12.5). In a proportion of cases, a thin residual layer of material was evident (Fig. 12.5). Compression of other plaque components, including lipid atheroma, has not been found to occur in an experimental angioplasty model[18] and the early theory that angioplasty increased lumen area as a result of the 'cold flow' compression of soft atheroma[19,20] is no longer accepted.

Acute myocardial infarction

Ultrasound observations in a series of 30 patients with acute myocardial infarction have been reported

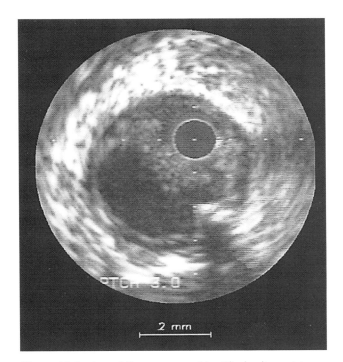

Figure 12.6. A mobile mass was identified adjacent to the catheter blank in the right coronary artery of a patient who developed multiple angiographic filling defects following balloon angioplasty of an unstable lesion. The scintillating ultrasonic texture of the mass and the resolution of angiographic filling defects following administration of intracoronary urokinase point to a thrombotic basis for these appearances. The blood pool distal to the mass appears relatively darker as a result of signal attenuation by the thrombus. Focal calcification is seen at 5 o'clock.

by Bokch and colleagues.[21] A distinctive, smooth-contoured imprint of the imaging catheter was seen in 68% of cases. Hypoechoic, mobile intraluminal masses, suggestive of loose or disrupted intraluminal thrombus, were seen in 88% of cases. The material thought to represent thrombus was less echogenic than the underlying plaque. Fissures were identified in only 28% of cases and dissection in 8%. The author and colleagues have noted appearances suggestive of loose intraluminal thrombus in a number of cases of both acute myocardial infarction and unstable angina (Fig. 12.6).

In infarct-related lesions, in which total occlusion is usual prior to imaging, a pattern of layering is seen that is similar to that seen in unstable lesions (Figs 12.3, 12.7), but a number of differences have also been observed. As illustrated in Fig. 12.8, proximal to the lesion, a bright, sharply demarcated inner layer was noted. Within the lesion, this density difference was less marked, and layer demarcation was made on the basis of a fine, circumferential echodense line and differences in echo texture rather than on differences in echodensity (Fig. 12.3). Although originally thought to represent differences in the constitution of the thrombus at the 'head' and the 'tail' of an acute thrombotic coronary lesion (platelet versus fibrin predominance), it now seems more probable that the echodense proximal layer results from a high concentration of rouleaux in static blood proximal to the occlusion, and that formed thrombus gives rise to the less well demarcated pattern within the occlusive lesion.

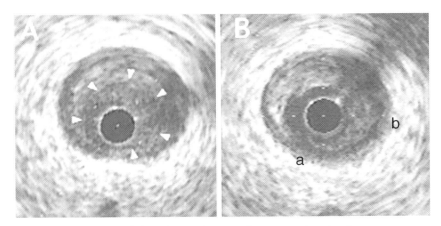

Figure 12.7. **(A)** A subtle echographic interface (arrowheads) demarcates an inner layer of probable thrombus. **(B)** Lumen area increase following angioplasty resulted from remodeling of the layer rather than vessel stretch. The plaque has torn at its thinnest point (a) and a subintimal dissection runs counterclockwise from 6 to 3 o'clock (as far as point b). Calibration 1 mm; 30 MHz transducer.

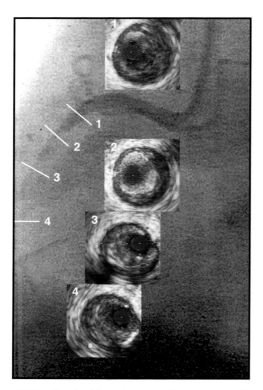

Figure 12.8. The highly echogenic layer proximal to infarct-related total occlusion, most probably arising from a high concentration of rouleaux in static blood rather than from formed thrombus.

Subacute lesions

Lesion layering has also been documented in a high-grade, angiographically smooth and concentric proximal right coronary artery stenosis three weeks following acute inferior myocardial infarction. In contrast to the behavior of more acute lesions undergoing balloon angioplasty, the inner layer appeared to be displaced to one side of the neolumen rather than being more comprehensively compressed or remodeled (Fig. 12.9). Directional atherectomy was subsequently performed to improve an inadequate angioplasty result. Histological analysis of the excised fragments revealed partially organized thrombus, which may have been less deformable than fresher thrombus occurring in acute lesions.

Identification of 'vulnerable' and ruptured plaques

By convention, relatively hypoechoic areas, thought not to result from attenuation or the effects of a limited dynamic range, have been called 'soft', on the basis of early work in which a correspondence between lipid-rich plaque or atheromatous collections and low echogenicity was made.[22] Subsequent work has emphasized the limited accuracy of intravascular ultrasound in detecting intramural lipid deposition.[23] To some extent, this discrepancy may relate to the histological definitions used by different investigators. Large atheromata or 'lipid abscesses', a likely example of which is seen in Fig. 12.10, are probably detected with greater accuracy. Our ability to study the phenomenon of 'plaque vulnerability' and to establish the capacity of ultrasound to predict which lesions are at risk of subsequent rupture depends on the reliable identification of such plaque types.

As image quality and resolution have improved, spontaneous intimal fissures and dissections that have led to an acute coronary event are detectable in a proportion of acute lesions (Fig. 12.11). This issue is addressed in detail in Chapter 14.

Implications for the pathophysiology of atherosclerosis

Features of the sub-acute case described above and the observations in acute lesions support the 'encrustation theory' of atherosclerosis originally espoused by von Rokitansky,[24] revived by Duguid[25] and more recently by Fulton,[26] who noted that '...the overwhelming majority of lesions which give rise to clinically important obliterative coronary artery disease not only have thrombosis as their fatal complication but lesser degrees of thrombosis in their earlier development.' Davies has argued that plaque growth following acute coronary events results from intraplaque hemorrhage by way of intimal fissures.[27] Falk has documented laminated thrombus of differing ages in unstable lesions leading to a fatal outcome.[14] Such a process may underlie stepwise plaque growth in survivors of episodes of intimal disruption and thrombosis that may or may not necessarily be clinically manifest, depending on the degree of associated lumen compromise.[28,29]

Technical and practical aspects

Although the risk of intravascular ultrasound imaging is marginally greater when performed in patients with unstable coronary disease, the absolute risk of significant complications remains very small.[30] No significant complications occurred in a

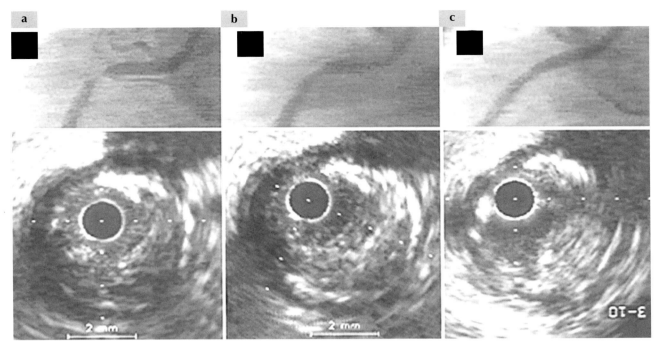

Figure 12.9. (a) In this patient three weeks after inferior wall myocardial infarction, angiography (upper left panel) revealed a high-grade concentric stenosis in the proximal right coronary artery. Intravascular ultrasound at the stenosis (lower panel) revealed wedging of the catheter blank within a large, eccentric lesion. A demarcated layer of probable organizing thrombus encircles the lumen. A focus of deep calcification is evident at 12 to 2 o'clock. **(b)** Following balloon angioplasty, angiography suggested a moderate residual stenosis. Ultrasound revealed inadequate lumen gain that appeared to be the result of vessel stretch and incomplete remodeling of the inner layer. **(c)** Directional coronary atherectomy gave rise to an excellent angiographic appearance (upper panel). Although intravascular ultrasound confirmed a doubling of lumen area, and showed a number of discrete 'bites' into the plaque from the atherectomy device (3 and 6 o'clock) residual plaque cross-sectional area nevertheless measured >60% of vessel area. 30 MHz transducer.

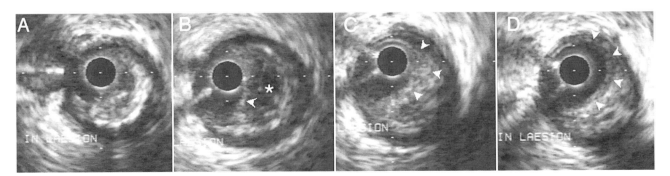

Figure 12.10. An example of a probable pool of lipid-rich material or 'atheroma' underlying a critical stenosis in a patient with unstable angina (a 'vulnerable plaque'). The series of images, A–D, is taken from a catheter pullback through the stenosis. Panel A shows the distal lesion at the origin of a diagonal branch. The catheter blank sits in a small, eccentrically placed lumen, the unoccupied portion of which is seen on its lower, left side. In B, the large eccentric plaque is made up of an echolucent core (asterisk) separated from the lumen by a thin cap (arrowhead). In C, subtle layering (possibly representing mural thrombus) is evident, the inner layer separated from the underlying lesion by a thin echolucent line (arrowheads). In D, the thin layer is better seen (arrowheads), appearing echolucent relative to the underlying plaque. Calibration 1 mm; 30 MHz transducer.

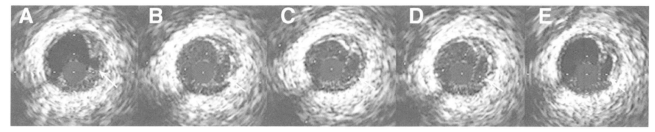

Figure 12.11. This series of images was acquired in the dominant left circumflex artery of a patient who had experienced an inferolateral myocardial infarction some months previously. Probable plaque ulceration was evident on the angiogram. The ultrasound images (proximal to distal, A to E) show a crescentic blood-filled space near the inner, endoluminal surface of the plaque, that communicates with the true lumen by way of a small communication, evident as a discontinuity in the 'fibrous cap' in panel A. Contrast injection (panels A and E) displaced echogenic blood from this space, confirming communication with the main lumen. These appearances are consistent with an emptied lipid pool, that may have triggered the previous acute event.

group of patients with unstable angina undergoing pre-interventional imaging (the author's study), although transient chest pain and ST-segment shift was not uncommon, limiting the time for which the probe could be left in place. Bokch et al.[21] reported that pre-interventional imaging was possible in 83% of infarction-related lesions compared with 50% of stable lesions, and did not lead to complications. Thus, despite the high-grade nature of these lesions, pre-interventional imaging has been performed without evidence of added risk in both unstable and acute infarction-related stenoses. Pre-interventional imaging is important, both to characterize the lesion accurately and to determine the true mechanism of angioplasty. A layered appearance may no longer be apparent on the postinterventional images; thus, in order to distinguish layer displacement from simple stretch, imaging prior to angioplasty is required (Fig. 12.1). In addition, a controlled, slow pullback of the catheter is essential to ensure complete characterization of the lesion, as tissue features such as layering may be subtle and easily missed if confined to a small number of frames on the video playback sequence.

A number of technical artifacts may introduce apparent layering within a lesion. A discrete circumferential line centered on the catheter blank may be seen when adjacent time gain controls are set to markedly different levels, but is recognized by its unnatural symmetry and position with respect to the center of the image. Temporal averaging of images obtained at the border of a high-grade lesion with an adjacent less stenosed segment can produce a 'layered' appearance but is excluded by switching

off the averaging process and by the demonstration of the phenomenon at different points throughout the lesion. The increased reflectivity of blood imaged at 30 MHz, particularly as flow becomes sluggish and rouleaux form, can be mistaken for a discrete tissue layer rather than the blood-filled lumen. As mentioned above, this phenomenon is seen proximal to total occlusions, typically in the context of acute myocardial infarction. Misinterpretation is guarded against by (a) injecting contrast or saline into the coronary to clear the lumen of blood speckle, and (b) by distinguishing the dynamic speckle generated by flowing blood on real-time viewing from the relatively static speckle of adjacent tissues or thrombus. The latter distinction is facilitated when the catheter blank does not completely occupy the lumen, allowing a small area of free lumen to be visualized and available for comparison with adjacent tissues (Fig. 12.1).

Conclusions

Although constrained by limited specificity for the identification of lipid and thrombus, intravascular ultrasound imaging clearly has the potential to provide important insights into the pathophysiology and natural history of the acute coronary syndromes. Using existing technology, a combination of morphological parameters may be used to characterize acute lesions. Fulfilling the potential of the technique in this area of research awaits the development of objective methods of tissue characterization.

References

1   Holmes D, Hartzler G, Smith H, Fuster V. Coronary artery thrombosis in patients with unstable angina. *Br Heart J* (1981) **45**:411–16.

2   Levin D, Fallon J. Significance of the angiographic morphology of localized coronary stenoses: histo-pathologic correlations. *Circulation* (1982) **66**:316–20.

3   Ambrose J, Winters S, Stern A et al. Angiographic morphology and the pathogenesis of unstable angina. *J Am Coll Cardiol* (1985) **5**:609–16.

4   Braunwald E. Unstable angina. A classification. *Circulation* (1989) **80**:410–14, or Ahmed WH, Bittl JA, Braunwald E. Relation between clinical presentation and angiographic findings in unstable angina pectoris, and comparisons with that in stable angina. *Am J Cardiol* (1993) **72**:544–50.

5   Vetrovec G, Leinbach R, Gold H, Cowley M. Intracoronary thrombolysis in syndromes of unstable ischemia: angiographic and clinical results. *Am Heart J* (1982) **104**:946–52.

6   Kalbfleisch S, McGillem M, Simon S, DeBoe S, Pinto I, Mancini G. Automated quantifiation of indexes of coronary lesion complexity—comparison between patients with stable and unstable angina. *Circulation* (1990) **82**:439–47.

7   Sherman C, Litvack R, Grundfest W et al. Coronary angioscopy in patients with unstable angina pectoris. *N Engl J Med* (1986) **315**:913–19.

8   Ramee S, White C, Collins T, Mesa J, Murgo J. Percutaneous angioscopy during coronary angioplasty using a steerable microangioscope. *J Am Coll Cardiol* (1991) **17**:100–5.

9   den Heijer P, Foley DP, Escanded J et al. Angioscopic versus angiographic detection of intimal dissection and intracoronary thrombus. *J Am Coll Cardiol* (1994) **24**:649–54.

10   Siegel R, Ariani M, Fishbein M et al. Histopathologic validation of angioscopy and intravascular ultrasound. *Circulation* (1991) **84**:109–17.

11   Jain A, Ramee S, Mesa J, Collins T, White C. Intracoronary thrombus: chronic urokinase infusion and evaluation with intravascular ultrasound. *Cathet Cardiovasc Diagn* (1992) **26**:212–14.

12   Hodgson J, Reddy D, Suneja R, Nair R, Lesnefsky E, Sheehan H. Intracoronary ultrasound imaging: correlation of plaque morphology with angiography, clinical syndrome and procedural results in patients undergoing coronary angioplasty. *J Am Coll Cardiol* (1993) **21**:35–44.

13   Kearney P, Erbel R, Rupprecht HJ et al. Differences in the morphology of unstable and stable coronary lesions and their impact on the mechanisms of angioplasty. An in vivo study with intravascular ultrasound. *Eur Heart J* (1996) **17**: 721–30.

14   Falk E. Unstable angina with fatal outcome: dynamic coronary thrombosis leading to infarction and/or sudden death. Autopsy evidence of recurrent mural thrombosis with peripheral embolization culminating in total vascular occlusion. *Circulation* (1985) **71**:699–708.

15   Davies MJ, Thomas A. Thrombosis and acute coronary artery lesions in sudden cardiac ischemic death. *N Engl J Med* (1984) **310**:1137–40.

16   Comess K, Fitzgerald P, Yock P. Intracoronary ultrasound imaging of graft thrombosis. *N Engl J Med* (1992) **327**:1691–2.

17   Mintz GS, Potkin BN, Cooke RH et al. Intravascular ultrasound imaging in a patient with unstable angina. *Am Heart J* (1992) **123**:1692–4.

18   Casteneda-Zuniga W, Formanek A, Tadavarthy M et al. The mechanism of balloon angioplasty. *Radiology* (1980) **135**:565–71.

19   Dotter C, Judkins M. Transluminal treatment of arteriosclerotic obstruction: description of a new technique and a preliminary report of its application. *Circulation* (1964) **30**:654–70.

20   Grüntzig A, Senning Å, Siegenthaler W. Non-operative dilatation of coronary-artery stenosis—percutaneous transluminal coronary angioplasty. *N Engl J Med* (1977) **301**:61–8.

21   Bokch WG, Schartl M, Beckmann SH, Dreysse S, Paeprer H. Intravascular ultrasound imaging in patients with acute myocardial infarction: comparison with chronic stable angina pectoris. *Coron Artery Dis* (1994) **5**:727–35.

22   Gussenhoven E, Essed C, Lancée C et al. Arterial wall characteristics determined by intravascular ultrasound imaging: an in vitro study. *J Am Coll Cardiol* (1989) **14**:947–52.

23   Peters RJ, Kok WE, Havenith MG, Rijsterborgh H, van der Wal A, Visser CA. Histopathologic validation of intracoronary ultrasound imaging. *J Am Soc Echocardiogr* (1994) **7**:230–41.

24   von Rokitansky K. *Lehrbuch der pathologische Anatomie*, Vol. 4. Vienna, 1841–46 (translated from the German by G Day). (London: Sydenham Society, 1852): 261.

25   Duguid JB. Thrombosis as a factor in the pathogenesis of coronary atherosclerosis. *J Pathol Bacteriol* (1946) **58**:207–12.

26   Fulton WF. Thrombosis and atherosclerosis. In: *The Coronary Arteries* (London: Charles C Thomas, 1965): 230–302.

27 Davies MJ, Thomas AC. Plaque fissuring—the cause of acute myocardial infarction, sudden ischaemic death, and crescendo angina. *Br Heart J* (1985) **53**:363–73.

28 Stary HC. Composition and classification of human atherosclerotic lesions. *Virchows Archiv A Pathol Anat* (1992) **421**:277–90.

29 Fuster V. The pathogenesis of coronary artery disease and the acute coronary syndromes. *N Engl J Med* (1992) **326**:242–50.

30 Hausmann D, on behalf of the SAFETY in ICUS group. The safety of intracoronary ultrasound. A multicentre survey of 2207 examinations. *Circulation* (1995) **91**: 623–30.

13 Intravascular ultrasound imaging of ruptured plaques

Junbo Ge and Raimund Erbel

Plaque rupture and the subsequent thrombus formation are major events which lead to progression of atherosclerosis and contribute significantly to the pathogenesis of acute coronary syndromes such as unstable angina, myocardial infarction, and sudden death.[1–5] After plaque rupture, the atheroma can be washed out and an emptied plaque be present.[1,5,6] Coronary angiography, which provides only the silhouette of the vessel lumen, is not suitable for defining plaque rupture or identifying plaque-at-risk (rupture-prone plaques). Only when an intraluminal thrombus formation is visualized as a filling defect protruding into the lumen or a deep ulceration causing contrast agent deposits can coronary angiography detect the indirect signs of plaque rupture.[7,8]

Table 13.1 **Clinical characteristics of the patients with (group A) and without (group B) plaque rupture.**

	Group A	Group B	P
Patients (n)	31	108	—
Sex (male)	27 (87%)	92 (85%)	NS
Age (years)	55.0 ± 8.5	57.7 ± 9.3	NS
Vessel			
LAD	15	56	—
LCX	0	11	—
RCA	14	32	—
LMCA	1	6	—
CABG	1	3	—
Hypertension	19 (61%)	49 (45%)	NS
Diabetes	7 (23%)	25 (23%)	NS
Smoking	21 (68%)	62 (57%)	NS
Hypercholesterolemia	23 (74%)	49 (45%)	<0.05
Family history	11 (35%)	44 (41%)	NS
Obesity	10 (32%)	38 (35%)	NS
Symptoms (UAP)	23 (74%)	19 (18%)	<0.001

LAD: left anterior descending artery; LCX: left circumflex coronary artery; RCA: right coronary artery; LMCA: left main coronary artery; CABG: coronary aorta bypass graft; UAP: unstable angina pectoris; NS: not significant.

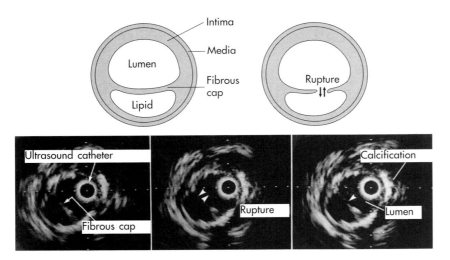

Figure 13.1. Schematic drawing (upper panel) and IVUS images of plaque rupture (lower panel). The ruptured plaque is characterized by a narrow tear in a thin fibrous cap and an emptied echolucent zone.

Intravascular ultrasound (IVUS) offers a new modality for visualizing the coronary artery wall, plaque morphology, and plaque composition,[9–14] and as such provides the potential for identifying plaque disruption, as a preliminary study has shown.[15] The authors examined 144 patients with IVUS; the IVUS images were suitable for analysis in 139 (97%). The patients were then divided into two groups according to whether or not a patient had plaque rupture. A total of 31 patients (22%) (group A) were found to have plaque rupture (Types I and II), of which 15 were found in the left anterior descending artery (LAD), 14 in the right coronary artery (RCA), one in the left main coronary artery (LMCA), and one in an LAD bypass. No plaque ruptures were found in the other 108 (78%) patients (group B). The clinical details and characteristics of both groups are listed in Table 13.1. Unstable angina was present in 23 (74%) of the 31 patients in group A, of whom two had had acute myocardial infarction within the previous two weeks. In contrast, only 19 (18%) of the 108 patients in group B presented with unstable angina ($P < 0.001$). No differences were found between the two groups concerning gender, age, and the risk factors, except hypercholesterolemia.

Plaque morphology

Ruptured plaques were characterized by a narrow tear in a thin fibrous cap with a deep echolucent zone within the plaque (Fig. 13.1). Communication between ulcerated emptied plaque and the lumen

Table 13.2 **Plaque dimensions and characteristics in patients with (group A) and without (group B) plaque rupture.**

	Group A	Group B	P
Thickness of fibrous cap (mm)	0.47 ± 0.20 (0.21–0.76)	0.96 ± 0.94 (0.4–1.7)	<0.01
Tear size (mm)	0.83 ± 0.29	—	—
Eccentricity	94%	64%	<0.01
Plaque size (mm²)	11.7 ± 7.0 (4.0–30.1)	13.4 ± 8.3 (4.0–26.2)	NS
Emptied plaque or lipid core size (mm²)	4.1 ± 3.2	1.32 ± 0.79	<0.001
Lipid/plaque ratio	38.5 ± 17.1%	11.2 ± 8.9%	<0.001
Percentage stenosis	56.2 ± 16.5%	67.9 ± 13.4%	<0.001
Superficial calcium deposits ($n = 29$)[a]	15 (52%)	54 (51%)	NS
Deep calcium deposits	5 (17%)	46 (43%)	0.019

Note: The values in the table indicate mean ± SD and range.
[a]The two patients with plaque ulceration were excluded.
NS: no statistical significance.

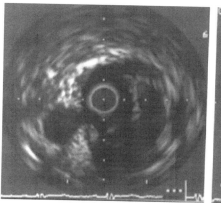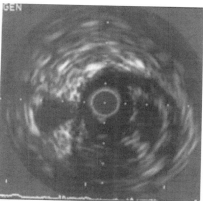

Figure 13.2. An IVUS image of plaque rupture. By injecting contrast material communication through the tear can be demonstrated (right). Calibration 1 mm, 20 MHz.

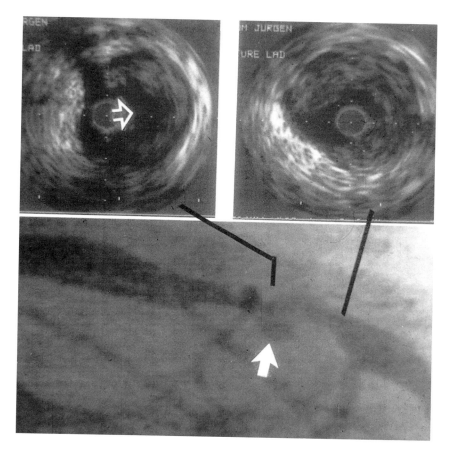

Figure 13.3. A patient with plaque ulceration which presents as aneurysmal bulging on angiography. IVUS demonstrated the bulging is actually a plaque ulceration. Calibration 1 mm, 20 MHz transducer, 3.5 F catheter.

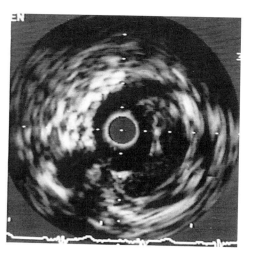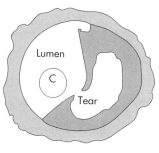

Figure 13.4. Schematic drawing of a ruptured plaque which was misdiagnosed as coronary aneurysm. Actually, the emptied plaque was filled with contrast agent which shows on focal dilation of the lumen. (From Ge et al.,[18] with permission.)

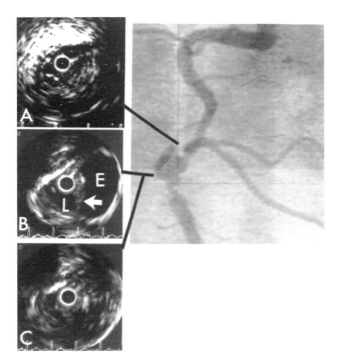

Figure 13.5. A patient was interpreted as having a coronary aneurysm in the right coronary artery by coronary angiography. IVUS showed that the angiographic aneurysm was actually an emptied plaque with a ruptured fibrous cap (arrow) and huge plaque formation proximally and distally to the tear. 3.5 F catheter, 20 MHz transducer. (From Ge et al.,[18] with permission.)

was demonstrated by injecting contrast material (Fig. 13.2). Plaque ulcerations presented as a sac in the plaque, which angiographically presented as a small aneursymal bulge (Fig. 13.3). An echolucent zone was present in 49 (45%) of the 108 patients without plaque rupture. Data on calcium deposits (superficial or deep) and plaque morphology (eccentric and concentric) in both groups are compared in Table 13.2. No differences were found between the two groups concerning superficial calcium deposits. Deep calcium deposits, however, were more common in group B (P = 0.019). Although eccentric plaques appear more frequently than concentric ones in both groups (94% versus 64%), they are more common in ruptured plaques (P < 0.01).

Frequently, ruptured plaques are misinterpreted as coronary aneurysms by contrast angiography because contrast agent fills the emptied plaque.[16] Figures 13.4 and 13.5 show the angiographic pseudo-aneurysms.[17] It is sometimes difficult to differentiate spontaneous dissection from plaque rupture at the early stage of atherosclerosis. Figure 13.6 shows an image of plaque rupture/intimal dissection. The former indicates plaque disruption with lipid washout; the latter indicates tear of the normal intima.

The location of the rupture is shown in Fig. 13.7. The tear was frequently located at the lateral part of the plaque. A central location was found in 26%.

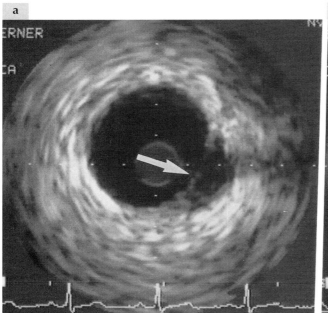
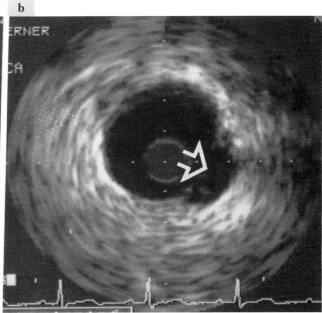

Figure 13.6. IVUS images of a patient with intramural haematoma. No obvious plaque formation was found apart from a small area of the proximal LA, Calibration 1 mm, 3.5 F, 30 MHz transducer. Arrows: fibrous cap.

Location of plaque rupture

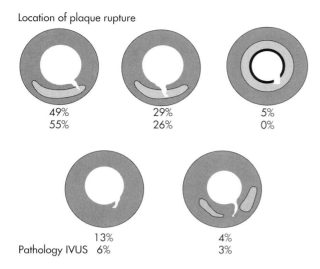

49%   29%   5%
55%   26%   0%

13%   4%
Pathology IVUS 6%   3%

Figure 13.7. IVUS location of the rupture in the plaques of 31 patients in comparison with the pathologic examination published previously.[17] (Modified from the schematic drawing of Richardson et al.,[17] with permission.)

Quantitative analysis of plaques

The vessel and plaque dimensions in both groups are listed in Table 13.2. No significant differences between the two groups were found concerning the vessel area or plaque area. The percentage stenosis in patients with plaque rupture (56.2 ± 13.5%) was significantly lower than in patients without plaque rupture (67.9 ± 13.4%) ($P < 0.001$). The emptied plaque cavity size (4.1 ± 3.2 mm^2) in patients with plaque rupture was significantly larger than the echolucent zone (0.7 ± 1.0 mm^2) in the 49 (45%) of the 108 patients without plaque rupture ($P < 0.001$). Similarly, the emptied plaque cavity/plaque size ratio in patients with plaque rupture (38.5 ± 17.1%) was larger than the echolucent zone/plaque ratio in patients without plaque rupture (11.2 ± 8.9%) ($P < 0.001$). The thickness of the fibrous cap in patients with plaque rupture (0.47 ± 0.20 mm) was thinner than that in patients without plaque rupture (0.96 ± 0.94 mm) ($P < 0.001$) (Table 13.2).

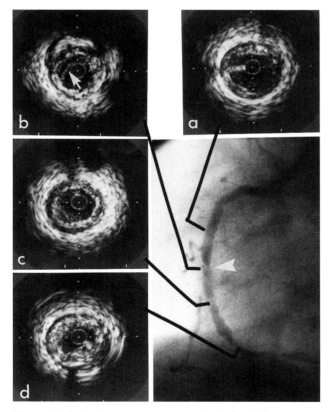

Figure 13.8. A plaque rupture (arrow) in the right coronary artery in a patient with unstable angina. Visible free floating intimal membrane. (From Ge et al.,[15] with permission.) 3.5 F, 20 MHz transducer, calibration 1 mm.

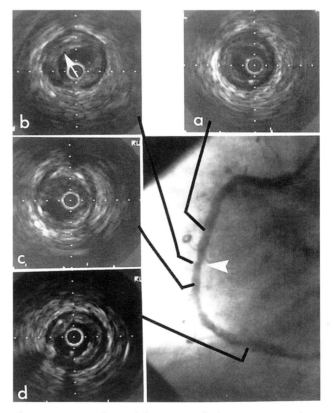

Figure 13.9. Healing of the ruptured plaque (arrow) of the same patient as shown in Fig. 13.8 10 days later. The layering effect can be visualized (arrow). No floating structure visualized. (From Ge et al.,[15] with permission.) 3.5 F, 20 MHz transducer, 1 mm calibration.

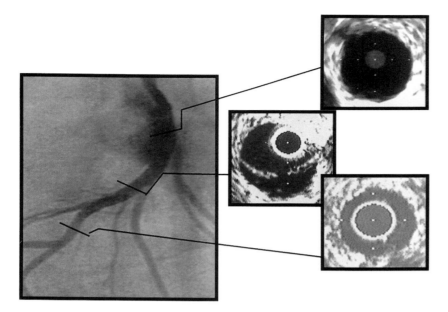

Figure 13.10. Normal coronary angiogram in a 42-year-old patient with a single episode of angina pectoris. Due to anterior hypokinesis an intracoronary ultrasound study was performed. In the middle of the LAD, IVUS revealed a spontaneous plaque rupture with a washed-out plaque and a rupture in the middle of the fibrous cap. Proximal and distal segments (upper and lower panel) were completely free of any atherosclerotic involvement. (From Baumgart et al.,[32] with permission.) 3.5 F, 20 MHz transducer, 1 mm calibration.

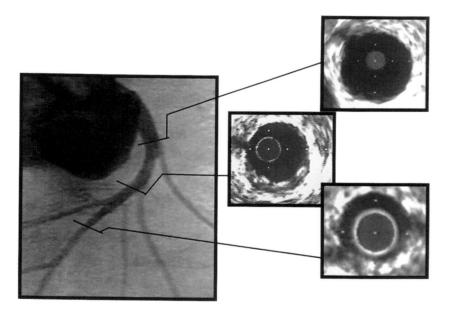

Figure 13.11. Angiographic and ultrasound control investigation 8 weeks later. Again, the angiogram was totally normal. IVUS investigation demonstrated a consolidation of the atherosclerotic site indicating a healed eccentric plaque (Stary III). This case uniquely demonstrates that plaque rupture occurring once or repetitively is involved in the development of atherosclerotic plaques. (From Baumgart et al.,[32] with permission.)

The site of the rupture

Plaque rupture is affected by numerous factors, including increased shear stress injury, turbulent plaque injury, transient collapse of the stenosis, rupture of the vasa vasorum, and circumferential stress within the plaque.[18–38] The site of rupture depends on the plaque morphology and its composition.[20,39,40] These findings are in agreement with the observations by Richardson et al. (Fig. 13.7). Discrepancies exist concerning the superficial tear and ulceration. IVUS found a lower percentage of superficial tears than pathology, whereas we found in 10% of patients with ulceration. This might be related to the resolution of current IVUS which is in the range of 150–200 µm. In another study, van der

Wal et al. reported that inflammation may destabilize the fibrous cap tissue and result in plaque rupture.[41] A recent study showed that macrophages play a significant role in plaque rupture because they may release lytic enzymes that degrade the fibrous cap, causing the atherosclerotic plaques to rupture.[42]

Role of plaque rupture in the process of plaque progression

Following plaque rupture blood enters the emptied plaque and the exposed subendothelial tissue (tissue factor) triggers the thrombotic process described above. Exposure of subendothelial tissue may result in platelet accumulation, which in turn may result

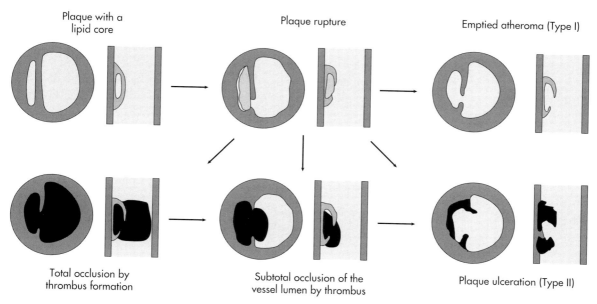

Figure 13.12. Schematic drawing of plaque rupture and the possibilities after plaque rupture in cross-sectional and longitudinal views. Grey: lumen; black: thrombus.

in release of platelet-derived growth factor (PDGF) and lead to smooth muscle cell proliferation.[34] The latter may account for progression of atherosclerosis. If the host wins in this battle, than in several episodes the plaques stabilize and there may be calcium deposits or fibrosis.[35] If the coagulation system wins, with the help of vascular spasm at that segment, then clinically acute coronary syndromes result.[23,33] The observation in the authors' study that percentage stenosis in patients with stable plaques is higher than in patients with unstable plaques may also address this hypothesis.

Once a plaque ruptures it may lead to unstable angina, acute myocardial infarction or sudden death, as stated above. The ruptured plaque may heal spontaneously, as reported by the authors' group.[15,32] Figures 13.8–13.11 show examples of healing of ruptured plaques. Again, it is difficult to differentiate plaque rupture from intimal dissection in Figs 13.10 and 13.11. Figure 13.12 summarizes the sequences after plaque rupture.

Limitations

In the IVUS study only the main epicardial coronary arteries and not the side-branches could be scanned, which may lead to underestimation of the true incidence of the plaque rupture. Nevertheless, coronary atherosclerosis involves most frequently the proximal portion of the coronary arteries, and usually occurs opposite the branches.[43] Thus the underestimation seems to be insignificant. With IVUS, it may be difficult to identify a ruptured plaque when the rupture is covered or filled by mural thrombi. This situation may be detected by the indirect sign of a layering appearance over the plaque.[28] Preliminary study of tissue characterization has demonstrated in vitro that thrombi result in a clearly different backscatter signal in comparison with fibrous tissue and lipid accumulation. This will enable the differentiation of different types of tissue.

Clinical implications

Plaque rupture is the key event leading to acute coronary syndromes. Identification of plaque rupture is therefore very important in patient management and for improving prognosis. For the first time the pathogenesis and natural history of plaque rupture can be studied in vivo. Future studies should be aimed at the identification of plaque at risk of rupturing before rupture occurs and should provide morphological evidence of the development of coronary syndromes.

References

1 Davies MJ, Thomas AC. Plaque fissuring – the cause of acute myocardial infarction, sudden ischemic death, and crescendo angina. *Br Heart J* 1985; **53**: 363–73.

2 Davies MJ, Bland MJ, Hangartner WR, Angelini A, Thomas AC. Factors influencing the presence or absence of acute coronary thrombi in sudden ischemic death. *Eur Heart J* 1989; **10**: 203–8.

3 Fuster V, Stein B, Ambrose JA, Badimon JJ, Chesebro JH. Atherosclerotic plaque rupture and thrombosis: evolving concepts. *Circulation* 1990; **82 (suppl II)**: 47–59.

4 Ridolfi RL, Hutchins GM. The relationship between coronary artery lesions and myocadial infarcts: ulceration of atherosclerotic plaques precipitating coronary thrombosis. *Am Heart J* 1977; **93**: 468–86.

5 Fuster V, Badimon L, Badimon JJ, Chesebro JH. The pathogenesis of coronary disease and the acute coronary syndromes. *New Engl J Med* 1992; **326**: 242–318.

6 Erbel R, Ge J, Görge G et al. Intravaskuläre Sonographie bei koronarer Herzkrankheit, Neue Aspekte zur Pathogenese. *Dtsch Med Wschr* 1995; **120**: 847–54.

7 Ambrose JA, Winters SL, Stern A et al. Angiographic morphology and the pathogenesis of unstable angina pectoris. *J Am Coll Cardiol* 1985; **5**: 609–16.

8 MacIssac AI, Thomas JD, Topol EJ. Toward the quiescent coronary plaque. *J Am Coll Cardiol* 1993; **22**: 1228–41.

9 Ge J, Erbel R, Gerber T et al. Intravascular ultrasound imaging of angiographically normal coronary arteries: a prospective study in vivo. *Br Heart J* 1994; **71**: 572–8.

10 Ge J, Erbel R, Zamorano J et al. Coronary artery remodeling in atherosclerotic disease: an intravascular ultrasound study in vivo. *Coron Artery Dis* 1993; **4**: 981–6.

11 Di Mario C, The SHK, Madretsma S et al. Detection and characterization of vascular lesions by intravascular ultrasound: an in vitro study correlated with histology. *J Am Soc Echocardiogr* 1992; **5**: 135–46.

12 Tobis JM, Mallery J, Mahon D et al. Intravascular ultrasound imaging of human coronary arteries in vivo. *Circulation* 1991; **83**: 913–26.

13 Fitzgerald PJ, Ports TA, Yock PY. Contribution of localized calcium deposits to dissection after angioplasty: an observational study using intravascular ultrasound. *Circulation* 1992; **86**: 64–70.

14 Honye J, Mahon DJ, Jain A et al. Morphological effects of coronary balloon angioplasty in vivo assessed by intravascular ultrasound imaging. *Circulation* 1992; **85**: 1012–25.

15 Ge J, Haude M, Görge G, Liu F, Erbel R. Silent healing of spontaneous plaque rupture demonstrated by intracoronary ultrasound. *Eur Heart J* 1995; **16**: 1149–51.

16 Braunwald E. Unstable angina, a classification. *Circulation* 1989; **80**: 410–14.

17 Richardson PD, Davies MJ, Born GVR. Influence of plaque configuration and stress distribution on fissuring of coronary atherosclerotic plaques. *Lancet* 1989; **2**: 941–4.

18 Ge J, Liu F, Kearney P et al. Intravascular ultrasound approach to the diagnosis of coronary aneurysms. *Am Heart J* 1995; **130**: 765–71.

19 Falk E. Why do plaques rupture? *Circulation* 1992; **86 (suppl)**: 30–42.

20 Fernandez OA, Badimon JJ, Falk E et al. Characterization of the relative thrombogenicity of atherosclerotic plaque components: implications for consequences of plaque rupture. *J Am Coll Cardiol* 1994; **23**: 1562–9.

21 Falk E. Plaque rupture with severe pre-existing stenosis precipitating coronary thrombosis: characteristics of coronary atherosclerotic plaques underlying fatal occlusive thrombi. *Br Heart J* 1983; **50**: 127–34.

22 Badimon L, Chesebro JH, Badimon JJ. Thrombus formation on ruptured atherosclerotic plaques and rethrombosis on evolving thrombi. *Circulation* 1992; **86 (suppl III)**: 74–85.

23 Falk E. Unstable angina with fatal outcome: dynamic coronary thrombosis leading to infarction and/or sudden death: autopsy evidence of recurrent mural thrombosis with peripheral embolization culminating in total vascular occlusion. *Circulation* 1985; **71**: 699–708.

24 Benson RL. The present status of coronary arterial disease. *Arch Pathol* 1926; **2**: 870–916.

25 Koch W, Kong LC. Über die Formen des Coronarverschlusses. Die Änderung im Coronarkreislauf und die Beziehung zur Angina pectoris. *Beitr Pathol Anat* 1932; **90**: 21–84.

26 Leary T. Experimental atherosclerosis in rabbit compared with human (coronary) atherosclerosis. *Arch Pathol* 1934; **17**: 453–92.

27 Clark E, Graef I, Chasis H. Thrombosis of aorta and coronary arteries, with special reference to 'fibrinoid' lesions. *Arch Pathol* 1936; **22**: 183–212.

28 Kearney P, Erbel R, Rupprecht HJ et al. Differences in the morphology of unstable and stable coronary lesions and their impact on the mechanisms of angioplasty. An in vivo study with intravascular ultrasound. *Eur Heart J* 1996; **17**: 721–30.

29 Sinapius D. Relationship between coronary artery thrombosis and myocardial infarction. *Dtsch Med Wochenschr* 1972; **97**: 433–8.

30 Zamorano J, Erbel R, Ge J et al. Spontaneous plaque rupture visualized by intravascular ultrasound. *Eur Heart J* 1994; **15**: 131–3.

31 Hort W. Der arteriosklerotische Polsterriß. *Versicherungsmedizin* 1991; **43**: 151–4.

32 Baumgart D, Liu F, Haude M, Görge G, Ge J, Erbel R. Acute plaque rupture and myocardial stunning in patient with normal coronary arteriography. *Lancet* 1995; **346**: 193–4.

33 Jorgensen L, Rowsell HC, Hovig T, Glynn MF, Mustard JF. Adenosine diphosphate-induced platelet aggregation and myocardial infarction in swine. *Lab Invest* 1967; **17**: 616–44.

34 Wilentz JR, Sanborn TA, Haudenschild CC, Valeri CR, Ryan TJ, Faxon DP. Platelet accumulation in experimental angioplasty: time course and relation to vascular injury. *Circulation* 1987; **75**: 636–42.

35 Gertz SD, Roberts WC. Hemodynamic shear stress force in rupture of coronary arterial atherosclerotic plaques. *Am J Cardiol* 1990; **66**: 1368–72.

36 Binns RL, Ku DN. Effect of stenosis on wall motion: a possible mechanism of stroke and transient ischemic attack. *Arteriosclerosis* 1989; **9**: 842–7.

37 Barger AC, Beeuwkes R, Lainey LL, Silverman KJ. Hypothesis: vasa vasorum and neovascularization of human coronary arteries: a possible role in the pathophysiology of atherosclerosis. *New Engl J Med* 1991; **88**: 8154–8.

38 Loree HM, Kamm RD, Atkinson CM, Lee RT. Turbulent pressure fluctuations on surface of model vascular stenosis. *Am J Physiol* 1991; **261**: H644–H650.

39 Loree HM, Kamm RD, Stringfellow RG, Lee RT. Effects of fibrous cap thickness on peak circumferential stress in model atherosclerotic vessels. *Circ Res* 1992; **71**: 850–8.

40 Ge J, Liu F, Görge G et al. Visualization of ulcerated unstable plaques by intracoronary ultrasound. *Z Kardiol* 1995; **84**: I86.

41 van der Wal AC, Becker AE, van der Loos CM, Das PK. Site of intimal rupture or erosion of thrombosed coronary atherosclerotic plaques is characterized by an inflammatory process irrespective of the dominal plaque morphology. *Circulation* 1994; **89**: 36–44.

42 Moreno RR, Falk E, Palacios IF, Newell JB, Fuster V, Fallon JT. Macrophage infiltration in acute coronary syndromes: implications for plaque rupture. *Circulation* 1995; **90**: 775–8.

43 Montenegro MR, Eggen DA. Topography of atherosclerosis in the coronary arteries. *Lab Invest* 1968; **18**: 586–93.

14 Coronary dissections: evaluation with intravascular ultrasound

Peter Kearney

Introduction

The term 'coronary dissection' has been used to describe angiographic appearances arising from a variety of different pathological entities.[1] The ambiguous and confusing terminology used to describe vessel wall disruption is contributed to in no small way by the significant limitations of contrast angiography in accurately characterizing such changes. Intravascular ultrasound imaging of the vessel wall offers the opportunity to describe vascular dissections in detail, and to understand better their etiology and prognostic significance.

Following a brief account of the different forms of dissection that occur in the coronary arteries, we summarize those difficulties encountered in characterizing dissections using contrast angiography, before moving on to review different aspects of imaging coronary dissections with intravascular ultrasound. For the purposes of this chapter, we define a dissection as a circumferential tear of the vessel wall.

Naturally occurring dissections

The rupture or fissuring of an atheromatous plaque is generally accepted to be one of the key initiating events in the generation of an acute coronary lesion.[2] Occasionally, such naturally occurring disruption in atheromatous vessels may extend circumferentially to form a dissection, an example of which is shown in Fig. 14.1.

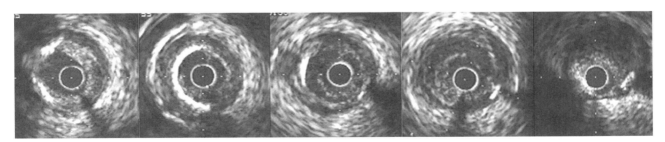

Figure 14.1. This series of ultrasound images was acquired in a man presenting with unstable angina. His angiogram showed a severe, complex stenosis in the proximal left anterior descending (LAD) artery. The ultrasound image within the stenosis (right-hand panel) reveals a large eccentric plaque surrounding the catheter blank. A small rim of free lumen is seen from 3 to 7 o'clock. Marked attenuation of the ultrasound signal is noted from 8 to 4 o'clock, and foci of calcification at 5 and 7 o'clock. A naturally occurring intimal dissection flap is seen in the images acquired more proximally (middle three panels), extending almost as far as the angiographically normal reference segment (left-hand panel). The dissection appears to have arisen at the junction of a plane of deep calcification (generating typical reverberations) with less dense tissue. Such a sequence of events has been well documented after angioplasty,[18] but not previously in spontaneous disruptions leading to acute coronary events. Calibration 1 mm; 30 MHz transducer.

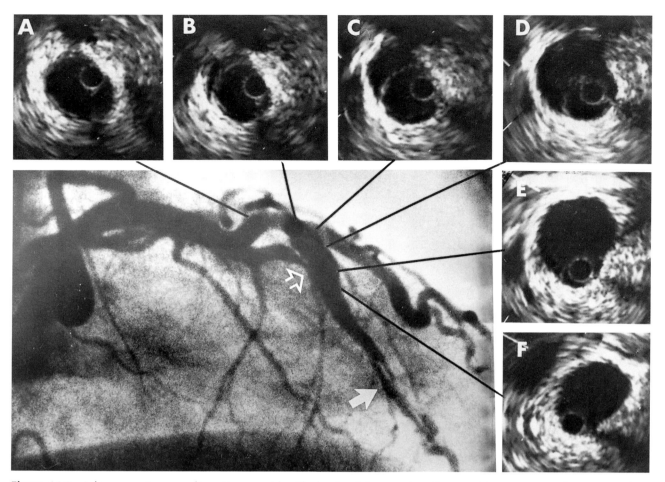

Figure 14.2. A long spontaneous dissection was identified using intravascular ultrasound in a woman who presented with unstable angina and an angiographically ambiguous lesion affecting her left anterior descending artery.[4] Angiogram (lower panel): the left anterior descending artery is seen in a right anterior oblique projection. A linear dissection, evident only in this projection at the junction of the mid and distal LAD (solid arrow), was easily missed. The true nature of the large, proximal false lumen (open arrow) was not readily apparent. ICUS: A. This image was acquired in the LAD immediately proximal to the dissection. The artery is normal with no intimal thickening. B to E. The semi-circular dissection membrane is seen as a very thin echodense line separating the false lumen (above) from the true lumen (below). The false lumen increases in size as the transducer is advanced from proximal (B) to distal (E). F. The true lumen has tapered to a diameter less than the catheter blank (<1.8 mm), which obscures the dissection membrane at this point. Only the false lumen is evident in this image at the distal end of the dissection. Calibration 1 mm, 20 MHz transducer.

Although rare, so-called 'spontaneous' coronary artery dissections, occurring in apparently disease-free vessels, account for a significant proportion of the ischemic coronary events that occur in young women (Fig. 14.2).[3] Most victims of the disorder die suddenly, but a clinical spectrum is seen including stable and unstable angina, myocardial infarction and cardiogenic shock. The classical histological finding is that of a large hematoma occupying the outer third of the media resulting in complete compression of the true lumen, but communicating dissections have been documented in vivo.[3,4]

Other naturally occurring coronary dissections include the proximal extension of type A aortic dissections,[5] and traumatic dissections in both atheromatous[6] and healthy[7] vessels as a result of blunt chest wall injury.

Iatrogenic dissection

Simple diagnostic catheterization may be complicated by coronary dissection.[8] The great majority of coronary dissections are now iatrogenic, generated during the performance of percutaneous coronary intervention. Most commonly the result of balloon dilatation, dissection may complicate the introduction of any of the hardware used for percutaneous intervention into the coronary arteries, including the guide wire alone.[9]

Table 14.1. **This table summarizes the findings of a study that aimed to determine the prognostic significance of different angiographic dissection patterns.[1] Over a 20-month period, 691 significant 'dissections' (type B–F) were detected in a series of 2133 procedures. A definition of each category of the NHLBI classification of intimal tears is provided in the second column, the number of each category in the next column, and the acute clinical success rate (as a percentage) associated with each category in the next column. The clinical success rate associated with type B dissections compared to all more severe dissection types is shown in column 5.**

Type	Description	No.	% success	
A	Radiolucent areas in lumen during contrast injection	N/A	N/A	N/A
B	Parallel tracts or double-lumen separated by a radiolucent area during contrast injection, with minimal or no persistence after dye clearance	543	93.7	93.7
C	Contrast outside the coronary lumen, with persistence of contrast in the area after clearance of dye from the coronary lumen	63	59.7	
D	Spiral luminal filling defects, frequently with extensive contrast-staining of the vessel	44	17.6	37.8
E	New, persistent filling defects (may represent thrombus)	18	55.6	
F	Total occlusion of the artery, without distal anterograde flow (also possibly thrombotic)	35	11.4	

Methods of evaluation

Angiographic evaluation

Until recently, contrast angiography has been the sole method to document coronary dissections in vivo. Waller et al. have highlighted the wide range of anatomical substrates presumed to underlie the angiographic appearances following coronary balloon angioplasty described by the term 'dissection' and the ambiguity of the term as used by different groups.[10] The standardized National Heart, Lung and Blood Institute (NHLBI) classification of angiographic appearances following coronary intervention (Table 14.1), often thought of as a classification of dissections, includes categories that range from nonobstructive filling defects (type A), to patterns that are likely to correspond with true dissection (types B to D), to obstructive lesions that are as likely to represent thrombus as dissection (types E or F). The imprecise nature of the terminology used to describe the angiographic appearances of vessel wall disruption is a natural consequence of the large assumptions that are made in attempting to characterize vessel wall anatomy from an angiographic lumenogram. Descriptions such as 'intimal' or 'sub-intimal' are necessarily imprecise, as the depth to which contrast extends on an angiogram cannot be identified.

A simple differentiation of dissection type into those with minimal or no contrast staining following clearance of the contrast injection (NHLBI type B) and all the other more severe dissection types (NHLBI types C–F) appears to allow stratification to low (type B) and high risk (types C–F) of subsequent abrupt vessel closure.[1] However, angiographic dissection morphology is not helpful in predicting late outcome as the data in this regard are highly contradictory. Studies can be cited that indicate a positive,[11] negative[12] or neutral[13] impact of the presence of dissection on the subsequent restenosis rate.

Ultrasonic evaluation

Methodological considerations

Intravascular tomography permits accurate and detailed scrutiny of coronary dissections, documenting in vivo the depth, circumferential distribution, and tissue plane of a dissection. Although dissections are usually readily identified as discrete, crescentic flaps of tissue, identification can sometimes be difficult, particularly in heavily diseased coronary arteries in which the lumen area is small. A number of maneuvers may be employed to confirm the presence of a dissection plane. A

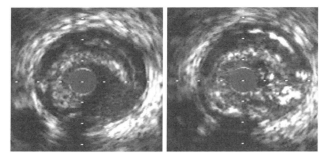

Figure 14.3. Injecting contrast medium or saline down the coronary during intravascular ultrasound imaging is an important maneuver to confirm the presence and extent of a dissection. This has a number of effects. When the blood pool is relatively echodense, clearance of the blood-related backscatter occurs, transiently introducing an echolucent area corresponding in its distribution to that occupied by blood. Microbubbles generate transient, prominent echodense signals that are variably confluent. In this example, such echodensities extend into a 'T' shaped subintimal dissection, one limb of which extends at least as far as 12 o'clock and the other to 7 o'clock.

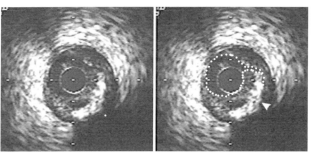

Figure 14.4. This image illustrates the difficulty of characterizing a dissection in the presence of acoustic shadowing. The same image of a dissected mixed plaque following angioplasty is shown without (left-hand panel) and with (right-hand panel) a dotted line to indicate the endoluminal border. The dissection ran behind a deep focus of dense fibrotic and calcific tissue (3 to 6 o'clock). Although its length could not be determined with confidence, discoordinate movement of the dense fibrous tissue and the underlying plaque on the real-time images suggested penetration of the dissection as far as the point indicated by the arrow.

dynamically changing speckle pattern within the body of the plaque, consistent with blood flowing within a dissection plane should be sought. An injection of contrast or saline results in the replacement of such a pattern by echolucent material and frequently introduces transient, coarse echodensities generated by microbubbles as seen in Fig. 14.3. Discoordinate movement of the dissection flap and the underlying plaque may be visible. A careful evaluation of adjacent segments to identify an entry or exit point or more apparent flap may also be helpful. An experimental technique has been developed to confirm the presence of communicating dissections. The highly variable nature of the backscatter signals generated by flowing blood can be distinguished from the more static radiofrequency pattern of adjacent tissues, allowing selective averaging and enhancement of blood-containing areas on sequential frames.[14]

In an in-vitro study, the sensitivity of IVUS for the detection of dissections was 79%.[15] Dissections were missed as a result of adherence of the dissection flap to the vessel wall, absence of a communication between true and false lumens, wall-wrapping of the dissection by the catheter, the inability to identify a dissection within a calcium-generated acoustic shadow (Fig. 14.4), and misdiagnosis (classifying a linear tear or rupture as a dissection). Although

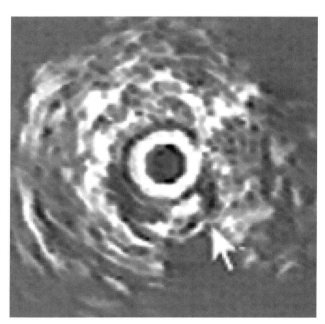

Figure 14.5. Previous generations of intravascular ultrasound scanners suffered from a narrow dynamic range. The high-contrast images were difficult to interpret, and detection of dissection planes was often difficult or impossible. A tentative diagnosis of dissection was made on this image on the basis of discordinate movement of adjacent segments of the plaque, but a false positive diagnosis could not be excluded. 20 MHz transducer.

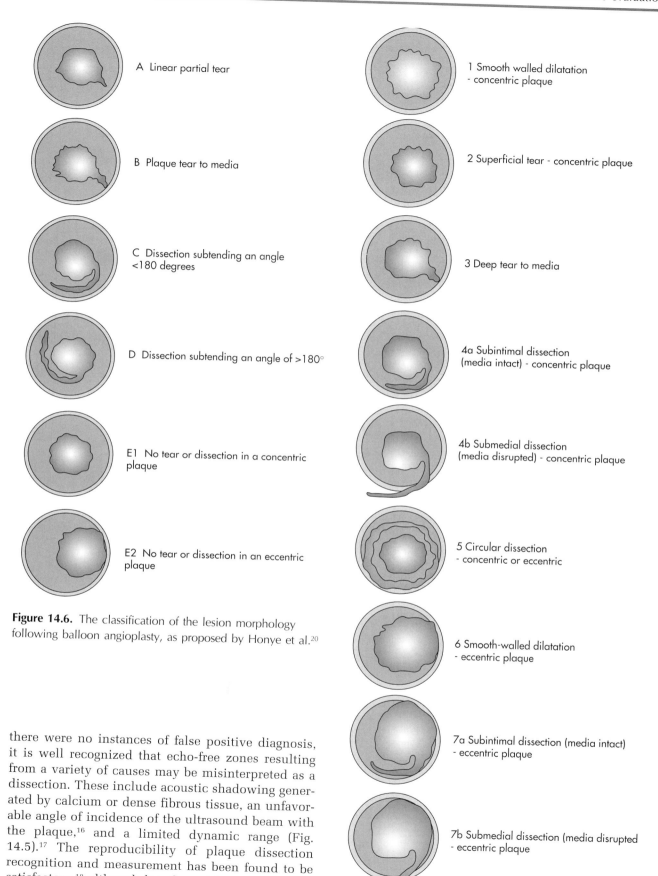

Figure 14.6. The classification of the lesion morphology following balloon angioplasty, as proposed by Honye et al.[20]

Figure 14.7. The classification of lesion morphology following balloon angioplasty, as proposed by Gerber et al.[21]

there were no instances of false positive diagnosis, it is well recognized that echo-free zones resulting from a variety of causes may be misinterpreted as a dissection. These include acoustic shadowing generated by calcium or dense fibrous tissue, an unfavorable angle of incidence of the ultrasound beam with the plaque,[16] and a limited dynamic range (Fig. 14.5).[17] The reproducibility of plaque dissection recognition and measurement has been found to be satisfactory,[18] although less favorable agreement has also been noted, despite the application of a well defined scoring and assessment system by all observers.[19]

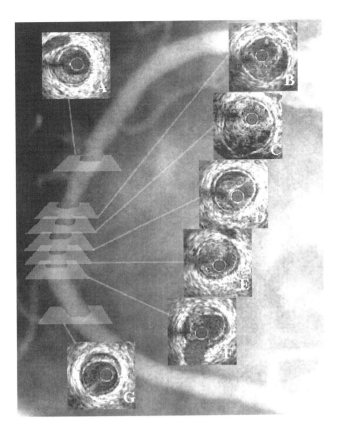

Figure 14.8a. Apart from mild intraluminal haziness at the angioplasty site in the mid part of the pars descendens of this right coronary artery, the angiographic result appeared very satisfactory. The series of ultrasound images illustrates both how a spiral dissection involving considerable residual lumen compromise may exist despite a satisfactory angiographic appearance, and how considerable variation in dissection morphology may occur along its length. Panel A shows the proximal reference segment and panel G the distal reference. In panel B, a dissection plane arising at 12 o'clock extends to 5 o'clock. In panel C it extends in an ill-defined manner behind the large eccentric plaque, and in panel D both the exit site at 12 o'clock, and a large dissection flap are clearly seen. Significant residual lumen stenosis and the exit site tear at 1 o'clock are visible in panel E. At the distal end of the dissection, at the origin of a marginal branch, the intima is disrupted but not dissected. The spiral morphology, typified by this lesion, is thought to be particularly at risk of acute closure. Calibration 1 mm, 30 MHz transducer.

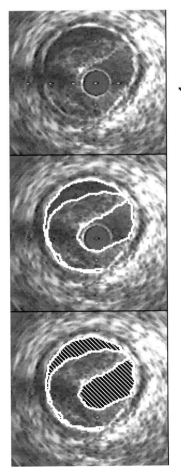

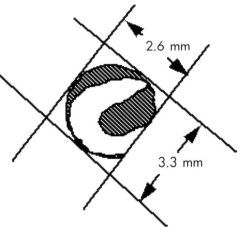

Angiographic dimensions
  Major diameter = 3.3 mm
  Minor diameter = 2.6 mm

True lumen
  Major diameter = 2.2 mm
  Minor diameter = 1.3 mm

Figure 14.8b. The extensive dissection seen on this image was angiographically 'silent' as a result of the almost complete circumferential passage of contrast in the subintimal dissection plane. The column of contrast medium, interpreted on the angiogram as the vessel lumen, measured 2.6 mm (minimum diameter) × 3.3 mm (maximum diameter). True lumen dimensions were 1.3 mm minimum diameter × 2.2 mm maximum diameter. 30 MHz transducer.

Classifications

It has been suggested that a dissection be classified as a 'mechanism of angioplasty' when less than 1 cm in length and/or less than 180° in circumferential extent, and a 'complication of angioplasty' if greater than 1 cm in length and/or 180° in circumference.[10] As yet, there has been no prospective validation of this histology-derived approach using intravascular ultrasound. At least two clinical classifications of intravascular ultrasound morphology after angioplasty have been proposed (Figs 14.6 and 14.7).[20,21] The categorical classification of morphology on the basis of the findings in one tomographic slice within the lesion (such as that at the site of minimum lumen area) is convenient and common practice, but fails to take into account both the variability of dissection morphology that may occur within a lesion (Fig. 14.8) and the longitudinal extent of the dissection. In an in-vitro study, only half of all dissections present within an angioplastied segment of vessel were detected when plaque morphology was evaluated solely at the site of greatest luminal stenosis (40% versus 79%).[15]

A simple approach to the evaluation of dissections is recommended in a recent account of the applications of intravascular ultrasound.[22] It is suggested that plaque disruption following intervention be classified as a rupture (linear tear) or dissection (circumferential tear). The following features should also be documented: the location of the dissection relative to the narrowest site within the lesion (proximal, distal or at the narrowest site), its axial length when a motorized pullback is available, its greatest circumferential extent, and its maximal depth ('partial' if short of the adventitia, and 'complete' if extending to the adventitia).

Pathophysiological insights

Intravascular ultrasound has contributed greatly to our understanding of dissection formation and the

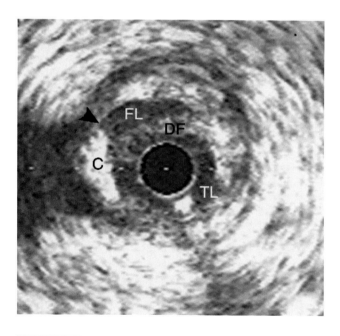

Figure 14.9a. Dissections frequently occur at the junction of fibrous plaque with focal calcific deposits, indicated in this image by the black arrowhead. TL: true lumen, FL: false lumen, DF: dissection flap, C: calcific deposit. Calibration 1 mm, 30 MHz transducer.

Figure 14.9b. This series of images was obtained during a catheter pullback through a lesion following angioplasty, in which a linear, type B dissection was evident angiographically. Dissection has occurred at the junction of fibrous and calcific tissue (left-hand panel). A very complex double lumen and significant residual lumen compromise, not evident angiographically, were evident at the distal end of the lesion (right-hand panel). Calibration 1 mm, 30 MHz transducer.

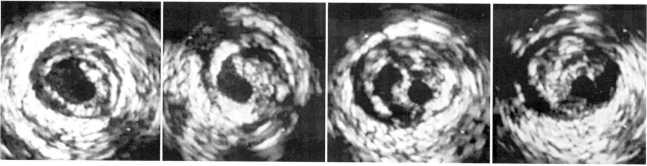

role played by dissection in achieving an increase in lumen area. Dissections tend to occur adjacent to areas of calcification where high shear stress occurs during vessel wall dilatation at the junction of the noncompliant calcific deposit and surrounding softer tissues (Fig. 14.9).[18] The tearing process appears to first develop at surprisingly low inflation pressures. In one study performed with a combined imaging-angioplasty catheter in peripheral arteries all dissections developed at an inflation pressure of under two atmospheres.[23] The important positive contribution of dissection to lumen gain, previously noted in histological studies[10] is supported by data documenting a 30% greater increase in lumen area in lesions with tears compared with those that appear to have a smooth-walled dilatation.[24] In an experimental model detailed geometric analysis of intravascular ultrasound images of plaques prior to dilatation was shown to identify stress points where plaque rupture and dissection were likely to occur.[25] Ultrasound reveals twice as many dissections following balloon angioplasty than is revealed by angiography.[24,26] A proportion of such cases are associated with clinical failure, and are classified as cases of 'restenosis' when angiography reveals apparent recurrence of a significant stenosis. It is now apparent that such cases have failed from the outset, and that the presence of a high-grade residual stenosis can be obscured by radial tracking of contrast medium into an extensive dissection (Fig. 14.8).

Despite the informative nature of these findings, evidence is not yet available that pre-interventional ultrasonic evaluation can reliably predict a potentially occlusive dissection, or indeed that postinterventional dissection morphology can predict the likelihood of acute vessel closure or late restenosis.[29] A number of small studies have produced conflicting results, one indicating a greater risk of restenosis in the absence of plaque wall tear or dissection,[20] while others have found that deep dissection correlates with an increased risk of late lumen loss.[30,31] Furthermore, the proportion of patients in which dissections have been identified after angioplasty using ultrasound is variable, ranging from 41%[32] to 83%[33] in different series.

Conclusions

The technology and methodology of intravascular ultrasound imaging have evolved rapidly and steeply over the past five years. Unhelpful inconsistencies such as those described in the preceding paragraph will be minimized as image quality continues to improve, operators are trained in a standard approach to examination and interpretation, and a consensus is reached on a 'common language' to document morphological findings. For the foreseeable future, intravascular ultrasound will remain the most informative method to study the pathophysiological and prognostic significance of different forms of coronary dissection.

References

1 Huber MS, Fishman Moody J, Madison J, Mooney MR. Use of a morphologic classification to predict clinical outcome after dissection from coronary angioplasty. *Am J Cardiol* (1991) **63**:467–71.

2 Davies MJ, Thomas AC. Plaque fissuring—the cause of acute myocardial infarction, sudden ischaemic death, and crescendo angina. *Br Heart J* (1985) **53**:363–73.

3 Kearney P, Singh H, Khan S, Lee G, Lucey J, Hutter J. Spontaneous coronary artery dissection: a report of three cases and review of the literature. *Postgrad Med J* (1993) **69**:940–5.

4 Kearney P, Erbel R, Ge J et al. Detection of spontaneous coronary artery dissection by intravascular ultrasound in a case of unstable angina. *Cathet Cardiovasc Diagn* (1994) **32**:58–61.

5 Wainwright CW. Dissecting aneurysm producing coronary occlusion by dissection of the coronary artery. *Bull Johns Hopk Hosp* (1944) **75**:81.

6 Roberts WC, Maron BJ. Sudden death while playing professional football. *Am Heart J* (1981) **102**:1062–3.

7 Kohli S, Saperia G, Waksmonski C, Pezzella S, Singh J. Coronary artery dissection secondary to blunt chest trauma. *Cathet Cardiovasc Diagn* (1988) **15**:179–83.

8 Prewitt KC, Wortham DC, Zen B, Pearson C. Increased risk of coronary artery dissection during coronary angiography with 6F catheters. *Angiology* (1993) **44**:107–13.

9 Farb A, Banks AK, Robinowitz M, Fistel S, Virmani R. Percutaneous transluminal coronary angioplasty guidewire-induced coronary artery dissection without balloon inflation. *Hum Path* (1991) **22**:97–8.

10 Waller BF, Orr CM, Pinkerton CA, van Tassel J, Peters T, Slack JD. Coronary balloon angioplasty dissections: 'The Good, the Bad and the Ugly'. *J Am Coll Cardiol* (1992) **20**:701–6.

11 Hirshfeld JW, Schwartz JS, Jugo R et al and the M-HEART investigators. Restenosis after coronary angioplasty: a multivariate statistical model to relate lesion and procedure variables to restenosis. *J Am Coll Cardiol* (1991) **18**:647–56.

12 Guiteras Val P, Bourassa MG, David PR et al. Restenosis after successful percutaneous transluminal coronary angioplasty: the Montreal Heart Institute experience. *Am J Cardiol* (1987) **60**:50B–55B.

13 Hermans WR, Rensing BJ, Foley DP et al on behalf of the MERCATOR study group. Therapeutic dissection after successful coronary balloon angioplasty: no influence on restenosis or on clinical outcome in 693 patients. *J Am Coll Cardiol* (1992) **20**:767–80.

14 Pasterkamp G, van der Heiden MS, Post MJ, Ter Haar Romeny BM, Mali WP, Borst C. Discrimination of the intravascular lumen and dissections in a single 30-MHz US image: use of 'confounding' blood backscatter to advantage. *Radiology* (1993) **187**:871–2.

15 van der Lugt A, Gussenhoven EJ, Stijnen T et al. Comparison of intravascular ultrasonic findings after coronary balloon angioplasty evaluated in vitro with histology. *Am J Cardiol* (1995) **76**:661–6.

16 Di Mario C, Madretsma S, Linker D et al. The angle of incidence of the ultrasonic beam: a critical factor for the image quality in intravascular ultrasonography. *Am Heart J* (1993) **125**:442–8.

17 Fitzgerald PJ, Brisken AF, Brennan JM, Hargrave VK, MacGregor JS, Yock PG. Errors in ultrasound image interpretation and measurement due to limited dynamic range. *Circulation* (1991) **84**:II438 (abstract).

18 Fitzgerald P, Ports T, Yock P. Contribution of localized calcium deposits to dissection after angioplasty: an observational study using intravascular ultrasound. *Circulation* (1992) **86**:64–70.

19 Peters RJ, Ge J, Linker DT, Visser CA, Yock PG. Observer agreement on qualitative analysis of intracoronary ultrasound images. *Circulation* (1994) **90**:I551 (abstract).

20 Honye J, Mahon D, Jain A et al. Morphological effects of coronary balloon angioplasty in vivo assessed by intravascular ultrasound imaging. *Circulation* (1992) **85**:1012–25.

21 Gerber T, Erbel R, Görge G, Ge J, Rupprecht H-J, Meyer J. Classification of morphologic effects of percutaneous transluminal coronary angioplasty assessed by intravascular ultrasound. *Am J Cardiol* (1992) **70**:1546–54.

22 Di Mario C, Görge G, Peters RJ et al. Clinical applications of intravascular ultrasound. *Eur Heart J* (1997) (in press).

23 Isner J, Rosenfield K, Losordo D et al. Combination balloon-ultrasound imaging catheter for percutaneous transluminal angioplasty—validation of imaging, analysis of recoil and identification of plaque fracture. *Circulation* (1991) **84**:739–54.

24 Fitzgerald PJ, Yock PG. Mechanisms and outcomes of angioplasty and atherectomy assessed by intravascular ultrasound imaging. *J Clin Ultrasound* (1993) **21**:579–88.

25 Lee R, Loree H, Cheng G, Lieberman E, Jaramillo N, Schoen F. Computational structural analysis based on intravascular ultrasound imaging before in vitro angioplasty: prediction of plaque fracture locations. *J Am Coll Cardiol* (1993) **21**:777–82.

26 Davidson CJ, Sheikh KH, Kisslo KB et al. Intracoronary ultrasound evaluation of interventional technologies. *Am J Cardiol* (1991) **68**:1305–9.

27 Peters RJ, on behalf of the PICTURE study group. Prediction of the risk of angiographic restenosis by intracoronary ultrasound imaging after coronary balloon angioplasty. *J Am Coll Cardiol* (1995) special issue: 35A (abstract).

28 Tenaglia A, Buller C, Kisslo K, Phillips H, Stack R, Davidson C. Intracoronary ultrasound predictors of adverse outcomes after coronary artery interventions. *J Am Coll Cardiol* (1992) **20**:1385–90.

29 Görge G, Erbel R, Gerber T, Ge J, Trauth B, Meyer J. Morphological findings by IVUS and clinical outcome after PTCA. *Circulation* (1992) **86**:518 (abstract).

30 Potkin BN, Keren G, Mintz GS et al. Arterial responses to balloon coronary angioplasty: an intravascular ultrasound study. *J Am Coll Cardiol* (1992) **20**:942–51.

15 The left main coronary artery

Junbo Ge and Raimund Erbel

Patients with left main coronary artery (LMCA) stenosis comprise a high-risk subgroup for acute coronary events (unstable angina, acute myocardial infarction, or sudden death), and in such cases coronary artery bypass grafting is strongly recommended.[1–4] The underlying reason for the poor prognosis in LMCA disease is related to the large amount of myocardium at risk. Coronary angiography, however, cannot provide early and accurate diagnosis of LMCA narrowing,[5–7] with multiple factors accounting for the suboptimal results. Angiography assesses only the luminal contour of the vessel and assumes adjacent segments to have normal values. Coronary artery remodeling in atherosclerosis and the anatomic characteristics of LMCA anatomy itself (for example, short and various courses) also add to the limitations on angiography.[1,6,8] Angiographic underestimation frequently occurs even when a significant stenosis is present.[6,8–10] Other factors directly related to the LMCA also play important roles in the incorrect assessments based on angiography. The LMCA is the shortest of the four coronary arteries, with a mean length of 1.35 cm.[1] When there is atherosclerotic plaque, the lesion is frequently diffused over the entire LMCA. Furthermore, the courses of LMCAs are more unpredictable, making more angiographic projections necessary for optimal study.

Intravascular ultrasound (IVUS) is a relatively new in-vivo imaging modality. It has proved sensitive and accurate in determining vessel dimensions and wall characteristics[11–15] in coronary arteries, including the LMCA.[8]

Angiographically normal left main coronary artery

In the authors' cardiovascular catheterization laboratory 92 consecutive patients (from April 1993 to December 1994, aged 22–75 years) were found to have angiographically normal coronary arteries (84/92 patients) or ambiguous coronary angiograms of the LMCA (8/92 patients). An ambiguous coronary angiogram was defined as showing no significant stenosis but with questionable lumen narrowing; this included hypodense regions of the LMCA or the LMCA being the same size as proximal left anterior descending coronary artery (LAD) or right circumflex coronary artery (RCX). Following diagnostic angiography, the LMCAs were studied with IVUS.

Morphologic observation

Atherosclerotic plaques were detected by IVUS in 31/92 (34%) patients with an angiographically normal or ambiguous LMCA. The patients were divided into two groups according to the presence or absence of plaque formation. Table 15.1 lists the clinical characteristics of the patients in both

Table 15.1 **Clinical characteristics of patients with and without plaques in the LMCA.**

Variables	Patients with LMCA plaques	Patients without LMCA plaques
No. of patients	31	61
Sex (M/F)	20/11	35/26
Age (years)	56.7 ± 9.1	54.8 ± 11.1
Vessel area (mm²)	23.3 ± 6.1	19.0 ± 6.5
LAD plaques	12/31(39%)	18/61(30%)

LMCA: left main coronary artery; LAD: left anterior descending coronary artery.

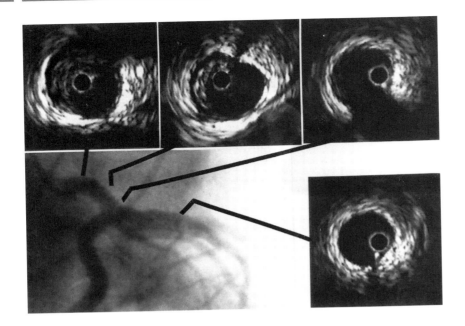

Figure 15.1. Coronary angiogram and intravascular ultrasound images of the LAD and LMCA. A large eccentric plaque is situated in the LMCA, causing a maximal area stenosis of 47.3%. No abnormality was found by coronary angiography. Intravascular ultrasound shows no plaque formation in the LAD.

groups. Eighty-three percent of the plaques were eccentric. Calcium deposits were detected in 17% of the plaques. In 66% of patients, no plaque formation in the LMCA was found by IVUS. Figure 15.1 is of a patient with a normal coronary angiogram of the LMCA but in whom IVUS demonstrated a severe stenosis (47.3%). In two patients with ambiguous angiograms of the LMCA, no abnormalities were found by IVUS (Fig. 15.2).

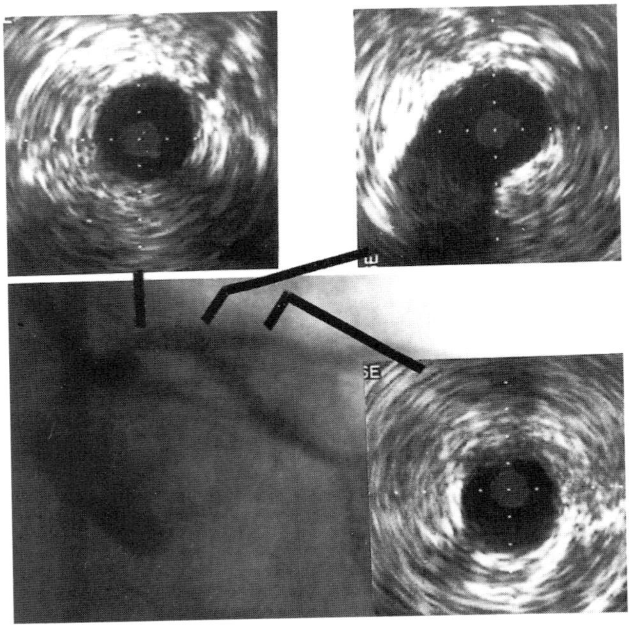

Quantitative analysis

In the patients with IVUS-detected plaques, the cross-sectional vessel area was 23.3 ± 6.1 mm^2. The plaque area was 6.3 ± 3.3 mm^2 (1.8–16.7 mm^2), and the area stenosis was $31.6 \pm 12.1\%$ (12–57.2%). The maximal lumen diameter was 4.5 ± 1.0 mm, the minimal 3.8 ± 0.8 mm. The diameter stenosis was $19.3 \pm 7.2\%$ (8.7–34.6%). The vessel area of the patients with LMCA plaque formation was larger than that of the patients without plaque formation (23.3 ± 6.1 mm^2 versus 19.0 ± 6.5 mm^2, $P < 0.01$) (Fig. 15.3). Four of the patients with a stenosis of more than 50% were advised to undergo bypass surgery based on the IVUS findings and clinical symptoms.

Clinical characteristics

Of the 92 patients, all had chest pain (typical or atypical) and normal or ambiguous coronary angiograms. Positive exercise electrocardiograms (ECGs) were found in 25 patients (27.2%), and positive thallium scintigraphy in 18 patients (19.6%). All four patients who had stenosis greater

Figure 15.2. Coronary angiogram and intravascular ultrasound images of the left coronary artery. Coronary angiography suspects an ambiguous lesion in the ostium while intravascular ultrasound showed that the whole left coronary artery is normal. The ambiguous angiogram is of an artifact.

than 50% and who were advised to undergo bypass surgery had positive exercise ECGs and three had positive thallium scintigraphy. After bypass surgery, all four patients remained uneventful. No interventions were performed in the other 27 patients, in whom the stenoses were less than 50%; however,

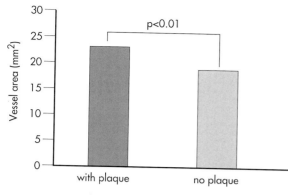

Figure 15.3. Comparison of cross-sectional vessel area between patients with plaque formation and those without plaque formation in the LMCA. The vessel area in the plaque formation group was significantly larger than that in the group without plaque formation, indicating that compensatory enlargement occurs in the plaque formation group.

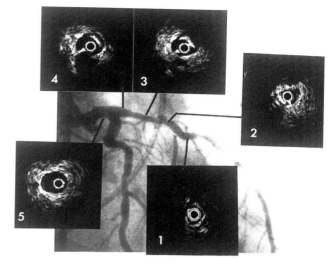

Figure 15.4. A patient with severe LAD stenosis underwent percutaneous transluminal coronary angioplasty. IVUS shows severe stenosis with severe calcification in the proximal LAD. No plaque was found in the LMCA.

these patients were advised to accept medical treatment and a close clinical follow-up.

Incidence and severity of LMCA stenosis in patients undergoing LAD interventions

Severe coronary stenosis can be ruled out when the left main coronary artery is free of atherosclerotic process imaged by transesophageal echocardiography and vice versa. The authors examined the LMCA in 132 patients who underwent LAD interventions with IVUS[22] and found atherosclerotic plaque in 96 patients (73%), of which 78% were eccentric and 24% were calcified plaques. The cross-sectional plaque area ranged from 1.5 to 21.0 mm^2 (8.4 ± 4.7 mm^2). The area stenosis was 34 ± 14% (8–66%). Diameter stenosis was 21 ± 8% (7–42%). Figure 15.4 shows a patient with severe LAD stenosis but with nearly normal LMCA. Figure 15.5 shows also a severe stenosis in the mid-LAD while only a plaque formation in the LMCA. Therefore, scanning the LMCA using transesophageal echocardiography is unable to rule out distal coronary artery disease.

Isolated LMCA stenosis

Coronary artery disease is usually diffuse; however, some patients have isolated LMCA stenosis or ostium stenosis. Figures 15.6 and 15.7 show two

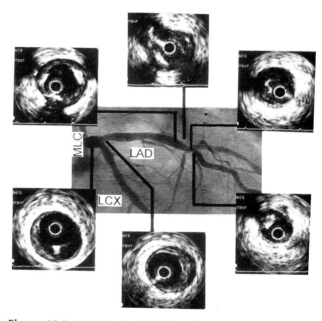

Figure 15.5. A patient with bifurcation stenosis in the mid-LAD. IVUS shows only a small plaque in the LMCA causing no hemodynamically significant lumen reduction.

patients with isolated LMCA stenosis visualized by IVUS, of whom one showed a normal coronary angiogram and the other showed angiographic high-degree stenosis. Frequently, ostium stenosis is very difficult to identify. Figure 15.6 shows a patient with suspected left coronary ostium stenosis because of pressure drop during diagnostic angiography. However, contrast coronary angiography is

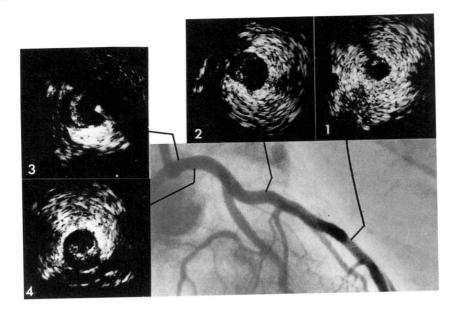

Figure 15.6. A 50-year-old patient with a normal coronary angiogram; however IVUS showed a large eccentric plaque in the ostium. A drop in catheter-tip pressure occurred when the angiography catheter was placed into the left main coronary ostium. No obvious abnormalities were documented on any projection of the angiogram. IVUS was performed just after angiography during which ischemic ECG changes occurred. IVUS demonstrated a large plaque in the ostium of the LMCA and, in view of this finding and an abnormal exercise ECG, bypass surgery was undertaken on this patient. (From Ge et al.,[22] with permission.)

Clinical significance

In clinical cardiology, angiographic findings are routinely used as the gold-standard in the diagnosis and management of patients with coronary artery disease. In view of the frequent errors based on angiographic findings, caution must be taken, particularly for patients with suspected LMCA disease. If the status of the LMCA is not clear after conventional angiography, IVUS should be performed to obtain a qualitative assessment of the atherosclerotic involvement and a quantitative analysis of the absolute luminal area and the percentage area stenosis of the vessel. The additional information provided by IVUS can help in decision-making.

Isolated LMCA stenosis is rare. Marked narrowing of the LMCA is usually indicative of severe diffuse coronary atherosclerosis.[1] A preliminary study has shown a high incidence of LMCA atherosclerosis (73%) in patients who underwent LAD interventions.[22] This also indicates that, although there is a high incidence of atherosclerotic involvement of LMCA, the stenosis seldom becomes a high-grade one requiring intervention. Although the underlying mechanism is still unknown, the special histology and anatomy of the LMCA may provide the explanation. Whether small plaques detected by IVUS really are clinically significant remains to be studied through long-term follow-up observation.

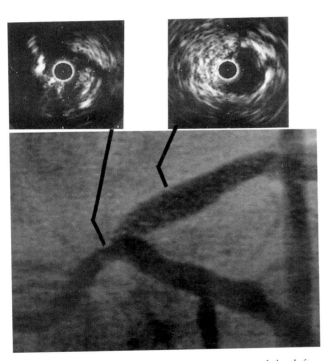

Figure 15.7. Left anterior oblique (LAO) view of the left coronary artery. High degree of the left main stenosis and the sinus nodal artery branching from the left circumflex artery. While advancing the IVUS catheter, asystole occurred (see also chapter 36).

not able to confirm this diagnosis. With IVUS, a high degree of ostium stenosis was identified.[23] Figure 15.7 shows a patient with angiographically indicated LMCA stenosis. Transient asystole occurred during IVUS examination.

Methodological considerations

Efforts have been made to assess the severity of coronary artery stenosis. Coronary angiography has been regarded as the most practical and reliable of these methods. However, studies have increasingly indicated that coronary angiography is associated with considerable error, in particular a frequent underestimation of the severity and extent of atherosclerotic lesions,[1,3,5,9,17,18] predominantly in vessels with severe disease.[9] Coronary angiography has the intrinsic limitation that is visualizes only the contour of the vessel lumen, not the morphology of the vessel wall. The luminal size of a certain segment is determined by using adjacent segments for reference. The experience of the angiogram reviewer also plays an important role. It is impossible to guarantee accurate assessment of lumen loss, even with the aid of quantitative computer processing. Isner et al.[17] compared the findings for the LMCA by angiography and histology in 28 patients; with angiography there was significant error (71%) in the evaluation of vessel stenosis.

In the authors' study, 37% of patients with a normal LMCA on angiography were found to have plaque formation. This incidence is high, considering the poor prognosis for LMCA stenosis. Furthermore, 4% of patients had LMCA stenosis of over 50% but were still regarded as 'normal' by coronary angiography. This is in agreement with other studies of the LMCA.[8,10,19] IVUS is able to overcome some of the limitations on coronary angiography in the study of the LMCA.[8,19] The additional information provided by IVUS proves to be valuable for clinical decision-making.[19]

References

1   Conti CR, Selby JH, Christie LG et al. Left main coronary artery stenosis: clinical spectrum, pathophysiology, and management. *Prog Cardiovasc Dis* 1979; **22**: 73–106.

2   Ge J, Liu F, Görge G et al. Angiographically 'silent' plaque in the left main coronary artery detected by intravascular ultrasound. *Coron Artery Dis* 1995; **6**: 805–15.

3   Lim JS, Proudfit WL, Sones FM. Left main coronary arterial obstruction: long-term follow-up of 141 nonsurgical cases. *Am J Cardiol* 1975; **36**: 131–5.

4   Takaro T, Peduzzi P, Deter KM et al. Survival in subgroups of patients with left main coronary artery disease. Veterans administration cooperative study of surgery for coronary arterial occlusive disease. *Circulation* 1982; **66**: 14–22.

5   Johnson DE, Alderman EL, Schröder JS et al. Transplant coronary artery disease: histopathologic correlations with angiographic morphology. *J Am Coll Cardiol* 1991; **17**: 449–57.

6   Glagov S, Weisenberg E, Zarins CK, Stankunavicius R, Koletti GJ. Compensatory enlargement of human atherosclerotic coronary arteries. *New Engl J Med* 1987; **316**: 1371–5.

7   Arnett EN, Isner JM, Redwood CR et al. Coronary artery narrowing in coronary heart disease: comparison of cineangiographic and necropsy findings. *Ann Intern Med* 1979; **91**: 350–5.

8   Gerber T, Erbel R, Görge G, Ge J, Rupprecht HJ, Meyer J. Extent of atherosclerosis and remodeling of the left main coronary artery determined by intravascular ultrasound. *Am J Cardiol* 1994; **73**: 666–71.

9   Schwartz JN, Kong Y, Hackel DB, Bartel AG. Comparison of angiographic and postmortem findings in patients with coronary artery disease. *Am J Cardiol* 1975; **36**: 174–8.

10   Porter T, Sears T, Xie F et al. Intravascular ultrasound study of angiographically mildly diseased coronary arteries. *J Am Coll Cardiol* 1993; **22**: 1858–65.

11   Pandian NG, Kreis A, Brokway B et al. Ultrasound angioscopy: real-time, two-dimensional, intraluminal ultrasound imaging of blood vessels. *Am J Cardiol* 1988; **62**: 493–4.

12   Ge J, Erbel R, Seidel I et al. Experimental evaluation of accuracy and safety of intraluminal ultrasound. *Z Kardiol* 1991; **80**: 595–601.

13   Tobis JM, Mallery J, Mathon D et al. Intravascular ultrasound imaging of human coronary arteries in vivo. *Circulation* 1991; **83**: 913–26.

14   Nissen SE, Gurley JC, Grines CL et al. Intravascular ultrasound assessment of lumen size and wall morphology in normal subjects and patients with coronary disease. *Circulation* 1991; **84**: 1087–99.

15   Ge J, Erbel R, Zamorano J et al. Coronary artery remodeling in atherosclerotic disease: an intravascular ultrasonic study in vivo. *Coron Artery Dis* 1993; **4**: 981–6.

16   Taylor HA, Deumite NJ, Chaitman BR, Davis KB, Killip T, Rogers WJ. Asymptomatic left main coronary artery disease in the coronary artery surgery study (CASS) registry. *Circulation* 1989; **79**: 1171–9.

17   Isner JA, Kishel J, Kent KM, Ronan JA, Ross AM, Roberts WC. Accuracy of angiographic determination of left main coronary arterial narrowing. Angiographic–histologic correlative analysis in 28 patients. *Circulation* 1981; **63**: 1056–64.

18 McPherson DD, Hiratzka LF, Lamberth WC et al. Delineation of the extent of coronary atherosclerosis by high-frequency epicardial echocardiography. *New Engl J Med* 1984; **316**: 304–9.

19 Nishimura RA, Higano ST, Holmes DR Jr. Use of intracoronary ultrasound imaging for assessing left main coronary artery disease. *Mayo Clin Proc* 1993; **68**: 134–40.

20 Ryan T, Armstrong WF, Feigenbaum H. Prospective evaluation of the left main artery using digital two-dimensional echocardiography. *J Am Coll Cardiol* 1986; **7**: 807–12.

21 Samdarshi TE, Nanda NC, Gatewood RP Jr et al. Usefulness and limitations of transesophageal echocardiography in the assessment of proximal coronary artery stenosis. *J Am Coll Cardiol* 1992; **19**: 572–80.

22 Ge J, Erbel R, Haude M, Görge G, Liu F, Meyer J. Incidence and severity of atherosclerosis in left main coronary artery in patients who undergo LAD interventions. *Z Kardiol* 1994; **83**: I49.

23 Ge J, Erbel R, Gerber T et al. Intravascular ultrasound imaging of angiographically normal coronary arteries: a prospective study in vivo. *Br Heart J* 1994; **71**: 572–8.

16 Myocardial bridging

Junbo Ge and Raimund Erbel

Introduction

Coronary arteries and their major branches usually run along the surface of the heart in the subepicardial tissue. Myocardial bridging (MB) is said to occur when a segment of a coronary artery travels through the myocardium. This phenomenon was first described by Grainicianu in the early 1920s.[1] In 1960, Portsmann and Iwig[2] first reported the angiographic appearance of transient occlusion in a segment of the left anterior descending coronary artery (LAD) during systole. A large discrepancy exists between pathological series, where the incidence has varied from 15% to 85%,[3,4] and angiographic series, where it is reported as being between 0.51% and 2.5%.[5–7] Reports have suggested that MB may be associated with myocardial ischemia,[5,8–10] myocardial infarction,[11–13] conduction disturbances,[14] and sudden death.[15,16] Although the systolic compression can be enhanced by nitroglycerin and positive inotropic drugs,[17,18] no signs of ischemia during stress testing have been detected by thallium scintigraphy.[19] Nevertheless, Noble and colleagues[5] observed that patients with a severe 'milking effect' (more than 75% narrowing during systole) can experience marked myocardial ischemia at rapid heart rates, as evidenced by ST-segment depression and increased left ventricular lactate products. Intravascular ultrasound imaging (IVUS) is a relatively new technique allowing accurate assessment of vascular anatomy. This technique is able to detect myocardial bridging and provide unique information concerning wall morphology in this condition.[20–22]

Morphologic observation

In all patients with angiographically typical milking effect with IVUS and intracoronary Doppler a highly characteristic systolic compression with delayed relaxation in diastole of the bridge segment was clearly visualized.[22] Figure 16.1 shows the angiographically characteristic milking effect in a bridge segment during a cardiac cycle. The lumen area decreased from 11.3 mm^2 to 6.1 mm^2; the lumen diameter decreased from 3.8 mm to 2.8 mm. The lumen compression was observed as being eccentric in 12/14 patients (86%) and concentric in 2/14 patients (14%). In 12 patients, atherosclerotic plaque was found in the segments proximal to the bridge (Fig. 16.2), and in four of these patients percutaneous transluminal coronary angioplasty (PTCA) was subsequently undertaken. The maximal plaque area ranged from 2 to 12 mm^2 (6.9 ± 3.9 mm^2). No atherosclerotic lesions were detected in the myocardial bridge segments and the segments distally in the eight patients in whom the IVUS catheter was successfully advanced through the entire bridge segment. Recently, a specific sign of myocardial bridging was detected by IVUS. This specific sign is called the 'half-moon' phenomenon (Fig. 16.3), which exists in all bridge patients. The width of the half-moon phenomenon is 0.40 ± 0.07 mm in systole and 0.41 ± 0.10 mm in diastole.

Quantitative analysis of the myocardial bridge and the normal segment proximal to the bridge

It was found that the lumen area of the bridge segments decreased from 8.1 ± 3.0 mm^2 to 5.0 ± 1.8 mm^2 ($P < 0.01$), and lumen diameter from 3.2 ± 0.6 mm to 2.6 ± 0.5 mm ($P < 0.001$) during the cardiac cycle. The corresponding angiographic values decreased from 5.7 ± 2.3 mm^2 to 2.1 ±

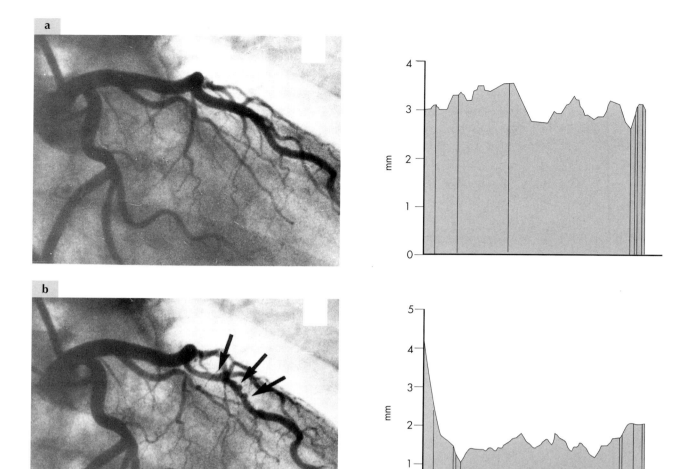

Figure 16.1. Coronary angiogram of the left coronary artery. A typical 'milking effect' is seen in the middle LAD (arrows). The right panel is based on quantitative coronary analysis. (From Ge et al.,[22] with permission.)

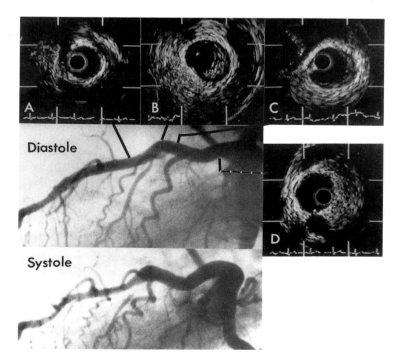

Figure 16.2. Intravascular ultrasonic appearance of the myocardial bridge segment and the LAD. An eccentric plaque formation is visualized in the segment proximal to the bridge (B). No abnormality was documented on angiography. 3.5 F catheter. (From Ge et al.,[22] with permission.)

Diastole   Systole

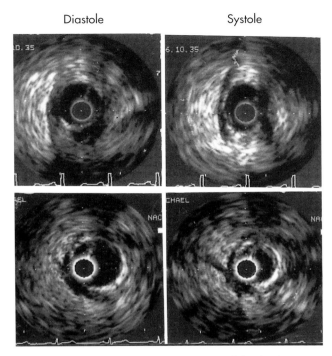

Figure 16.3. Characteristic appearance of the bridge segment during diastole and systole. A specific 'half-moon' phenomenon is seen around the bridge segment. 3.5 F catheter, 1 mm calibration.

0.8 mm² ($P < 0.001$) and from 2.7 ± 0.6 mm to 1.7 ± 0.3 mm ($P < 0.001$). In addition, the difference in measurements based on IVUS and angiography was statistically significant (all $P < 0.01$). In the normal segment proximal to the bridge the maximal lumen area can be seen in very early diastole while the minimal lumen area is at the beginning of systole (Fig. 16.4, lower panel). The cyclic changes are illustrated in Fig. 16.4, where the largest lumen of the selected myocardial bridge segment is seen in mid-diastole and the smallest lumen between end-systole and early diastole (Fig. 16.4, lower panel). The cross-sectional lumen area variation during the cardiac cycle was 40 ± 25% in the MB segments and 9 ± 7% in the normal segments ($P < 0.01$) (Fig. 16.4, upper panel).

Coronary flow mapping and flow reserve

In this group of patients, it was found that coronary flow reserve (CFR) was 2.2 ± 0.7, significantly decreased in comparison with the normal values.[23] A highly characteristic flow pattern showing a

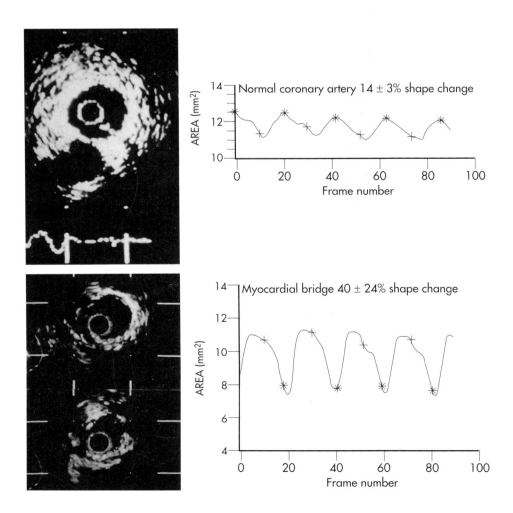

Figure 16.4. Computer-analyzed cross-sectional area variation of the myocardial bridge during the cardiac cycle. The upper panel shows the area variation at a normal segment proximal to the bridge segment (systolic area increase). The lower panel shows the area variation of the bridge segment during the cardiac cycle. 4.8 F catheter, 1 mm calibration (systolic area decrease).

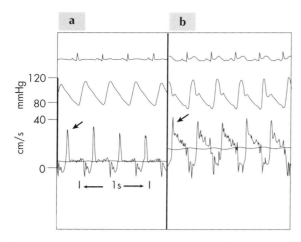

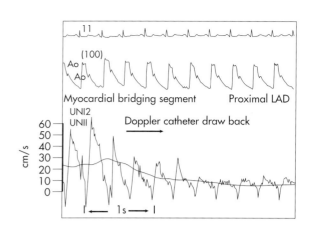

Figure 16.5. Intracoronary Doppler recording in a vessel with a myocardial bridge at rest (left) and after injection of papaverine (right). A prominent peak in velocity in early diastole is a pattern typical of myocardial bridging (arrow). 3 F Millar Doppler catheter, 20 MHz transducer. (From Ge et al.,[22] with permission.)

Figure 16.6. Doppler flow pattern during pullback of the Doppler transducer. The characteristic flow pattern disappeared when the Doppler transducer was pulled back to the normal segment proximal to the myocardial bridging. 3 F Millar Doppler catheter, 20 MHz transducer. (From Ge et al.,[22] with permission.)

prominent peak in coronary flow in early diastole was observed in 86% of patients (Fig. 16.5). This characteristic flow pattern was abolished as the Doppler transducer was pulled back to the normal segment (Fig. 16.6).

Using intracoronary Doppler flow wire, apart from the typical flow pattern observed with the Doppler catheter, a characteristic retrograde flow was detected in the bridge segment and the proximal segment in a large proportion of patients, especially under nitroglycerin provocation (Fig. 16.7). This flow pattern correlated with the pressure gradient during intracoronary double-tip pressure measurement (see below).

Pressure measurement: evidence of atherogenesis in the proximal segment

Intracoronary pressure was measured in a patient with angiographically typical bridging, by use of a double-tip catheter. A pressure drop in the distal segment (Fig.16.8) and a pressure gradient phenomenon in the bridge segment (Fig. 16.9) were found. The pressure in the proximal segment was 160/26 mmHg, much higher than that of the aortic pressure of 128/68 mmHg.[24] This addresses the

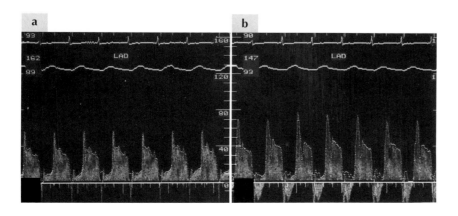

Figure 16.7. Coronary flow velocity recorded by Doppler flow wire. A typical 'fingertip' phenomenon is seen at the beginning of diastole. After intracoronary administration of 0.2 mg nitroglycerin, a retrograde flow is seen during end-systole (b). Doppler flow wire, 15 MHz, 0.014 inch (Cardiometrics).

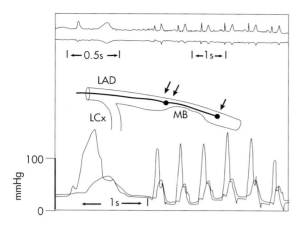

Figure 16.8. Pressure measurement with double-tip pressure catheter. The proximal sensor is located in the proximal segment of the bridge (160/26 mmHg) and the distal sensor in the segment distal to the bridge (68/30 mmHg). (From Ge et al.,[24] with permission.)

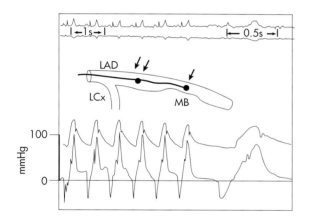

Figure 16.9. Double-tip pressure catheter with the proximal sensor located in the normal segment (126/68 mmHg) and the distal sensor in the distal bridge segment (102/20 mmHg). A pressure gradient is clearly seen. (From Ge et al.,[24] with permission.)

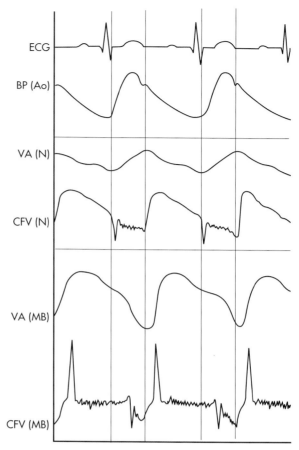

Figure 16.10. The contrasting patterns of variation in vessel area and coronary flow velocity are outlined for a normal vessel (VA(N) and CFV(N)) and in a muscle bridge segment (VA(MB) and CFV(MB)). The timing of events in the cardiac cycle is apparent from the dotted lines at the end of the QRS (the start of isometric contraction of the left ventricle and the point of opening of the aortic valve) and at the end of the T-wave (the end of systole and the point of closure of the aortic valve).

mechanism of the previous pathologic observations that atherosclerotic lesions seldom involve the bridge segment[25,26] so much as the wall stress and subsequent injury to which the segment proximal to the MB is particularly prone.[27]

Risse et al.[28] reported that the intima of the MB segment (66.3 μm) was thinner than that of the proximal part (406.6 μm). The currently used IVUS catheter (20 MHz) is not able to determine the thickness of the intima and media of the MB segment because the resolution is too low at approximately 150 μm.

The reduction of CRF in patients with MB may be due to a moderate increase in resting flow velocity and a limited hyperemic response as a result of reduced mid to late diastolic flow velocity, due to prolonged relief of the myocardial compression, and marked reduction in systolic flow velocity, as demonstrated in Fig. 16.5. These results may help to explain the previous observations that this syndrome is associated with myocardial ischemia, myocardial infarction, and conduction system disturbances.[5,8–16] Alternatively, the reduced CFR may be a reflection of the presence of atherosclerosis in the segment proximal to the MB.

A sharp acceleration of flow is seen in early diastole, followed by immediate marked deceleration. Flow velocity plateaus for the remainder of diastole prior to a drop in systole. In contrast to the normal pattern of vessel area change during the cardiac cycle, in which an increase in area is seen throughout systole in conjunction with the rise in aortic root pressure, MB segments undergo a marked decrease in area, particularly in the second half of systole. Importantly, this vessel compression persists into early diastole. The hemodynamic consequences of these changes in vessel area can be seen in the coronary flow velocity traces in the schematic drawing in Fig. 16.10. In early diastole, as the intraventricular pressure quickly drops during the slower decline in aortic root pressure, maximal coronary perfusion pressure occurs. In normal coronaries this results in a typical acceleration in coronary flow followed by a gradual decline. The rate of deceleration may be attenuated by the simultaneous gradual decrease in vessel area. In contrast, the very sharp increase in velocity in the bridge segment is the result of a high pressure gradient due to compression and low distal pressure which is slowly released. The sudden deceleration appears to be the result of the rapid increase in vessel area that occurs during relaxation of the bridge in diastole which abolishes the pressure gradient. This hypothesis is supported by simultaneous intracoronary pressure measurements.[24]

References

1   Grainicianu A. Anatomische Studien über die Coronararterien und experimentelle Untersuchugen über ihre Durchgängigkeit. *Virchows Arch A Pathol Anat Histopathol* 1922; **238**: 1–8.

2   Portsmann W, Iwig, J. Die intramurale Koronarie im Angiogramm. *Fortschr Rontgenstr* 1960; **92**: 129–32.

3   Polachek P. Relation of myocardial bridges and loops on the coronary arteries to coronary occlusions. *Am Heart J* 1961; **61**: 44–52.

4   Edwards JC, Burnsides C, Swarm RL, Lansing AJ. Arteriosclerosis in the intramural and extramural portions of coronary arteries in human heart. *Circulation* 1956; **13**: 235–41.

5   Noble J, Bourassa MG, Petitclerc R, Dyrda I. Myocardial bridging and milking effect of the left anterior descending coronary artery: normal variant or obstruction? *Am J Cardiol* 1976; **37**: 993–9.

6   Ishimori T, Raizner AF, Chabine RA, Awdeh M, Luchi R. Myocardial bridges in man: clinical correlations and angiographic accentuation with nitroglycerin. *Cathet Cardiovasc Diagn* 1977; **3**: 59–65.

7   Voss H, Kupper W, Hanrath P, Mathy D, Montz R, Buecking J. Klinik, Laktatmetabolismus, Koronarvenenflow und biphasisches 201-Thallium-Myokardszintigramm bei Myokardbrücken des Ramus descendens anterior: Verlaufsvariante oder Obstruktion? *Z Kardiol* 1980; **69**: 347–52.

8   Ciampricotti R, El Gamal M. Vasospastic coronary occlusion associated with a myocardial bridge. *Cathet Cardiovasc Diagn* 1988; **14**: 118–20.

9   Rossi L, Dander B, Nidasio GP et al. Myocardial bridges and ischemic heart disease. *Eur Heart J* 1980; **1**: 239–45.

10   Kramer JR, Kitazume H, Proudfit WL, Sones FM Jr. Clinical significance of isolated coronary bridges: benign and frequent condition involving the left anterior descending artery. *Am Heart J* 1982; **103**: 282–8.

11   Vasan RS, Bahl VK, Rajani M. Myocardial infarction associated with a myocardial bridge. *Int J Cardiol* 1989; **25**: 240–1.

12   Feldman AM, Baughman KL. Myocardial infarction associated with a myocardial bridge. *Am Heart J* 1986; **111**: 784–7.

13   Endo M, Lee YW, Hayashi H, Wada J. Angiographic evidence of myocardial squeezing accompanying tachyarrhythmia as a possible cause of myocardial infarction. *Chest* 1978; **73**: 431–3.

14   Den Dulk K, Brugada P, Braat S, Heddle B, Wellens HJJ. Myocardial bridging as a cause of paroxysmal atrioventricular block. *J Am Coll Cardiol* 1983; **1**: 965–70.

15   Morales AR, Romanelli R, Boucek RJ. The mural left anterior descending coronary artery, strenuous exercise and sudden death. *Circulation* 1980; **62**: 230–7.

16   Bestetti RB, Costa RS, Zucolotto S, Oliveira JSM. Fatal outcome associated with autopsy proven myocardial bridging of the left anterior descending coronary artery. *Eur Heart J* 1989; **10**: 573–6.

17   Erbel R, Treese N, Alken G, Bollenbach E, Meyer J. Provocation of myocardial bridging in patients with normal coronary arteries by nitroglycerin and orciprenalin. *Eur Heart J* 1985; **6 (suppl I)**: 71.

18   Diefenbach C, Erbel R, Treese N, Bollenbach E. Frequency of myocardial bridging after adrenergic stimulation and after load reduction in patients with

angina pectoris, but normal coronary arteries. *Z Kardiol* 1994; **83**: 809–15.

19 Faruqui AMA, Maloy WC, Feiner JM, Schlent RC, Logan WD, Symbas P. Symptomatic myocardial bridging of a coronary artery. *Am J Cardiol* 1978; **41**: 1305–10.

20 Ge J, Erbel R, Gerber T, Görge G, Meyer J. Value and limitation of intravascular ultrasound in the evaluation of myocardial bridging. *Z Kardiol* 1992; **81 (suppl 1)**: 189.

21 Erbel R, Rupprecht HJ, Ge J, Gerber T, Görge G, Meyer J. Coronary artery shape and flow changes induced by myocardial bridging. *Echocardiography* 1993; **10**: 71–7.

22 Ge J, Erbel R, Rupprecht HJ et al. Comparison of intravascular ultrasound and angiography in the assessment of myocardial bridging. *Circulation* 1994; **89**: 1725–32.

23 Erbel G, Ge J, Kearney P et al. Value of intracoronary ultrasound and Doppler in the differentiation of angiographically normal coronary arteries: a prospective study in patients with angina pectoris. *Eur Heart J* 1996; **17**: 880–9.

24 Ge J, Erbel R, Görge G, Haude M, Meyer J. High wall shear stress proximal to myocardial bridging and atherosclerosis: intracoronary ultrasound and pressure measurements. *Br Heart J* 1995; **73**: 462–5.

25 Scholte M, Weis P, Prestele H. Die Koronare Muskelbrücke des Ramus descendens anterior. *Virchows Arch A Pathol Anat Histopathol* 1977; **375**: 23–36.

26 Lee SS, Wu TL. The role of the mural coronary artery in prevention of coronary atherosclerosis. *Arch Pathol* 1972; **93**: 32–5.

27 Willis GC. Localizing factors in atherosclerosis. *Can Med Assoc J* 1954; **70**: 1–8.

28 Risse M, Weiler G. Die koronare Muskelbruecke und ihre Beziehungen zu lokaler Koronarsklerose, regionaler Myokardischaemie und Koronarspasmus, Eine morphometrische Studie. *Z Kardiol* 1985; **74**: 700–5.

17 Ambiguous lesions

Dietrich Baumgart

Introduction

Until recently coronary angiography has been regarded as the 'gold standard' for visualizing and quantifying coronary artery disease. However, coronary angiography portrays only the contrast-filled lumen of the coronary artery, with almost no information on the vessel wall. Coronary angiography can relatively accurately determine changes in lumen diameter with respect to a reference segment. In recent years it was supposed that these reference segments represented normal arterial segments with little or no arteriosclerotic involvement. However, pathological and recent studies by intravascular ultrasound (IVUS) have demonstrated that only the minority of 'normal' reference segments are truly normal.[1]

The interpretation of coronary angiographic images is limited; Glagov et al. and Ge et al. demonstrated that arteriosclerotic coronary arteries enlarge to maintain the vessel lumen with increasing plaque area.[2,3] By this compensatory process, lumen reduction will not occur unless plaque area exceeds 40–45%; that is, angiography will show a 'normal' lumen in the early stage of coronary artery disease. Thus it is not surprising that a number of discrepancies exist between angiographic imaging and pathologic findings.

Intravascular ultrasound is a relatively new imaging modality allowing insight into the coronary arterial wall. It provides information on both the vessel wall structure and the characteristics of the atherosclerotic plaques or thrombus formation. In addition, accurate quantification of vessel lumen and plaque dimensions as well as lumen, vessel, and plaque areas are possible. Recently intravscular ultrasound has been intensively used to guide coronary interventions. In this respect IVUS has on the one hand served to confirm the indication for coronary angioplasty, and has helped to select the appropriate angioplasty procedure based on the lesion morphology as well as the presence or absence of calcification. On the other hand, IVUS guidance has prevented coronary angioplasty in lesions that were not suitable for current devices or not as severe as angiographic measurements predicted. Whereas the extreme ends of the spectrum, that is, from normal coronary arteries to severely stenosed segments, can be discriminated with good predictability by angiography, intermediate lesions ranging from approximately 40% to 70% diameter stenosis are difficult to quantify. Some of these lesions can be classified as ambiguous. This ambiguity can be regarded with respect to the identification and characterization of lesions or plaques and to the decision-making process of the operator.

Ambiguous lesions are intermediate lesions with unclear stenosis severity judged by coronary angiography. Sometimes the angiographic picture disagrees with the overall clinical picture and the symptoms of the patient. Furthermore, ambiguous lesions

---

Lesions classfied as ambiguous from coronary angiography

- Intermediate lesions with unclear stenosis severity
- Aneurysmatic widening of the coronary segment
- Ostial lesions
- Branching vessels
- Vessel tortuosity
- Main stem lesions
- Focal spasm
- Sites of plaque rupture
- Dissections following coronary angioplasty
- Unclear haziness
- Contrast density changes

relate to unclear morphological structures that cannot readily be identified by angiography, including ostial lesion and branching vessels. A third category of ambiguous lesions consists of unclear filling defects or haziness of either spontaneous or interventional origin. The box gives an overview of the most commonly encountered ambiguous lesions.

Intermediate lesions with unclear stenosis severity

With the use of biplane angiography and multiple projections it is possible to obtain an angiogram perpendicular to the maximal thickness of the plaque. However, only in less than 50% of cases can appropriate orthogonal projections be achieved for exact quantification of the luminal area in the reference and the diseased segments.[4] In carefully selected patient populations the regression coefficient of the correlation between intravascular ultrasound and coronary angiography was close to one. Only Tobis et al. demonstrated a poor correlation, with large mean differences between intravascular ultrasound and coronary angiography.[5] As mentioned above, the reference segment of the 'normal' angiographic segment is frequently diseased due to intimal thickening or more severe plaque involvement. Thus, vessel cross-sectional area of the reference segment measured by angiography is smaller than that measured by intravascular ultrasound. These methodological limitations of coronary angiography result in less severe percentage diameter and cross-sectional area stenoses than would be obtained with intravascular ultrasound. In contrast, intravascular ultrasound directly visualizes the plaque size as well as the eccentricity of the plaque from inside the vessel (Fig. 17.1).

Apart from these inherent methodological differences, artifacts caused by flow-mediated phenomena of the contrast medium can alter the perception of the stenosis. Large caliber changes due to significant atherosclerotic involvement, preferentially in large coronary arteries, for example, large right coronary arteries, may cause flow turbulences which in turn may mimic a high-grade stenosis. With IVUS the area stenosis comparing the reference lumen to the stenosis area lumen can be determined; but also the relation of the luminal area to the vessel area including the plaque area and the echolucent zone up to the border of the external elastic lamina can be assessed. Thus a more objective cross-sectional estimate of the disease process is possible.

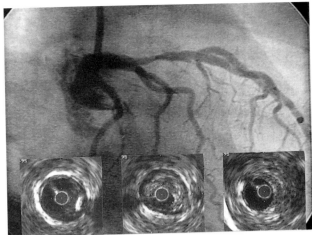

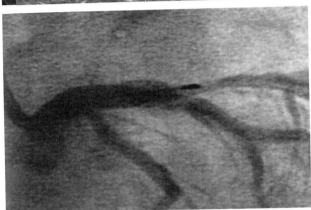

Figure 17.1. Upper panel: angiographic view in right anterior oblique (RAO) projection of the left anterior descending coronary artery with an intermediate type stenosis just distal to a large diagonal side-branch. Stenosis severity by quantitative coronary angiography is only 53%. In contrast, stenosis severity by IVUS amounts to 84% (central IVUS image). Furthermore, the IVUS examination reveals atherosclerotic involvement proximal to the lesion site. Lower panel: magnified angiographic view of lesion site with the intravascular catheter in place. Note that the actual lesion site lies just distal to the tip of the IVUS catheter as the ultrasonic beam using a mechanically rotated system is angled (108), giving a somewhat forward view. (3.5 F catheter; 30 MHz transducer; 1 mm calibration.)

Aneurysmatic widening of the coronary segment

One of the major drawbacks of coronary angiography is the fact that changes in luminal size can only be assessed in relation to a 'normal' reference segment. Thus, changes in caliber size are judged only in relative terms. Given a normal, truly undiseased reference segment, any increase in luminal size would be

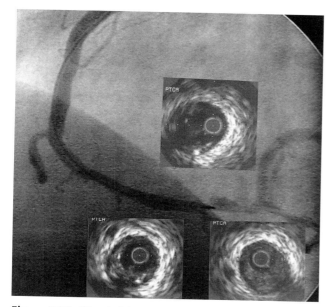

Figure 17.2. Distal right coronary artery (RCA) with aneurysmatic widening just proximal to the branching point of the RCA at the crux cordis. Given the IVUS examination, the angiographic image is misleading. IVUS clearly identifies the lesion as an ulcerated plaque (middle upper IVUS scan) that has been washed out in the course of degeneration. Due to heavy atherosclerotic involvement of the RCA proximally and distally, the lesion appears as an aneurysm-like structure. Without IVUS a clear delineation between true and false aneurysms is not possible.

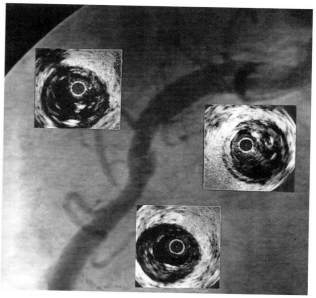

Figure 17.3. Unclear haziness in the proximal part of the right coronary artery involving also the ostial part. IVUS examination reveals a degenerated concentric plaque with multiple dissections as well as flaps which float in the lumen. Further distal caliber changes are due to various degrees of atherosclerotic involvement.

anticipated to be an aneurysm of the coronary arterial wall. However, as pointed out earlier, most of the so-called normal reference segments are diseased themselves. In these cases, increases in luminal size only extremely rarely indicate a coronary aneurysm. Instead, such aneurysmatic widening of the coronary artery mostly represents a contrast-filled emptied plaque following an acute plaque rupture—otherwise known as a pseudoaneurysm. On the other hand, such contrast fillings outside the regular contour of the coronary artery can be the expression of plaque ulceration. As coronary angiography will not help to differentiate these entities further, intravascular ultrasound is the only way to elucidate these clearly ambiguous lesions. Intravascular ultrasound will clarify the status of the adjacent reference segments and will quantify the degree of the atherosclerotic involvement, and for the first time is able to differentiate true from false aneurysms and pseudoaneurysms (Fig. 17.2).[6]

Ostial lesions

The severity of ostial lesions is difficult to assess. First, the mostly rectangular branching of the major coronary arteries from the aorta causes a turbulent flow at the site of the ostia during contrast injection. Such turbulent flow may itself lead to a number of flow-mediated phenomena which hamper the assessment of coronary lesions located adjacent to the ostium. Secondly, the coronary diagnostic or guiding catheter cannot always be positioned in such a way as to render optimal conditions for contrast medium injection. On the one hand, the catheter may be positioned only adjacent to the coronary ostium without sufficient back-up. In this case a cloud of contrast medium will blur the picture during contrast injection making the correct diagnosis, especially in the ostial region, difficult. On the other hand, the catheter may be positioned to some extent within the coronary artery without necessarily causing a significant drop in perfusion pressure. In this case, the luminogram of the first part of the right coronary artery or the main stem will be governed by the shape of the catheter partially masking the actual coronary lesion. Again, under these circumstances correct diagnosis is possible using IVUS with a 20 and 30 MHz transducer. IVUS is regularly able to visualize the coronary artery up to the aorta and even through the guiding catheter (Fig. 17.3).

Branching vessels

Branching points of coronary vessels are usually predestined locations for the manifestation of atherosclerosis. Thus in interventional cardiology these target sites are generally of crucial interest for the operator. At the same time, these branching points divide the stream of contrast medium, again causing turbulent flow with a number of known flow-related phenomena. Such phenomena are especially encountered when the branching involves large-caliber changes, for example, in the proximal part of the left anterior descending artery (LAD) with smaller septal or diagonal branches. With additional IVUS investigation some atherosclerotic involvement at the branching point is generally found. However, additional flow phenomena tend to overestimate the degree of stenosis of the smaller branching vessel (Fig. 17.4).

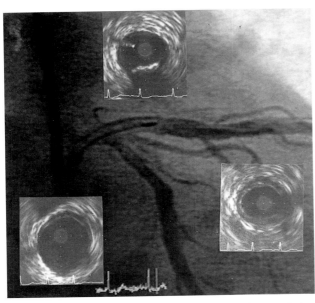

Figure 17.4. Unclear haziness in the proximal part of the left coronary artery. A short and rather large main stem divides into a relatively large LAD and a smaller LCX. IVUS examination reveals a large main stem with only a little intimal thickening (left lower panel). The proximal part of the LAD shows a distinct focal plaque with typical calcification. As in this case, this type of plaque is seldom visualized with coronary angiography. One centimeter distal to the calcification a soft concentric plaque can be seen, indicating early atherosclerosis. From IVUS examination, no indication for an interventional procedure could be deduced. Instead, the unclear haziness seems to be related to the turbulent flow, given the large main stem and the branching of the two major vessels.

Vessel tortuosity

Vessel tortuosity may be a projection-dependent phenomenon. Whereas in one projection the vessel seems extremely tortuous due to foreshortening of the specific projection, usually the orthogonal projection will render a clearer picture of the lesion site. However, such vessel tortuosity may obscure the true severity of the lesion, particularly in type B_2 or type C lesions. Vessel tortuosity is a phenomenon usually encountered in severe and extensive coronary artery disease. Such vessel tortuosity is a typical sign of long-lasting arterial hypertension.

Independent of the nature of the tortuosity, however, the phenomenon makes the estimation of the degree of stenosis extremely difficult from the angiographic image. With additional IVUS examination the perception of the stenosis becomes much clearer. However, caution has to be exercised when analyzing the IVUS images. The tortuosity leads inevitably to eccenteric positions of the IVUS catheter giving rise to distorted IVUS images and tangential cross-sections underestimating stenosis severity. A special problem is the nonuniform rotation which is quite often seen in tortuous vessels due to the increased friction during catheter transducer rotation. Nevertheless, the asssessment of plaque burden at the site of the stenosis is far more accurate than with conventional angiography (Fig. 17.5).

Main stem lesions

Main stem lesions can be very difficult to assess from angiography. Part of the reason relates to the ostial nature of such lesions, as mentioned above. Another reason relates to the actual size of the main stem and the nature of the plaque. Significant main stem disease is accurately diagnosed when the size of the main stem is reduced below the size of the proximal LAD or left circumflex coronary artery (LCX). However, the main stem can already be significantly diseased when the main stem equals the size of the proximal LAD and LCX. The diagnosis of main stem disease is complicated by the fact that most of the plaque involves the main stem concentrically. As with other parts of the epicardial coronary arteries, the main stem also undergoes considerable remodeling to maintain a patent lumen.[7] From the author's experience with 92 patients 35% were found to have a considerable plaque burden of more than 40% area stenosis on IVUS examination. Of these, 89% of the plaques were concentric, the remaining 11% having an eccentric shape. Based solely on the IVUS

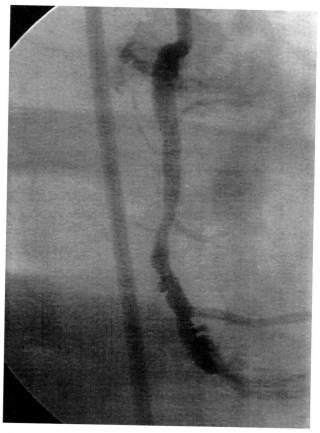
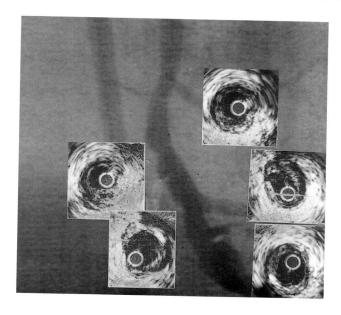

Figure 17.5. Left panel: right coronary artery with little angiographic change in the proximal and mid-portion of the artery. The distal segments, however, show a complex atherosclerotic lesion with multiple degenerated plaques. Right panel: further insight into the nature of the underlying plaque is provided by IVUS examination. Overall the whole segment contains a thick layer of atherosclerotic plaque of concentric or eccentric nature. Parts of the plaques have degenerated and been washed out leaving bizarre angiographic structures. In other regions (upper left) unstable plaques remain with a lipid core and the propensity to rupture.

examination four patients were identified as high-risk patients with severe main stem disease and consequently were sent for bypass surgery and not for interventional cardiology.[6]

Focal spasm

Coronary spasm is usually a dynamic phenomenon that can be diagnosed using conventional angiography. Usually the right coronary artery is prone to spasm upon catheter or guide wire insertion and such spasm can be reversed with intracoronary nitroglycerin injection. In these cases the whole coronary artery is usually involved. Focal spasm, however, is a phenomenon that may be difficult to diagnose from angiography. Focal spasm may occur at sites of atherosclerotic damage of the endothelium allowing local α-adrenergic coronary constriction to

override vasodilatory factors. Such spasm can mimic a significant stenosis and may not be readily reversible with nitroglycerin. Particularly in an ostial position of the right and left coronary arteries, catheter-induced spasm is difficult to differentiate from atherosclerosis. In some patients only additional IVUS examination can give information regarding the degree of plaque burden at the site and can help to decide whether an interventional procedure is indicated. It has to be remembered, however, that 90% of focal spasms occur at the site of the plaque formation as an overshoot reaction to extrinsic or intrinsic stimuli.

Sites of plaque rupture

IVUS can differentiate between plaque rupture and spontaneous dissection. With plaque rupture an emptied plaque with remnants of plaque material, thrombi, and adjacent atherosclerotic plaque may be seen. From a pathophysiologic view such plaque material can lead to distal embolization. Depending on the size of the plaque and location of the rupture site, such an event may lead to the manifestation of ischemic syndromes or remain clinically silent. Often the tear in the fibrous cap can be visualized when the plaque ulcer develops. Most frequently these tears occur in the outer third of the fibrous cap. From the author's observation probably a number of such plaque ruptures will cause only minor clinical consequences.[8] If coronary angiography is indicated these rupture sites may remain undetected. They are superimposed on plaques otherwise described as type C lesions, or unstable lesions, or may occur without angiographically visible luminal narrowing.[8] Only additional IVUS investigation will enable the correct differential diagnosis to be made. Additional signs of plaque rupture are the complete or incomplete vessel occlusions found in acute unstable angina pectoris. The typical sign is a layering phenomenon which may even be multiple and seems to be a sign of thrombus formation.

With spontaneous dissection only the intimal membrane or an intimal flap can be detected. At the site of dissection atherosclerotic involvement is unusual. Within the false lumen no remnants of plaque material are seen. However, on injection of contrast medium the false lumen will be filled with contrast medium and can easily be visualized by IVUS.[9]

Dissections following coronary angioplasty

Dissections following coronary angioplasty are a hazard that may be underestimated by conventional angiography. In part, this may be a projection-dependent problem. But in a number of cases even severe dissections may remain undiscovered by angiography. Thus additional IVUS examination may not only help to identify dissections but also helps to classify the type of dissection.[10] In 40 patients with dissections detected by IVUS, angiography was correct in 25% and showed haziness only in another 25%. Significantly, IVUS failed to identify dissections that were visible in angiography in 10% of the cases. Apparently the IVUS catheter or the guide wire adheres flaps and may wrap flaps back to the wall once they have protruded into the lumen. IVUS is therefore not the perfect method for identifying dissections. Nevertheless, IVUS represents a refinement of dissection stratification. It can guide the subsequent angioplastic approach and can be decisive for additional stent placement (Fig. 17.6).

Unclear spontaneous or postinterventional haziness

Haziness is an angiographic phenomenon describing regions of the coronary artery which appear lighter than the rest of the contrast-filled lumen. Haziness is a rather ambiguous phenomenon as it does not correlate to any particular pathophysiological entity. Basically, luminal haziness documents significant flow disturbances causing areas of high and low flow in which contrast medium is unequally distributed. Some of the pathological findings in the coronary arteries that may also cause some degree of haziness have been mentioned above. Usually we relate to the

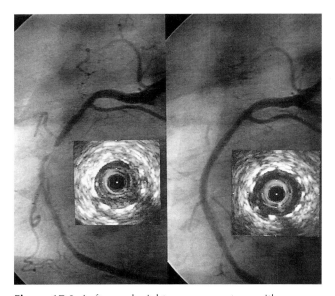

Figure 17.6. Left panel: right coronary artery with severe restenosis in the middle segment following stent implantation six months earlier. From the angiographic image and the previous catheter report it was unclear whether the restenosis was mainly due to insufficient stent expansion or exclusively to intimal hyperplasia. In the first case, a de novo balloon angioplasty with an upsized balloon would be indicated. In the latter case, laser angioplasty should be performed. IVUS examination revealed a sufficient stent expansion of the Palmaz–Schatz stent with excellent alignment of the stent struts. Thus, restenosis was merely due to intimal hyperplasia. Right panel: excellent result in angiography and in IVUS following laser angioplasty. Almost no residual intimal hyperplasia is seen.

phenomenon of haziness postinterventionally when a minor dissection, otherwise known as type A, has occurred. This type of dissection is usually benign in nature with little propensity for causing acute or subacute vessel closure. In this case the haziness is caused by turbulent flow due to small intimal tears, which are inherent with conventional balloon angioplasty. Nevertheless, as haziness is such a poorly defined entity and largely dependent on the subjective view of the operator, IVUS may sometimes detect major dissections. Based on the author's experience, the combination of haziness and a suboptimal contrast medium run-off should indicate the necessity for subsequent IVUS examination in order properly to assess the type of dissection and to prevent adverse events.

Haziness can sometimes also be encountered during diagnostic angiography. In these cases interpretation of the finding may be difficult as no obvious manipulation has preceded the investigation. Again, any obstacle that disturbs laminar coronary flow may be responsible. Commonly, spontaneous dissections or spontaneous plaque ruptures, as well as spontaneous thrombus formations, are encountered (Figs 17.7 and 17.8).

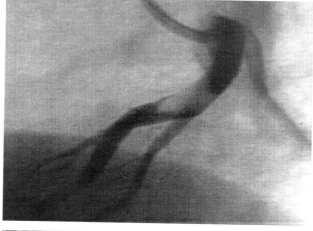

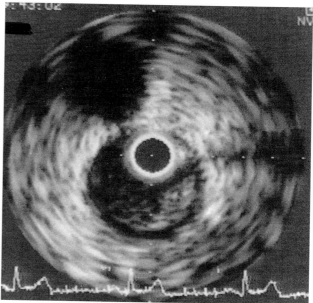

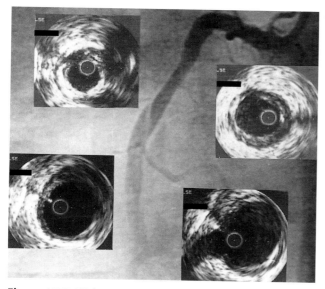

Figure 17.7. Right coronary artery with no severe coronary stenosis. No previous interventional procedure was performed. However, in the mid-part of the RCA the angiographic picture resembles that of a spontaneous dissection. As the patient was symptomatic with angina pectoris under moderate exercise, IVUS examination was performed for further clarification of the lesion. Although angiography showed only minor irregularities of the proximal RCA, IVUS revealed concentric as well as eccentric atherosclerotic plaque along the entire RCA. The degree of atherosclerotic involvement varied significantly. As a consequence, drastic caliber changes occurred, resulting in turbulent flow. Such flow-related phenomena mimic the picture of a spontaneous dissection in angiography. IVUS helped to establish the correct diagnosis. No intervention was performed.

Figure 17.8. Upper panel: large epicardial coronary arteries with unclear haziness in the LAD upon diagnostic angiography. The patient was catheterized for acute onset of angina pectoris and significant ST-segment depressions in the inferior leads. Lower panel: IVUS revealed a large LAD, however, with the absence of any atherosclerosis. Around the IVUS catheter a large mass of echodense material was found that turned out to be thrombus material. This spontaneous thrombus could be dissolved by conventional balloon angioplasty and additional application of thrombolytic therapy.

References

1 Mintz GS, Painter JA, Pichard AD et al. Atherosclerosis in angiographically 'normal' coronary artery reference segments: an intravascular ultrasound study with clinical correlation. *J Am Coll Cardiol* 1995; **25**: 1479–85.

2 Glagov S, Weisenberg E, Zarins CK, Stankunavicius R, Kolettis GJ. Compensatory enlargement of human atherosclerotic coronary arteries. *N Engl J Med* 1987; **316**: 1371–5.

3 Ge J, Erbel R, Zamorano J et al. Coronary artery remodeling in atherosclerotic disease: an intravascular ultrasound study in vivo. *Coronary Artery Dis* 1993; **4**: 981–6.

4 Blanckenhorn DH, Krausch DM. Reversal of atherosclerosis and sclerosis: the two components of atherosclerosis. *Circulation* 1989; **79**: 1–7.

5 Tobis JM, Mallery J, Mahon D et al. Intravascular ultrasound imaging of human coronary arteries in vivo. *Circulation* 1991; **83**: 913–26.

6 Ge J, Liu F, Kearney P et al. Intravscular ultrasound diagnosis of a coronary pseudoaneurysm following percutaneous transluminal coronary angioplasty. *Am Heart J* 1995; **130**: 765–71.

7 Gerber T, Erbel R, Görge G, Ge J, Rupprecht H, Meyer J. Extent of atherosclerosis and remodeling of the left main coronary artery determined by intravascular ultrasound. *Am J Cardiol* 1994; **73**: 666–71.

8 Baumgart D, Liu F, Haude M, Görge G, Ge J, Erbel R. Acute plaque rupture and myocardial stunting in patient with normal coronary arteriography. *Lancet* 1995; **346**: 193–4.

9 Kearney P, Erbel R, Ge J et al. Assessment of spontaneous coronary artery dissection by intravascular ultrasound in a patient with unstable angina. *Cathet Cardiovasc Diagn* 1994; **32**: 58–68.

10 Gerber TC, Erbel R, Görge G, Ge J, Rupprecht HJ, Meyer J. Classification of morphologic effects of percutaneous transluminal coronary angioplasty assessed by intravascular ultrasound *Am J Cardiol* 1992; **70**: 1546–54.

18 Coronary artery disease in transplanted hearts

Junbo Ge, Dietrich Baumgart, Michael Haude and Raimund Erbel

Introduction

Although survival after heart transplantation has improved over the past decade,[1] rejection and infection continue to be considered to influence early survival. Nevertheless, the major cause of late death is the development of cardiac allograft vasculopathy, which manifests as an accelerated form of coronary atherosclerosis.[2] The incidence of this vasculopathy has been reported to range from 5 to 25% at 1 year and from 50 to 60% at 5 years, resulting in up to 30% of late allograft failures.[3,4] The absence of afferent autonomic innervation results in allograft recipients being unable to experience classic symptoms of ischemia; as a result, the onset of allograft vasculopathy is frequently silent. Coronary angiography is not able to detect the early signs of vasculopathy. Moreover, there is no method available for the assessment of coronary perfusion.

Whether the coronary atherosclerotic process is the continuation of pre-existing atherosclerotic lesions from the donor or a new onset which occurs after operation in the recipient remains unknown. Combining intravascular ultrasound and Doppler flow mapping may provide detailed information concerning coronary morphology and function.

Table 18.1. Intravascular ultrasound variables. (From Rickenbacher et al.,[5] with permission.)

Years after transplantation	Pts (no.)	Intimal thickness (mm)	Intimal index	Stanford class	Ecc (%)	Calc (%)
Baseline (<2 mo)	50	0.09 ± 0.02*	0.07 ± 0.01†	1.5 ± 0.02*	18	8
1	52	0.16 ± 0.02†	0.14 ± 0.02	2.3 ± 0.2	44	2
2	47	0.23 ± 0.03	0.17 ± 0.02	2.5 ± 0.2	43	9
3	33	0.26 ± 0.04	0.20 ± 0.03	2.7 ± 0.2	39	6
4	34	0.27 ± 0.03	0.21 ± 0.03	2.5 ± 0.2†	35	12
5	35	0.33 ± 0.04	0.24 ± 0.03	3.2 ± 0.2	51	6†
6–10	42	0.33 ± 0.04	0.25 ± 0.03	3.0 ± 0.2	38	24
11–15	11	0.30 ± 0.06	0.27 ± 0.05	2.8 ± 0.3	27	46

*$p < 0.01$, †$p < 0.05$ versus value in succeeding year. Data are expressed as mean value ± SEM or percent of studies. Calc = studies showing calcification; Ecc = studies showing eccentric lesions; Pts = patients; Stanford class = Stanford classification of lesion severity.

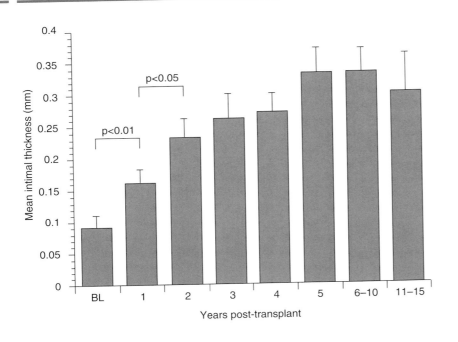

Figure 18.1. Bar graphs showing the correlation of mean intimal thickness with time after transplantation. Data are expressed as mean ± standard error of mean. BL: baseline (< 2 months after transplantation). (From Rickenbacher et al.,[5] with permission.)

Allograft coronary vasculopathy

The Stanford group[5] studied heart transplant patients serially with coronary angiography and intravascular ultrasound (IVUS) and found that intimal thickness was significantly greater at 1 year than at baseline (Table 18.1). Based on the intimal thickness and vessel circumference involved, they classified lesion severity as follows:

- class 0 = no measurable intimal layer by ultrasound
- class 1 (minimal) = an intimal layer <0.3 mm thick involving <180° of the vessel circumference
- class 2 (mild) = an intimal layer <0.3 mm thick involving >180° of the vessel circumference
- class 3 (moderate) = an intimal layer 0.3–0.5 mm thick or an intimal layer >0.5 mm thick involving <180° of the vessel circumference
- class 4 (severe) = an intimal layer >0.5 mm involving <180° of the vessel circumference or an intimal layer >1 mm thick at any point of the vessel circumference

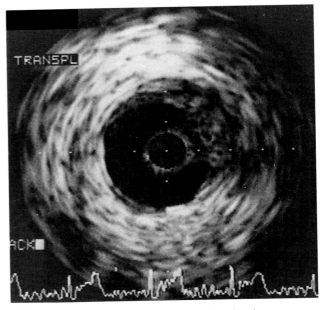

Figure 18.2. Plaque formation 1 month after heart transplantation.

They reported that the most striking progression of disease occurred during the first 2 years after transplantation (Fig. 18.1). In a serial examination of 21 patients with IVUS of all three vessels (a total of 63 coronary arteries), the present authors found plaque formation in 18 vessels (Fig. 18.2) although all the coronary arteries presented normal coronary angiograms.[6] Intracoronary flow mapping using Doppler FloWire (Cardiometrics, Mountain View,

CA, USA) was available in 56 vessels, of which coronary flow reserve was found to be reduced in 34 vessels (61%) (Fig. 18.3). Reports indicate that decreased coronary flow reserve might be an early sign of rejection.

In a serial follow-up study, it was found that coronary flow reserve can be normalized after transplantation. Figure 18.4 shows coronary Doppler flow

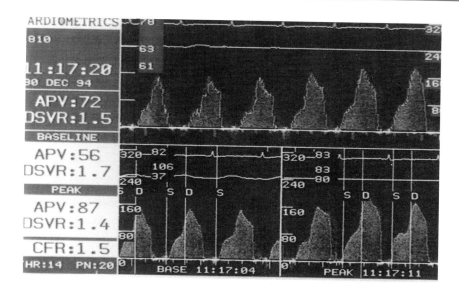

Figure 18.3. Intracoronary flow mapping of an LAD 3 years after transplantation in a patient with IVUS-detected plaque formation. Intracoronary Doppler shows a decreased coronary flow reserve (CFR) in the corresponding vessel of 1.5 after intracoronary administration of 18 µg adenosine. Myocardial bridging also exists in the LAD of the patient. A typical 'no systolic antegrade flow' phenomenon is also demonstrated. Values given as cm/s except the ratio CFR from peak to baseline velocity.

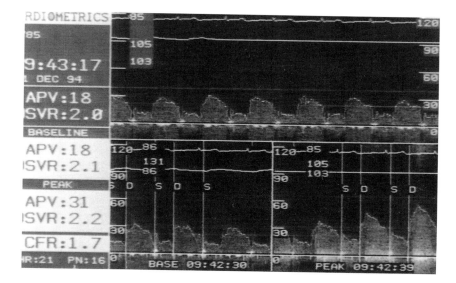

Figure 18.4. Coronary flow mapping 5 years after heart transplantation. A coronary flow reserve (CFR) of 1.7 was found in the left circumflex coronary artery. Values given as cm/s except the ratio CFR from peak to baseline velocity.

APV = average peak velocity
DSVR = diastolic/systolic velocity ratio.

mapping of a patient 5 years after transplantation; a reduced coronary flow reserve of 1.7 was found in the left circumflex coronary artery. Figure 18.5 shows the coronary Doppler flow registration of the same patient 1 year later. Normalization of the coronary flow reserve was found.

Transplanted coronary diseases

Transplanted coronary diseases are those coronary disorders obtained from the donor, such as pre-existing atherosclerosis, coronary dysfunction, myocardial bridging, etc. The Stanford group found that

only 22% of the patients studied during the first 2 months after transplantation had no evidence of intimal thickening and that 26% already had class 3 and 4 changes.[5] The present authors also found plaque formation in a patient 2 months after heart transplantation from a 19-year-old donor (Fig. 18.6). Whether the plaque formed after transplantation is not known.

However, pre-existing atherosclerotic lesions might be reversible. The authors have demonstrated this in a patient who underwent urgent heart transplantation with an atherosclerotic donor heart because of severe congestive heart failure due to idiopathic dilated cardiomyopathy and who showed plaque regression 5 years after heart transplantation (Figs 18.7 and 18.8).[7] Moreover, myocardial bridging was found in two of the 22 patients (9%) in the authors' center. Both of them presented with a typical 'fingertip' flow velocity profile in the segment proximal to the bridge (see chapter 16). All the patients showed normal or nearly normal coronary angiograms.

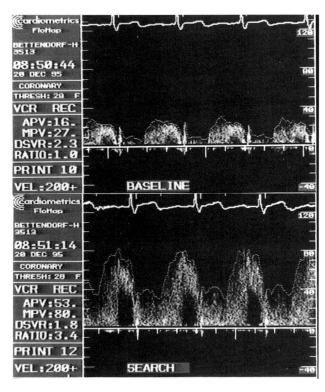

Figure 18.5. Coronary flow mapping of the same vessel in the patient shown in Fig. 21.4 one year later. Normalization of coronary flow reserve (CFR) (3.4) was found. APV = average peak velocity, MPV = mean peak velocity, DSVR = diastolic/systolic velocity ratio.

Follow-up of coronary artery morphology and function in transplanted hearts

As pointed out above, coronary angiography frequently underestimates coronary artery disease and does not allow detection of the early signs of atherosclerosis, especially in transplanted hearts.[8] In addition, it provides little information concerning coronary function. Combining IVUS and Doppler flow mapping techniques offers detailed information regarding coronary morphology and function. It has been reported that IVUS in cardiac transplant patients does not accelerate the progression of angiographically quantifiable coronary artery disease.[9] Therefore it is necessary to use IVUS and Doppler to detect early allograft vasculopathy so as to guide clinical management. Coronary arteries should be studied before transplantation to rule out coronary artery disease in the future. In one patient, 2 months after transplantation from a 14-year-old donor, reduced coronary flow reserve was found in all three coronary arteries. Whether this reduced coronary flow reserve will normalize in the same way as plaque regression remains unknown. Serial studies should be performed in order to answer this question.

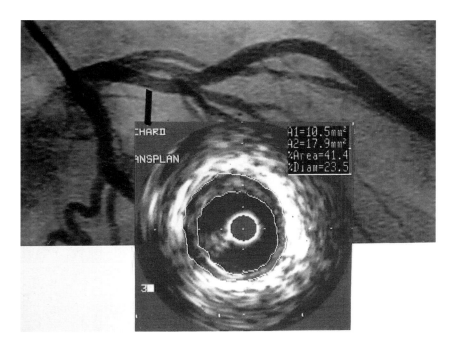

Figure 18.6. Coronary angiogram and IVUS imaging of a patient 2 months after heart transplantation. Concentric intimal thickening produces a lumen area narrowing of 41% and a diameter narrowing of 23%. Coronary angiography does not show any abnormality of the vessel. Calibration 1 mm; 30 MHz transducer.

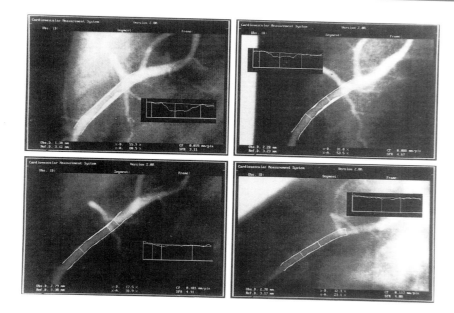

Figure 18.7. Serial quantitative angiographic evaluation of an allograft atherosclerotic lesion 1 year (top left), 2 years (top right), 3 years (bottom left), and 5 years (bottom right) after urgent cardiac transplantation. (From Haude et al.,[7] with permission.)

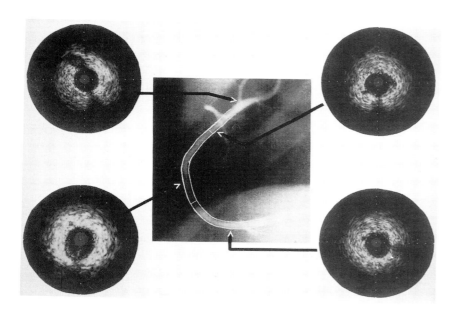

Figure 18.8. Coronary angiogram and IVUS images 5 years after heart transplantation of the same patient as Fig. 18.4. IVUS shows a class 4 intimal thickening in the proximal segment without luminal narrowing. Coronary angiogram shows atherosclerosis regression in comparison with the examination performed serially. (From Haude et al.,[7] with permission.)

References

1 Kriett JM, Kaye MP. The registry of the International Society for Heart and Lung Transplantation: seventh official report – 1990. *J Heart Transplant* (1990) **9**:323–30.

2 Miller LW. Transplant coronary artery disease. *J Heart Lung Transplant* (1992) **3**:51–4 (edit).

3 Uretsky BF, Murali S, Reddy PS et al. Development of coronary artery disease in cardiac transplant patients receiving immunosuppressive therapy with cyclosrine and prednisone. *Circulation* (1987) **76**:827–33.

4 Ventura HO, Smart FW, Stapleton DD, Toups T, Price HL. Cardiac allograft vasculopathy: current concepts. *J La State Med Soc* (1993) **145**:195–202.

5 Rickenbacher PR, Pinto FJ, Chenzbraun A et al. Incidence and severity of transplanted coronary artery disease early and up to 15 years after transplantation as detected by intravascular ultrasound. *J Am Coll Cardiol* (1995) **25**:171–7.

6 Ge J, Haude M, Caspari G et al. Detection of occult coronary artery disease in patients with heart transplantation. *Z Kardiol* (1996) **85**:II66.

7   Haude M, Ge J, Machraoui A, Erbel R, Zerkowski HR. Regression of pre-existing coronary artery disease in a donor heart after cardiac transplantation. *Eur J Cardiothorac Surg* (1995) **9**:399–402.

8   Ventura HO, White CJ, Jain SP et al. Assessment of intracoronary morphology in cardiac transplant recipients by angioscopy and intravascular ultrasound. *Am J Cardiol* (1993) **72**:805–9.

9   Pinto FJ, St Goar FG, Gao SZ et al. Immediate and one-year safety of intracoronary ultrasonic imaging: evaluation with serial quantitative angiography. *Circulation* (1993) **88**:1709–14.

19 Intravascular ultrasound imaging of saphenous vein grafts

Fengqi Liu, Raimund Erbel, Junbo Ge and Günter Görge

Introduction

Since its introduction, coronary artery bypass graft surgery has been increasingly used and has significantly contributed to the improvement of angina pectoris and an increase in survival of patients with obstructive coronary artery disease.[1] However, the long-term patency of bypass grafts remains a serious problem. Besides the progression of disease in the native coronary circulation, the ubiquity of atherosclerosis in the grafts, especially in saphenous vein grafts, gives rise to the recurrence of ischemic symptoms in about 4–8% of patients annually.[2,3] This subgroup has severe native coronary disease and is prone to acute coronary events when the grafts deteriorate. Transcatheter vessel angioplasty is playing a more and more important role in the management of these patients, because reoperation is not only technically more difficult but also carries higher risks of morbidity and mortality. An understanding of the changes in vein bypass grafts during life is essential for an accurate diagnosis and optimal treatment. Histologic studies demonstrate that there is usually extensive and diffuse pathology in vein bypass grafts. Studies at variable intervals after graft implantation have indicated that there is no significant correlation between angiographic and histologic findings.[4–7] Thus it appears that angiography is limited in evaluating such vessels. Intravascular ultrasound has advantages over angiography for the study of saphenous vein grafts and the findings correlate well with histologic findings.[4,5] A number of medical centers are integrating this new imaging modality into their approach in the diagnosis of and intervention in vein-graft stenosis. As the saphenous veins are the most widely used grafts and more often develop stenosis or occlusion than other grafts, such as the internal mammary artery, this chapter will discuss the study of saphenous vein grafts with intravascular ultrasound imaging.

Histologic findings

The pathogenesis of saphenous vein graft disease can be classified as acute (< 1 month), subacute (1–12 months), intermediate (1–5 years), and long term (> 5 years).[8] In the majority, acute thrombosis is the cause of graft occlusion during the first month after surgery. Subacute occlusion has contributed to fibrointimal hyperplasia, with or without concomitant thrombosis. The long-term pathologic changes are a process of progressive atherosclerosis. Despite some morphologic differences between vein grafts and native coronary artery atherosclerosis, the resulting pathology is the same, either (a) high-grade stenosis or (b) plaque rupture or ulceration precipitating thrombosis and acute occlusion. The latter is especially frequent in saphenous vein grafts as a major mechanism of late occlusion leading to recurrent symptoms or even death.[9] Detailed histologic analysis of grafts excised at the time of reoperation or autopsy has revealed that there are seven morphologic alterations that can occur in autogenous vein grafts after implantation into the arterial circulation (Table 19.1).[10,11]

Table 19.1. **Histologic alterations of saphenous vein bypass grafts and diagnostic value of intravascular ultrasound.**

Endothelial damage
Medial hypertrophy
Medial necrosis
Graft wall fibrosis (media and adventitia)
Intimal hyperplasia[a]
Atherosclerosis
  Plaque tissue features
      Lipid,[a] fibrosis,[a] calcification[b]
  Plaque morphology
      Concentric,[b] eccentric[b]
      Plaque rupture[b] or ulceration[b]
      Rupture-mediated thrombosis[b] and closure
Aneurysmal dilation[b]

[a] Sensitive and specific by intravascular ultrasound study.
[b] Highly sensitive and specific by intravascular ultrasound study.

Clinical and angiographic studies of the vein graft natural history

Studies indicate that there is a progressive deterioration of saphenous vein grafts.[12,13] Almost 50% of vein grafts have significant stenosis at 6-year follow-up with angiography, of which 21% are totally occluded grafts. Saphenous graft loss is approximately 7% during the first week, 15–20% during the first year, 1–2% per year from 1 to 6 years, and 4% per year from 6 to 10 years. There is an increasing population of bypass patients who need revascularization of vein grafts. Nonoperative angioplasty for vein bypass grafts plays a growing role in the management of this subgroup of patients. This calls for an imaging approach such as intravascular ultrasound together with angiography to guide optimal diagnosis and treatment of vein grafts.

Intravascular ultrasound studies of saphenous vein bypass grafts

Intravascular ultrasound (IVUS) is a superior imaging modality for the study of vessel topography, as compared with angiography and angioscopy.[4–6] Comparative studies with pathology in vitro have confirmed that IVUS is capable of accurate measurements of lumen dimensions of saphenous vein grafts. IVUS imaging also provides morphologic features of the vessel wall which agree with histologic data. In-vivo observations have demonstrated that IVUS provides more valuable information than angiography and allows detailed study of vein graft disease. Saphenous vein graft lesions are high-risk lesions for transcatheter angioplasty.[14] In the experience of the authors and others, vein graft lesions show more elastic recoil after angioplasty than lesions in native coronary arteries. Stenting is

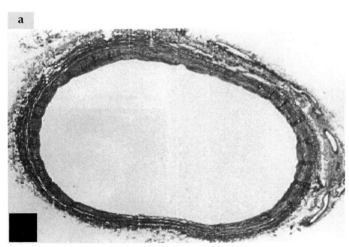
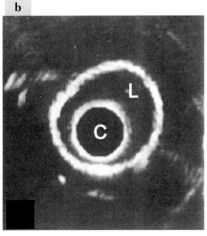

Figure 19.1. Comparison between IVUS and histologic findings. Panel a, histologic cross-sectional view of a freshly harvested saphenous vein (stained with Verhoeff–van Gieson stain, original magnification × 6.25). A normal thin-walled vein with a widely patent lumen is demonstrated. The dark black fibers represent elastin, which accounts for the bright echogenic appearance on IVUS imaging (panel b). Note the absence of echoreflectance within the vessel lumen. C: IVUS catheter; L: vessel lumen. (Reproduced, with permission, from ref. 5.)

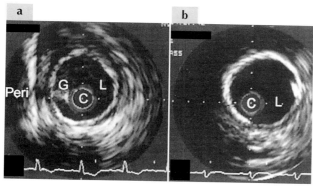

Figure 19.2. These two cross-sectional images from one saphenous vein graft were found to be normal by angiography. The bypass operation was performed four years ago. Panel a shows a large vessel with a regular lumen free of plaque. The vein wall is echogenically strong although it is not thick. The vessel wall cannot be divided as three layers from IVUS imaging. Panel b: the vein wall is very strongly echogenic from seven o'clock to three o'clock. C: IVUS catheter; L: lumen; G: guide wire; Peri: assumed to be the pericardium.

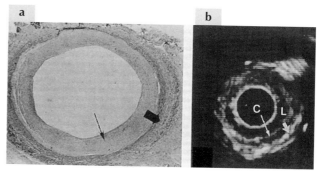

Figure 19.4. Panel a: histologic cross-sectional view of a long-term implanted saphenous vein graft (stained with Verhoeff–van Gieson stain, original magnification × 6.25). Concentric thickening and sclerosis of the vein wall (thick arrow) and narrowing of the vessel lumen (L) by intimal hyperplasia (thin arrow) are evident. Panel b: IVUS imaging revealed a bright, highly reflective region that correlates with the thickened vein wall (thick arrow) and a faint echolucent band (thin arrow) that correlates with the intimal hyperplasia observed on histologic study. C: IVUS catheter; L: lumen. (Reproduced, with permission, from ref. 5.)

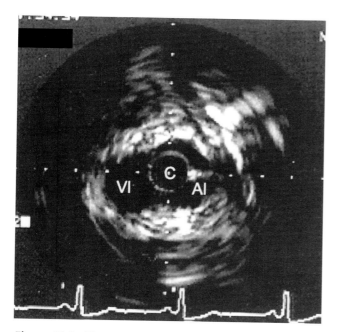

Figure 19.3. The anastomosis between a saphenous vein graft and the first diagonal artery. The figure shows two vessels merging into one. The IVUS catheter is located in the arterial lumen. There is no plaque formation. The artery wall is thicker than that of the vein. C: IVUS catheter; Vl: vein lumen; Al: artery lumen. 3.5 F catheter, 20 MHz transducer, 1 mm calibration.

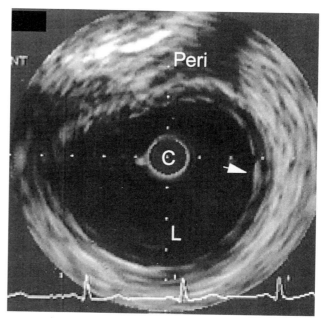

Figure 19.5. An in-vivo example of IVUS imaging of a saphenous vein graft with possible intimal hyperplasia. The patient was a 59-year-old man who had the graft to the left anterior descending artery five years ago. The vessel appears to be a three-layered structure with a thin wall. The intima is thickened overall (arrow) and its echoreflection is weak. C: IVUS catheter; L: lumen; Peri: possibly the pericardium. 3.5 F catheter, 20 MHz transducer, 1 mm calibration.

frequently necessary. IVUS can guide the interventional procedure to obtain optimal acute results as well as reduce late restenosis. There is a high reproducibility of IVUS assessment of stent implantation in saphenous vein grafts.[15] There follows an introduction to intravascular ultrasound imaging of saphenous vein grafts in normal and disease conditions.

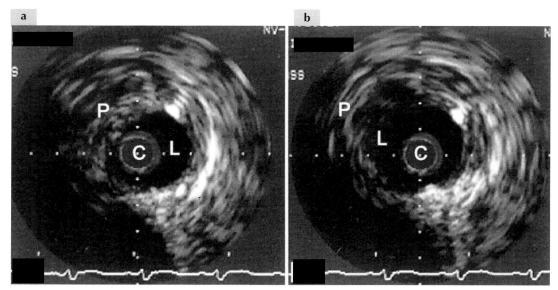

Figure 19.6. In vein grafts no active vessel pulsation is observed. However, at the anastomosis with the aorta or coronary artery there may be obvious passive vein pulsation caused by aorta or artery. This phenomenon should be taken into account when stenosis severity is estimated. The images were taken from a five-year-old vein graft at the site of anastomosis between saphenous graft and aorta. Panel a: an image taken during systole. The vessel area percentage stenosis is over 60%. Panel b: the diastolic cross-sectional imaging . C: IVUS catheter; L: lumen; Pla: plaque; Peri: pericardium. 3.5 F catheter, 20 MHz transducer, 1 mm calibration.

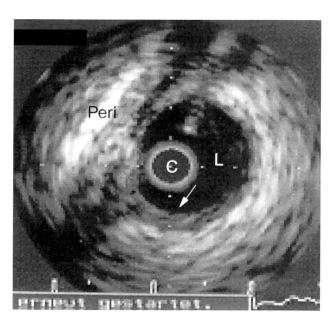

Figure 19.7. Intravascular ultrasound imaging shows a diseased saphenous vein graft with a small eccentric soft plaque (arrow) occupying less than 20% of the lumen. The soft plaque is characterized as having an echo signal intensity lower than that of the adventitia. In this image the plaque is homogeneous without calcium deposit. C: IVUS catheter; L: lumen; Peri: pericardium. 3.5 F catheter, 20 MHz transducer, 1 mm calibration.

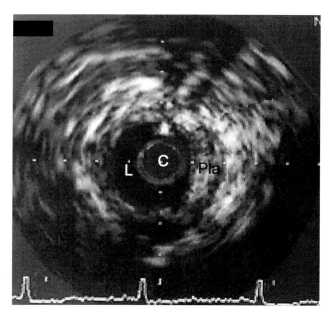

Figure 19.8. An advanced plaque in a venous graft (eight years after bypass operation). The lesion is concentric with soft and fibrous compositions. The arrow indicates a possible lipid-pool between five and seven o'clock. C: IVUS catheter; L: lumen; Pla: plaque. 3.5 F catheter, 20 MHz transducer, 1 mm calibration.

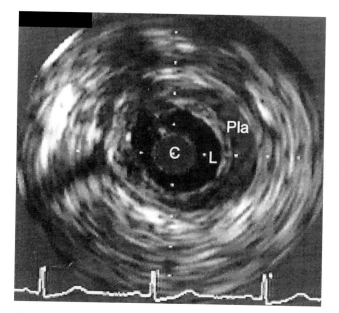

Figure 19.9. The patient had the saphenous vein graft to the right coronary artery 11 years ago and has returned for catheterization because of renewed angina pectoris. IVUS examination detected a circular soft plaque formation with a percentage area loss of over 60%. Balloon dilatation and stenting were performed. The patient is asymptomatic at follow-up. C: IVUS catheter; L: lumen; Pla: plaque. 3.5 F catheter, 20 MHz transducer, 1 mm calibration.

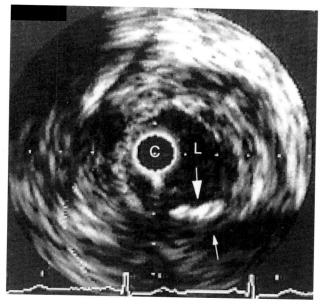

Figure 19.10. IVUS imaging illustrating a calcified plaque in the venous bypass graft to the right coronary artery. The calcium occupies about 45° of the arch (arrow), casting acoustic shadowing (arrow) on the structures behind it. Most of the plaque is probably of fibrous composition. Lesion calcification in vein grafts is not as common as in native arteries. C: IVUS catheter; L: lumen. 3.5 F catheter, 20 MHz transducer, 1 mm calibration.

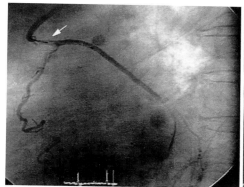 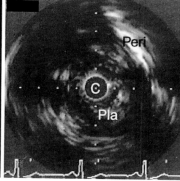

Figure 19.11. High-grade ostium stenosis of the saphenous vein graft to the first diagonal branch of the left anterior descending artery (five years after operation). The vessel is almost occluded by a very large mixed plaque (soft and fibrous). A 4 mm stent was implanted into the ostium. C: IVUS catheter; Pla: plaque; Peri: pericardium. 3.5 F catheter, 20 MHz transducer, 1 mm calibration.

Normal vein graft

A vein graft segment with a regular lumen and without obvious intimal thickening is considered normal. A typical appearance of a normal vein graft is a thin-walled vessel. The vessel wall is seen as a relatively homogeneous echogenic structure with absence of echoreflectance within the vessel lumen. In vein grafts the three-layer appearance is rare. A three-layer appearance indicates intimal thickening as suggested by histologic and IVUS study.[5,16] There is usually no obvious pulsatile variation during the cardiac cycle. Extravascular structures (possibly pericardium) are commonly visualized and are highly echogenic. Figures 19.1 and 19.2 show examples of IVUS images of normal saphenous vein grafts. There is no intimal thickening, nor plaque formation. Figure 19.3 shows the image of a normal anastomosis between a vein graft and the native coronary artery.

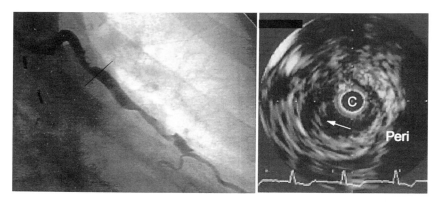

Figure 19.12. A 54-year-old man was referred to the cardiac catheterization laboratory for unstable angina pectoris. Angiography showed diffuse disease in the four-year-old saphenous graft to the first diagonal artery. Before intervention, IVUS examination detected a spontaneous dissection (arrow) in the eccentric hard plaque. The flap can be seen fluttering during real-time imaging. The dissection was thought to be one of the reasons for unstable angina. The patient was free of angina after multiple stent implantation. C: IVUS catheter; Peri: pericardium. 3.5 F catheter, 30 MHz transducer, 1 mm calibration.

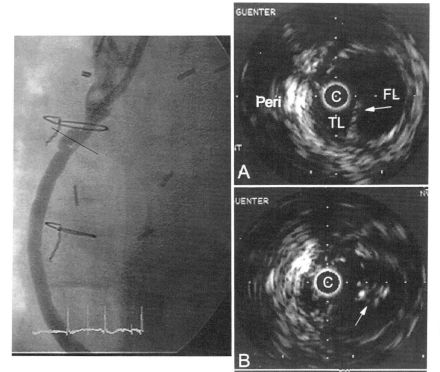

Figure 19.13. A case of spontaneous plaque rupture in a saphenous vein bypass to the right coronary artery. The patient had the bypass four years previously and recently suffered from unstable angina. Angiography indicated an ambiguous lesion in the proximal segment of the vein graft. IVUS imaging demonstrated a spontaneous plaque rupture. Panel A: a large vein graft with plaque formation. However, the plaque ruptured and most of the content within the plaque was washed away, leaving a thin plaque cap (arrow) and a large empty lumen. Panel B: the imaging during contrast medium injection into bypass. Contrast medium appears in the false lumen (arrow). C: IVUS catheter; TL: true lumen; FL: false lumen; Peri: pericardium. 3.5 F catheter, 30 MHz transducer, 1 mm calibration.

Diseased vein grafts

A vein segment showing eccentric or concentric atherosclerotic plaque should be considered diseased. Intravascular ultrasound allows the visualization of the pathologic changes in chronically implanted vein grafts, which are similar to coronary artery atherosclerosis[17,18] including intimal proliferation. Atheromatous plaque is classified in the following four categories:

1) Soft plaque, when the echoreflectance of the atheroma is lower than that of the adventitia, including:
   a) loose and cellular fibrous tissue – medium or low echoreflections in the atheroma
   b) lipid – extremely low echoreflectance or an echolucent space which is usually surrounded by echodense regions or covered by a fibrous cap (see below).

2) Fibrous plaque, when the echoreflectance of the plaque is similar to that of the adventitia, including:

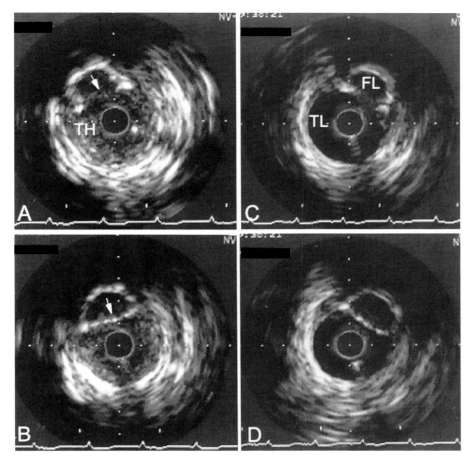

Figure 19.14. The serial images illustrate a case of spontaneous plaque rupture complicated by thrombosis in the vein grafts and subsequently treated with balloon angioplasty. The patient had saphenous vein bypass grafts 15 years ago. He had angina pectoris between CCS III and VI. Angiography found a high-grade stenosis in the middle segment of the vein graft to the right coronary artery. IVUS shows a high-grade obstructive lesion. Furthermore, careful study of the images shows that there is a small eccentric ruptured plaque. The small plaque has a thin cap and a false lumen. Panels A and B are images before intervention. Panels C and D are images after 4 mm balloon dilatation. Panel A: a wide opening of the plaque rupture into the vessel lumen (arrow). Blood flow signal is seen in the false lumen. At both sides of the opening there are calcium deposits. Around the IVUS catheter are speckled materials, which are assumed to be thrombi. In the false lumen some speckled reflection can be seen. Panel B: the imaging of the same lesion at the site a little proximal to the opening. The plaque has the same shape but with a complete cap (arrow) on the surface side towards the lumen. No opening can be detected in the cap from this section. Panel C: imaging after 4 mm balloon dilatation at the same section as in panel A. The speckled materials have almost all gone, which indicates that this is most probably a case of thrombosis after plaque rupture. Both the false lumen and true lumen are free of thrombus. Panel D shows the image at the same section as panel B. The thin cap of plaque is still the same as seen in panel B, suggesting a cap with dense fibrous tissue. TL: true lumen; FL: false lumen; TH: thrombus. 3.5 F catheter, 30 MHz transducer, 1 mm calibration.

a) fibrous cap – intense ultrasound reflectance at the lumen surface of the atheroma with 'softer' echoes behind, indicating densely packed tissue with high collagen content
b) dense fibrous tissue – highly echogenic intense ultrasound reflectance without deep acoustic shadows
3) Calcium deposit – intense echoreflections with clearly defined acoustic shadows.
4) Thrombus – speckled low and medium echoreflectance at the surface of atheroma plaque.

Thrombus is positively identified when mobility of the thrombus is present. In the subgroup of patients undergoing vein graft angioplasty, IVUS shows that soft plaques are common while calcified plaques are infrequent. Plaque ulceration or rupture is frequently detected, often complicated by thrombosis. In such situations, prompt intervention is indicated. Intravascular ultrasound can provide exact information on the lesion and guide the appropriate angioplastic approach. Figures 19.2–19.16 illustrate the clinical use of

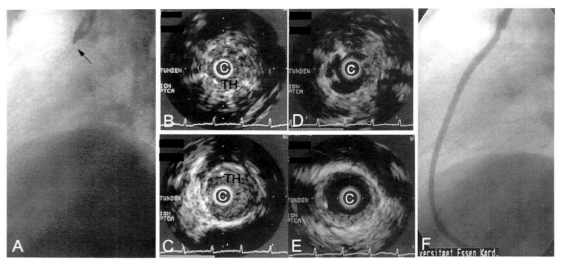

Figure 19.15. A case of acute occlusion by thrombus documented by serial studies. The patient is a 66-year-old man who had saphenous vein grafts eight years ago. His condition was stable until three days previously when he suffered a recurrent angina. Angiography at a local hospital found a long high-grade stenosis at the proximal segment of the bypass to the right coronary artery. As the angina was getting worse he was transferred for interventional therapy. Repeated angiography discovered that the bypass was already occluded. The bypass was reopened after balloon dilatation and stent implantation. The patient improved. Antithrombotic drugs were administered. However, 10 hours later the symptoms deteriorated and repeated angiography showed that the recanalized graft was again closed (panel A). IVUS detected thrombus within the stent and the segment distal to it (panels B and C). The bypass was reopened by repeated balloon angioplasty. The final results are shown in panels D and E for IVUS images and panel F for angiography. C: IVUS catheter; TH: thrombus. 3.5 F catheter, 30 MHz transducer, 1 mm calibration.

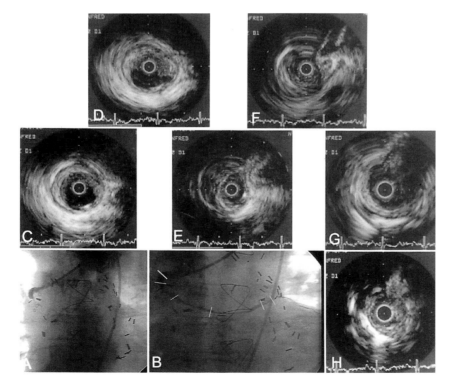

Figure 19.16. The vein bypass to the first diagonal artery was occluded two months before admission and an attempt at recanalization failed. ReoPro was administered for two days to prevent further thrombus formation. Then a new approach with Angiojet catheter was successfully used to reopen the vessel. Panels A and B show the angiograms before and after Angiojet thrombectomy. IVUS shows the acute results after Angiojet procedure (panels C–H, from proximal to distal segments). Angiojet produced irregular lumen without severe dissection. Multiple stent implantation achieved a good final result. (The Angiojet system utilizes high-velocity sterile saline jets for percutaneous break-up and removal of unorganized thrombus.)

IVUS imaging and atherosclerotic manifestations of diseased saphenous vein grafts. The abnormalities of saphenous vein grafts demonstrated by IVUS are: intimal thickening (Figs 19.4, 19.5); early plaque formation (Fig. 19.7); advanced plaques (Figs 19.8–19.11); special manifestations such as spontaneous dissection (Fig. 19.12), spontaneous plaque rupture (Fig. 19.13) and rupture complicated by thrombus (Figs 19.14–19.16).

References

1 Nwasokwa ON, Koss JH, Friedman GH, Grunwald AM, Bodenheimer MM. Bypass surgery for chronic stable angina: predictors of survival benefit and strategy for patient selection. *Ann Intern Med* 1991; **114**: 1035–49.

2 Cameron A, Kemp HG, Shimomura S et al. Aortocoronary bypass surgery, a 7-year follow-up. *Circulation* 1979; **60(supple I)**: I9–I13.

3 The VA Coronary Artery Bypass Surgery Cooperative Study Group. Eighteen-year follow-up in the Veterans Affairs Cooperative Study of coronary artery bypass surgery for stable angina. *Circulation* 1992; **86**: 121–30.

4 Keren G, Douek P, Oblon C et al. Atherosclerotic saphenous vein grafts treated with different interventional procedures assessed by intravascular ultrasound. *Am Heart J* 1992; **124**: 198–206.

5 Willard JE, Netto D, Demian SE et al. Intravsacular ultrasound imaging of saphenous vein grafts in vitro: comparison with histologic and quantitative angiographic findings. *J Am Coll Cardiol* 1992; **19**: 759–64.

6 Spray TL, Roberts WC. Changes in saphenous veins used as aortocoronary bypass grafts. *Am Heart J* 1977; **94**: 500–16.

7 Smith SH, Geer JC. Morphology of saphenous vein–coronary artery bypass. *Arch Pathol Lab Med* 1983; **107**: 13–18.

8 Cox JL, Chiasson DA, Gotlieb AI. Stranger in a strange land: the pathogenesis of saphenous vein graft stenosis with emphasis on structural and functional differences between veins and arteries. *Prog Cardiovasc Dis* 1991; **34**: 45–68.

9 Walts AE, Fishbein MC, Matloff JM. Thrombosed, ruptured atheromatous plaques in saphenous vein coronary artery bypass grafts: a ten years' experience. *Am Heart J* 1987; **114**: 718–23.

10 Lawrie GM, Lie JT, Morris GC, Beazley HL. Vein grafts patency and intimal proliferation after aortocoronary bypass: early and long-term angiographic correlations. *Am J Cardiol* 1976; **38**: 856–62.

11 Waller BF, Roberts WC. Amount of narrowing by atherosclerotic plaque in 44 nonbypassed and 52 bypassed major epicardial coronary arteries in 32 necropsy patients who died within one month of aortocoronary bypass grafting. *Am J Cardiol* 1980; **46**: 956–62.

12 Campos EE, Cinderella JA, Fahin ER. Long-term angiographic follow-up of normal and minimal diseased saphenous vein grafts. *J Am Coll Cardiol* 1993; **21**: 1175–80.

13 Douglas JS. Percutaneous intervention in patients with prior coronary bypass surgery. In: Topol EJ ed. *Textbook of Interventional Cardiology*, 2nd edn (Philadelphia: WB Saunders, 1993): 339–54.

14 Ellis SG. Coronary lesions at increased risk. *Am Heart J* 1995; **130**: 643–6.

15 Mintz GS, Griffin J, Chuang YC et al. Reproducibility of the intravascular ultrasound assessment of stent implantation in saphenous vein grafts. *Am J Cardiol* 1995; **75**: 167–9.

16 Fitzgerald PJ, St Goar FG, Connolly AJ et al. Intravascular ultrasound imaging of coronary arteries. Is three layers the norm? *Circulation* 1992; **86**: 154–8.

17 Stary HC. Evolution and progression of atherosclerotic lesions in coronary arteries of children and adults. *Atherosclerosis* 1989; **9(suppl I)**: 19–32.

18 Stary HC, Chandler AB, Dinsmore et al. A definition of advanced types of atherosclerotic lesions and a histological classification of atherosclerosis. A report from the Committee on Vascular Lesions of the Council on Arteriosclerosis, American Heart Association. *Circulation* 1995; **92**: 1355–74.

20 Mechanisms of percutaneous transluminal coronary balloon angioplasty assessed by ultrasound imaging: prediction of immediate results

Robert Gil, Carlo Di Mario, Francesco Prati, Clemens von Birgelen, Jos R T C Roelandt and Patrick W Serruys (with the technical assistance of W M van Swijndregt and J Ligthart)

Introduction

Although percutaneous transluminal balloon angioplasty (PTCA) is now widely applied for treatment of coronary artery disease, the knowledge concerning the mechanism of angioplasty is still limited and is mainly derived from in-vitro studies.[1–4] Intracoronary ultrasound (ICUS) offers a unique opportunity to study plaque composition in vivo, with a good correlation between ultrasonic and histologic plaque characteristics.[5–7] It has been shown that most qualitative and quantitative measurements of lumen and plaque dimensions have low intra- and interobserver variability.[8] The measurements of lumen and plaque areas before and after coronary intervention provide the opportunity to assess the mechanisms of immediate postprocedural lumen enlargement.[9,10]

The elucidation of the operative mechanisms of PTCA in plaques with different preprocedural composition potentially may lead to an optimized strategy for treatment of individual stenosis.

In this study serial ultrasound examinations were performed before and immediately after PTCA in order to assess the relations between lesion composition and distribution and mechanisms of acute lumen enlargement after PTCA.

Methods

Study group

Seventy-seven primary lesions in 77 patients (66 with one-vessel disease and 11 with two-vessel disease) treated with PTCA were examined in this study. There were 62 men and 15 women. Their age ranged from 29 to 77 years (mean 58.1±10.8). Forty-two (54.5%) patients were treated because of unstable angina pectoris. PTCA procedure was considered successful when residual diameter stenosis, measured with on-line quantitative angiography, was less than 50%. In this study an angiographically successful result was achieved in all patients. PTCA was performed in 37 left anterior descending artery lesions, in 17 circumflex artery lesions and in 23 right coronary artery lesions. All patients signed a written informed consent form approved by the Medical Ethical Committee, Erasmus University/Dijkzigt Hospital.

Basal demographic and angiographic characteristics are shown in Table 20.1.

Angiographic assessment

Baseline angiograms were recorded in at least two orthogonal projections before and after PTCA. An

Table 20.1. Demographic and angiographic characteristics of the study patients.

Patients/lesions	77/77
Gender (M/F)	62/15
Mean age (range)	58.1±10.8 (29–77)
Previous MI	8 (10.4%)
Diabetes mellitus	7 (9.1%)
Hypercholesterolemia	22 (28.6%)
Single/multivessel disease	66/11
Coronary syndrome: stable/unstable	35/42
Vessel dilated:	
LAD	37
LCX	17
RCA	23

MI: myocardial infarction; LAD: left anterior descending; LCX: left circumflex artery; RCA: right coronary artery.

intracoronary bolus of isosorbide dinitrate (1–3 mg) was injected immediately before angiography. Quantitative coronary arteriography was performed using a previously described computer-assisted automatic quantitative analysis system (CAAS, Pie Data, Maastricht, The Netherlands).[11,12] The presence or absence of calcium by fluoroscopy was noted. The presence and characteristics of angiographic dissections were defined according to the criteria of the National Heart, Lung and Blood Institute PTCA Registry.[13]

Ultrasound assessment

Intracoronary ultrasound examinations were performed before and after PTCA using a 4.3 F or 2.9 F mechanical ultrasound catheter operating at 30 MHz (CVIS, Sunnyvale, CA).

The imaging probe was positioned distal to the target stenosis and then a manual continuous pullback was performed to obtain an initial assessment of the lesion. In 27 (35.1%) patients, a second withdrawal of the ultrasound catheter was performed using a motorized pullback device at a constant speed of 1.0 mm/s. By using reproducible anatomic landmarks as the side-branches or calcifications comparable cross-sectional slices within the treated segment could be obtained before and after PTCA.

There were no complications related to ultrasound imaging.

Ultrasonic image analysis

Qualitative and quantitative characteristics of the ultrasonic images were assessed by a consensus of two experienced observers. The plaque classification was based on its prevalent composition. Four types of plaque were distinguished:

Soft plaque: more than 80% of the plaque area is composed of tissue with an echogenicity lower than the echogenicity of the adventitia (arc of lesion calcium less than 90°).
Fibrous plaque: more than 80% of the plaque area is composed of tissue producing echoes as bright or brighter than the adventitia but without acoustic shadowing (arc of lesion calcium less than 90°).
Diffuse calcified plaque: bright echoes within a plaque demonstrating acoustic shadowing and occupying more than 180° of vessel wall circumference.
Mixed plaque: a plaque involving bright echoes with acoustic shadowing encompassing more than 90° but less than 180° of vessel wall circumference or a mixture of soft and fibrous plaque with each component occupying less than 80% of the plaque area.

The total circumferential calcium arc was measured (Fig. 20.1) and calcium localization was distinguished between subendothelial (no plaque visible between calcium deposits and lumen) and deep (calcium deposits central and at the base of the plaque) (Fig. 20.2).

An eccentricity index was calculated as the ratio between minimal and maximal wall thickness assessed before PTCA (not necessarily along the same diameter). Eccentric lesions were defined as lesions with an index smaller than 0.5.[14]

Total vessel area was defined as the integrated area central to the medial–adventitial boundary. The boundary between the lumen and intima (leading edge) was used to define the lumen area. In case of wedging of the ultrasound probe in the stenosis before PTCA, a cross-sectional area of 1.61 mm^2 or of the 4.3 F and 2.9 F ultrasound probes was used, respectively. Plaque area was defined as the difference between total vessel and lumen area.[15] Figure 20.3 presents measurements performed before and after PTCA in soft lesion.

The presence and characteristics of wall disruption after PTCA were classified according to previously described criteria.[14] Plaque fracture was classified as a rupture in a radial direction and wall dissection was defined as a plaque rupture in a tangential direction (Fig. 20.4). The presence of blood speckles inside the newly formed lumen and the effect of

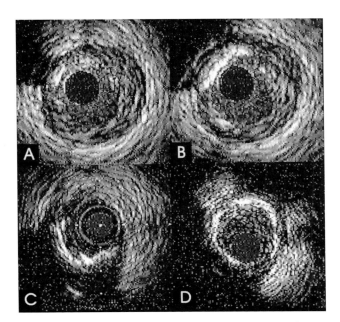

Figure 20.1. Preprocedural cross-sectional images of lesions with different amounts of calcium. Increasing total arc of calcium allows one to distinguish soft (A), mixed (B, C) and severely calcified (D) lesions.

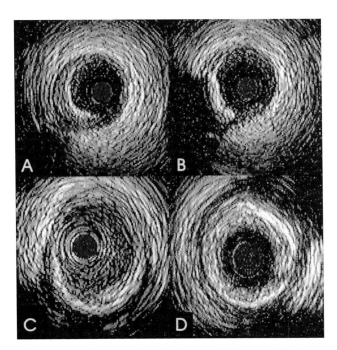

Figure 20.2. Cross-sectional ultrasound images of lesions with different localization of calcium: A: thin layer of subendothelial calcium deposits; B: 80° arc of superficial–central calcium deposits; C: deep–central position of the calcium deposits; D: calcium deposits located mainly at the base of the plaque.

vigorous flushing with contrast medium or saline were used to distinguish artifacts from true wall disruptions.

Statistical analysis

Data are presented as mean±1 SD. A two-tailed Student's *t*-test for paired data was used to compare differences in the parameters characterizing the mechanisms of acute results after PTCA according to preintervention plaque composition and presence of fracture/dissection after PTCA. A chi-square test was used to compare differences among qualitative variables. Regression analysis was used to assess the correlation between quantitative ultrasonic measurements and acute changes after PTCA. A *p*-value of less than 0.05 was considered significant.

Results

Procedure

There was no significant difference in terms of balloon-to-artery ratio and time of balloon inflation among plaques of different ultrasonic characteristics. However, a trend towards longer duration of balloon inflation and significantly higher balloon pressure was found for diffusely calcified lesions (Table 20.2). No clear influence of balloon-to-artery ratio, time of balloon inflation and maximal balloon pressure on vessel lumen and plaque after PTCA was found. Only significant correlations between balloon-to-artery ratio and postprocedural total vessel and plaque area changes were found for mixed lesions ($r = -0.58$ and $r = 0.61$, respectively; $p < 0.05$).

Angiographic analysis

Calcium was identified in the target stenosis by angiography in eight (10.4%) cases. The preprocedural minimal lumen diameter and percentage area stenosis (1.11±0.3 mm and 82.6±10%, respectively) were significantly improved ($p < 0.000\,01$) after PTCA (1.98±0.4 mm and 50.7±16.4%, respectively).

A National Heart, Lung and Blood Institute Registry class B or C angiographic dissection was present in 17/77 (22.1%) patients.

Qualitative ultrasound analysis

Using ultrasound 42 lesions (54.5%) were classified as soft, none as fibrous, 11 (14.3%) as diffuse calcific and 24 (31.2%) as mixed. Twenty-three (29.9%) lesions were concentric. Fifty-nine of 77 lesions (76.6%) showed focal or diffuse areas of calcification.

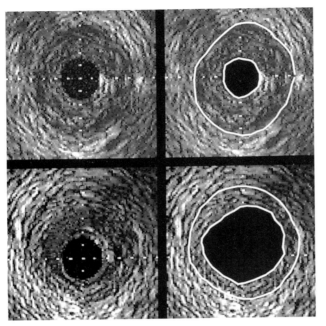

PRE-PTCA
LA=1.61 mm²
TA=13.7 mm²
PLA=12.1 mm²
AS=88%

POST-PTCA
LA=7.2 mm²
TA=14.8 mm²
PLA=7.6 mm²
AS=51%

Figure 20.3. Cross-sectional ultrasound images of the target stenosis in the left anterior descending coronary artery classified as soft before (upper panel) and immediately after PTCA (lower panel). The lumen area and the total vessel area are contoured in white. The corresponding measurements (mm²) are reported. Note the significant plaque reduction and practically no change in total vessel area. LA, TA, PLA: lumen, total vessel and plaque areas; AS: percentage area stenosis.

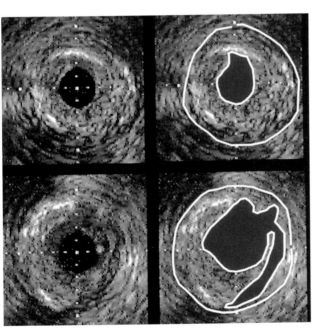

PRE-PTCA
LA=2.8 mm²
TA=17.0 mm²
PLA=14.2 mm²
AS=84%

POST-PTCA
LA=7.7 mm²
TA=20.4 mm²
PLA=12.7 mm²
AS=62%

Figure 20.4. Cross-sectional ultrasound images of the target stenosis in the left circumflex coronary artery classified as mixed before (upper panel) and immediately after PTCA (lower panel). The lumen area and the total vessel area are contoured in white. The corresponding measurements (mm²) are reported. Note the relatively larger increase in total vessel area, partially related to the presence of plaque dissection and only minimal plaque reduction. LA, TA, PLA: lumen, total vessel and plaque areas; AS: percentage area stenosis.

Table 20.2. Plaque composition and procedural variables.

Plaque type	n	Inflation time (s)	Maximal BA pressure (atm)	BA/A ratio	ICUS presence of wall disruption
Soft	42	332.2±203.7	9.0±3.15	1.07±0.23	18 (42.0%)
Calcific	11	414.2±349.9	11.3±3.75*	1.12±0.18	11 (100.0%)
Mixed	24	279.4±184.5	9.81±2.70	1.03±0.11	17 (70.8%)

*p <0.05 calcific vs soft.
BA: angioplasty balloon; BA/A: balloon-to-artery ratio.

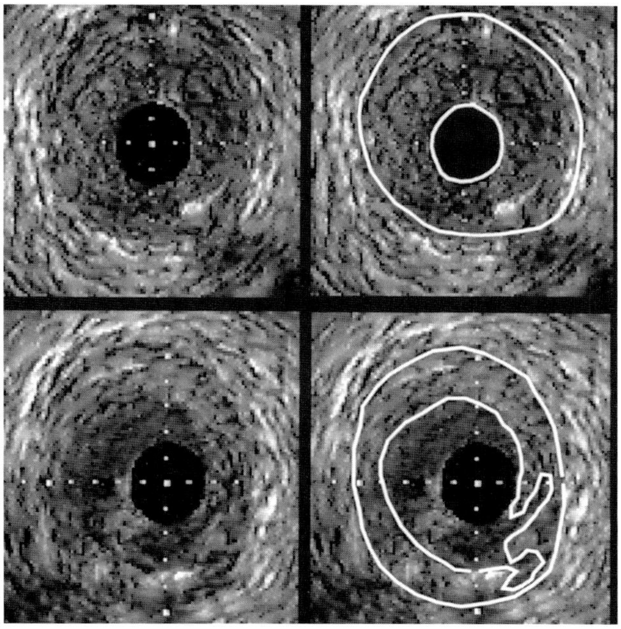

PRE-PTCA
LA=1.61 mm²
TA=17.4 mm²
PLA=15.8 mm²
AS=91%

POST-PTCA
LA=7.3 mm²
TA=18.1 mm²
PLA=10.8 mm²
AS=60%

Figure 20.5. Cross-sectional ultrasound images of the target stenoses in the left anterior descending coronary artery classified as soft (but with small deposit of calcium at 5 o'clock) before (upper panel) and immediately after (lower panel) PTCA. The lumen area and the total vessel area contours are traced in white. The corresponding measurements (mm²) are reported. Note that despite a small vessel disruption, plaque reduction was the main operative mechanism in lumen enlargement. LA, TA, PLA: lumen, total vessel and plaque areas; AS: percentage area stenosis.

In 21 cases (35.6%) calcium localization was defined as subendothelial and in 38 (64.4%) cases as deep.

The presence of fracture and dissection was found in 9 (11.7%) and 37 (48%) of cases, respectively. All of the 11 diffusely calcific plaques (100%), 17/24 (70.8%) mixed plaques and 18/42 (42.8%) soft plaques developed fractures or dissections after PTCA (Table 20.2). Focal deposits of calcium were present in all but three of the predominantly soft plaques which developed fracture or dissection after PTCA. Figure 20.5 presents the measurements performed before and immediately after PTCA in a soft lesion with a small deposit of calcium.

Quantitative ultrasound analysis

Table 20.3 reports the changes in lumen, total vessel and plaque areas before and after PTCA. Before PTCA, the ultrasound probe was wedged in the lesion in 75.3% of cases (58/77). After PTCA, minimal cross-sectional lumen area of the target stenosis increased significantly for all treated lesions. Total vessel area for the studied group increased significantly by 1.7±1.66 mm², which accounts for 48.9% of the immediate lumen gain. Plaque area decreased significantly by 1.75±1.89 mm², accounting for the remaining 51.1% of the immediate lumen gain (Fig. 20.6).

Table 20.3. Intracoronary ultrasound area measurements before and after balloon angioplasty.

Parameter	Pre-PTCA	Post-PTCA	*P*-value
LA ref. (mm²)	9.08±3.04	9.29±3.03	NS
TA ref. (mm²)	17.33±5.09	17.61±5.07	NS
PLA ref. (mm²)	8.24±3.42	8.32±3.52	NS
AS ref. (%)	46.50±12.29	46.25±12.35	NS
LA stenosis (mm²)	1.94±0.81	5.40±1.59	0.000 001
TA stenosis (mm²)	15.40±4.68	17.1±4.77	0.03
PLA stenosis (mm²)	13.44±4.59	11.74±4.77	0.02
AS (%)	86.45±5.99	67.21±8.79	0.000 001

LA, TA, PLA: lumen, total vessel and plaque area, respectively; ref.: reference segment; AS: area stenosis.

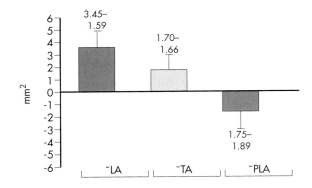

Figure 20.6. The lumen area (LA), total area (TA) and plaque area (PLA) changes before and after PTCA in the studied population. It is clear that plaque reduction and vessel expansion played almost equal roles in postprocedural lumen enlargement.

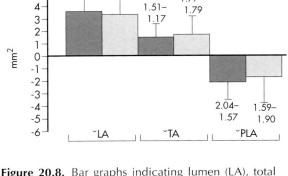

Figure 20.8. Bar graphs indicating lumen (LA), total vessel (TA) and plaque area (PLA) changes before and after PTCA in arteries with and without vessel wall disruptions. Note no significant differences in immediate lumen gain and plaque reduction between both groups.

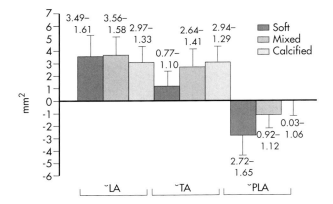

Figure 20.7. The lumen area (LA), total area (TA) and plaque area (PLA) changes before and after PTCA are distinguished according to the prevalent plaque composition. Although no significant differences in acute lumen gain were observed, soft plaques appear to have a larger plaque reduction and smaller vessel expansion compared with mixed and calcified plaques.

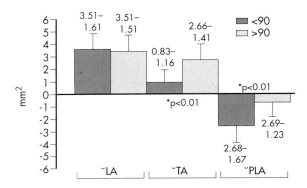

Figure 20.9. Bar graphs indicating lumen (LA), total area (TA) and plaque area (PLA) changes before and after PTCA in arteries with total arc of lesion calcium larger than and equal to or smaller than 90°. Note the significantly larger increase in total area in the group with a total arc exceeding 90°.

There was no significant difference in acute lumen gain according to plaque composition, although a smaller lumen enlargement was achieved in diffusely calcified lesions than in soft or mixed lesions (Fig. 20.7). A greater acute lumen gain was obtained in concentric than in eccentric lesions but the difference was not significant (3.60±1.57 versus 3.37±1.40, respectively; NS). Postprocedural lesion morphology (presence of fracture and/or dissection) could not be demonstrated to affect significantly the mechanisms of acute lumen enlargement (Fig. 20.8).

In soft lesions lumen gain was predominantly associated with plaque reduction (77.9%) whereas in calcified and mixed lesions the main operative mechanism was vessel expansion (99.1 and 74.2%, respectively; NS) (Fig. 20.7). There was no significant difference in acute lumen gain in plaques with subendothelial and deep calcifications (3.37±1.57 mm² versus 3.55±1.56 mm², respectively; NS). In the lesions with total arc of calcium greater than 90° the main contribution to post-PTCA lumen enlargement was vessel expansion (79.3%). On the contrary, in lesions with a smaller total arc of calcification, plaque reduction (76.2%) was the predominant mechanism (Fig. 20.9). The magnitude of total arc of lesion calcification showed a positive correlation with the increase in

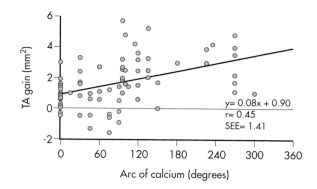

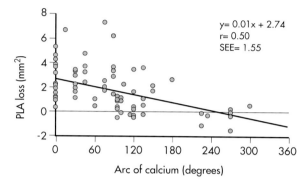

Figure 20.10. Plots of changes in total vessel (upper panel) and plaque (lower panel) areas depending on total arc of lesion calcium. TA gain: difference between post- and pre-PTCA total vessel areas; PLA loss: difference between post- and pre-PTCA plaque areas.

total vessel area ($r = 0.45$, $P < 0.05$) and an inverse correlation with plaque reduction ($r = -0.50$, $p < 0.05$) (Figs 20.10).

There was no significant correlation between lesion eccentricity and total vessel, lumen and plaque area changes after PTCA for all the lesions studied. However, a trend towards a greater plaque reduction in concentric lesions was found when compared with eccentric lesions (acute lumen gain of 58.3% versus 48.5%, respectively).

Discussion

Since its introduction into clinical practice, many theories regarding the operative mechanism of coronary balloon angioplasty have been proposed. Initially, compression and redistribution of the atherosclerotic plaque was postulated as the main mechanism of lumen enlargement after PTCA.[16,17] Histology studies indicated that rupture of vessel wall components and overstretching of the arterial wall were almost invariably associated with balloon dilatation.[1-3]

For a long time these hypotheses were based on animal studies[18,19] or in-vitro studies on post-mortem specimens.[1-3] However, plaque characteristics in experimental atherosclerosis are very different from the characteristics of human plaques and pathologic specimens obtained from patients with an unfavorable outcome after coronary interventions are not representative of the entire spectrum of morphological changes that occur after PTCA. Although coronary quantitative angiography has been established as a 'gold standard' for the assessment of coronary stenosis severity, this technique has clear limitations for the assessment of coronary interventions since the presence of complex wall injury modifies the circular geometry of the lumen which is a prerequisite for precise measurements.[20,21] ICUS is the only coronary imaging technique which can directly study plaque composition and distribution in vivo.[5,6] Moreover, this technique is more sensitive than angiography in the detection of the presence of calcification and vessel wall disruption[4,7,22,23] and can quantitatively assess the changes in lumen and plaque area before and after intervention.[9,10,14] Because of these features ICUS may permit the identification of high-risk lesions and predictors of restenosis.[4,24] ICUS has also the potential to elucidate the mechanisms of successful coronary intervention. Recent studies have confirmed that PTCA induces vessel wall fractures or dissections in the majority of cases and that the main mechanism of lumen enlargement is total vessel area expansion.[25-28] The study of Botas et al.[29] has shown that coronary distensibility increases after PTCA as a result of releasing the outer vessel wall from the cicatrizing effects of the noncompliant atherosclerotic intimal plaque.

This study showed that vessel expansion is responsible for half the lumen enlargement after PTCA (Fig. 20.6). More interestingly, in this study the authors observed a correlation between the composition of atherosclerotic plaque and the mechanisms of balloon dilatation. A reduction in plaque area was the main operative mechanism in lesions with soft plaque, whereas expansion of the total vessel area was the predominant mechanism of lumen area increase in lesions with calcified and mixed plaques (Fig. 20.7). In particular, as shown in previous studies,[4,30] the presence and amount of calcium deposits significantly influenced the development of vessel wall disruptions. In lesions with an extensive amount of calcium, a partial vessel rupture is essential for a successful balloon dilatation, as the rigid plaque structure does not allow compression as occurs in the presence of thrombi or fibrofatty lesions.

Despite these different mechanisms, the final lumen enlargement was similar in soft and mixed lesions and only slightly smaller in diffusely calcified plaques. Plaque calcification, therefore, appears to be only a partial contraindication to PTCA, but does require higher balloon pressures to achieve results comparable to the results obtained in noncalcified plaques and is associated with a high prevalence of wall fractures and/or dissections.

This study has shown also that despite a satisfactory immediate postprocedural lumen gain an enormous residual plaque burden remains, helping to explain why restenosis is so frequent after PTCA.[4,24]

Conclusion

Plaque composition is a major determinant of the mechanisms of PTCA. Plaque compression and/or axial redistribution is the main mechanism of PTCA in soft plaque while wall disruption and total vessel expansion are predominant in mixed and calcified plaques.

References

1   Lyon RT, Zarins ChK, Lu Ch-T et al. Vessel, plaque, and lumen morphology after transluminal balloon angioplasty. Quantitative study in distended human arteries. *Arteriosclerosis* 1987; **7**: 306–14.

2   Waller BF, Gorfinkel HJ, Rogers FJ et al. Early and late morphologic changes in major epicardial coronary arteries after percutaneous transluminal coronary angioplasty. *Am J Cardiol* 1984; **53 (suppl C)**: 42–7.

3   Farb A, Virmani R, Atkinson JB et al. Plaque morphology and pathologic changes in arteries from patients dying after coronary balloon angioplasty. *J Am Coll Cardiol* 1990; **16**: 1421–9.

4   Virmani R, Farb A, Burke AP. Coronary angioplasty from the perspective of atherosclerotic plaque: morphologic predictors of immediate success and restenosis. *Am Heart J* 1994; **127**: 163–79.

5   Di Mario C, The SHK, Madretsma S et al. Detection and characterization of vascular lesions by intravascular ultrasound: an in vitro study correlated with histology. *J Am Soc Echocardiogr* 1992; **5**: 135–46.

6   Gussenhoven EJ, Essed CE, Lancée CT et al. Arterial wall characteristics determined by intravascular ultrasound imaging: an in vitro study. *J Am Coll Cardiol* 1989; **14**: 947–52.

7   Friedrich GJ, Moes NY, Mühlberger VA et al. Detection of intralesional calcium by intracoronary ultrasound depends on the histologic pattern. *Am Heart J* 1994; **128**: 435–41.

8   Hausmann D, Lundkvist A-JS, Friedrich GJ, Mullen WL, Fitzgerald PJ, Yock PG. Intracoronary ultrasound imaging: intraobserver and interobserver variability of morphometric measurements. *Am Heart J* 1994; **128**: 674–80.

9   Losordo DW, Rosenfield K, Pieczek A et al. How does angioplasty work? Serial analysis of human iliac arteries using intravascular ultrasound. *Circulation* 1992; **86**: 1845–58.

10   The SHK, Gussenhoven EJ, Zhong Y et al. Effect of balloon angioplasty on femoral artery evaluated with intravascular ultrasound imaging. *Circulation* 1992; **86**: 483–93.

11   Gronenschild E, Janssen J, Tijdens F. CAAS II: a second generation system for off-line and on-line quantitative coronary angiography. *Cathet Cardiovasc Diagn* 1994; **33**: 61–75.

12   Haase J, Di Mario C, Slager CJ et al. In-vivo validation of on-line and off-line geometric coronary measurements using insertion of stenosis phantoms in porcine coronary arteries. *Cathet Cardiovasc Diagn* 1992; **27**: 16–27.

13   Dorros G, Cowley MJ, Simpson J et al. Percutaneous transluminal coronary angioplasty: report of complications from the National Heart, Lung and Blood Institute PTCA registry. *Circulation* 1983; **67**: 723–30.

14   Honye J, Mahon DJ, White CJ et al. Morphological effects of coronary balloon angioplasty in vivo assessed by intravascular ultrasound imaging. *Circulation* 1992; **85**: 1012–25.

15   Hodgson McJB, Reddy KG, Suneja R et al. Intracoronary ultrasound imaging: correlation of plaque morphology with angiography, clinical syndrome and procedural results in patients undergoing coronary angioplasty. *J Am Coll Cardiol* 1993; **21**: 35–44.

16   Dotter CT, Judkins MP. Transluminal treatment of atherosclerotic obstructions: description of a new technique and preliminary report of its application. *Circulation* 1964; **30**: 654–70.

17   Gruentzig AR. Transluminal dilatation of coronary artery stenosis. *Lancet* 1978; **1**: 263–7.

18   Sunborn TA, Faxon DP, Haudenschild Ch et al. The mechanism of transluminal angioplasty: evidence for formation of aneurysm in experimental atherosclerosis. *Circulation* 1983; **68**: 1136–40.

19   Fischell TA, Grant G, Johnson DE. Determinants of smooth muscle injury during balloon angioplasty. *Circulation* 1990; **82**: 2170–84.

20 Haase J, Ozaki Y, Di Mario C et al. Can intracoronary ultrasound correctly assess the luminal dimensions of coronary artery lesions? A comparison with quantitative angiography. *Eur Heart J* 1995; **16**: 112–19.

21 De Scheerder I, De Man F, Herregods MC et al. Intravascular ultrasound versus angiography for measurement of luminal diameters in normal and diseased coronary arteries. *Am Heart J* 1994; **127**: 2243–51.

22 Mintz GS, Douek P, Pichard AD et al. Target lesion calcification in coronary artery disease: an intravascular ultrasound study. *J Am Coll Cardiol* 1994; **22**: 1149–55.

23 Mintz GS, Popma JJ, Pichard AD et al. Patterns of calcification in coronary artery disease. A statistical analysis of intravascular ultrasound and coronary angiography in 1155 lesions. *Circulation* 1995; **91**: 1959–65.

24 Jain SP, Jain A, Collins TJ et al. Predictors of restenosis: a morphometric and quantitative evaluation by intravascular ultrasound. *Am Heart J* 1994; **128**: 664–73.

25 Nakamura S, Mahon DJ, Maheswaran B et al. An explanation for discrepancy between angiographic and intravascular ultrasound measurements after percutaneous transluminal coronary angioplasty. *J Am Coll Cardiol* 1995; **25**: 633–9.

26 Tenaglia AN, Buller CE, Kisslo KB et al. Mechanisms of balloon angioplasty and directional coronary atherectomy as assessed by intracoronary ultrasound. *J Am Coll Cardiol* 1992; **20**: 685–91.

27 Braden GA, Herrington DM, Downes TR et al. Qualitative and quantitative contrasts in the mechanisms of lumen enlargement by coronary balloon angioplasty and directional coronary atherectomy. *J Am Coll Cardiol* 1994; **23**: 40–8.

28 Di Mario C, Gil R, Camenzind E et al. Quantitative assessment with intracoronary ultrasound of the mechanisms of restenosis after percutaneous transluminal balloon angioplasty and directional coronary atherectomy. *Am J Cardiol* 1995; **75**: 772–7.

29 Botas J, Clark DA, Pinto F et al. Balloon angioplasty results in increased segmental coronary distensibility: a likely mechanism of percutaneous transluminal coronary angioplasty. *J Am Coll Cardiol* 1994; **23**: 1043–52.

30 Fitzgerald PJ, Ports TA, Yock PG. Contribution of localized calcium deposits to dissection after angioplasty in vivo assessed by intravascular ultrasound imaging. *Circulation* 1992; **86**: 64–70.

21 Mechanisms of percutaneous transluminal coronary angioplasty assessed by intravascular ultrasound

Günter Görge, Michael Haude, Junbo Ge, Fengqi Liu and Raimund Erbel

Introduction

Since its introduction by Grüntzig et al. in the late Seventies, percutaneous transluminal coronary angioplasty (PTCA) has gained explosive interest and clinical impact.[1,2] It is today's most commonly used intervention in cardiology and its use exceeds the number of bypass grafts in many countries. Although acute complications such as flow-limiting coronary artery dissections, acute myocardial infarcts or vessel perforation may occur, PTCA is surprisingly safe if performed by experienced operators.

Mechanisms of PTCA

Despite its widespread use, the mechanisms of PTCA are not well understood. The main reason for this is that the target of PTCA, the vessel wall and the underlying plaque, cannot be imaged by angiography directly.[3,4] Angiography is a silhouette method which is unable to provide sufficient information about the vessel wall.[5,6] The pioneers of angioplasty in peripheral vessels and the coronary arteries, Dotter, Judkins, and Grüntzig, suggested plaque compression or plaque remodeling as the major effects leading to luminal enlargement.[2,7] However, the composition of most coronary plaques, with high amounts of fibrotic or calcified lesions, makes this theory unlikely to be the predominant mechanism. The reason for the propagation of the compression and remodeling theory was that most of the animal models were based on a lipid-rich diet, leading to relatively soft lipid-rich plaques with little fibrotic or calcified material.

Post-mortem studies have had a tremendous impact on our knowledge and understanding of PTCA mechanisms. Waller et al. showed that fissures, plaque fracture, and dissections are the main mechanisms of lumen enlargement after PTCA.[8] Düber et al. and Jungbluth et al. showed in post-mortem cases that most of the PTCA-induced dissections in eccentric lesions occurred at the plaque–vessel conjunction, a region with high shear stress.[9,10] Nevertheless, it is unclear whether post-mortem studies in patients who died due to complications after PTCA are representative for the effects of PTCA in all patients.

Role of intravascular ultrasound (IVUS)

Because of these fundamental limitations it is not surprising that a large number of studies have identified a wide range of clinical, anatomical, and procedural factors influencing both the acute and the long-term outcome after PTCA (for a review see refs 11–13). One can speculate that a technique providing better evaluation of the acute effects of PTCA on the vessel wall and the underlying plaque would be very helpful in assessing and optimizing the effects of PTCA.[14–16]

IVUS, a catheter-based method for obtaining on-line cross-sectional images of peripheral and coronary artery vessels, allows the in-vivo assessment of the effects of various interventional procedures, including PTCA. In ex-vivo studies, Gussenhoven et al. evaluated the effects of PTCA on vessel segments using high-frequency intravascular ultrasound.[17–20] In this experimental study in 250 coronary segments, fissures and dissections were the main mechanisms of luminal enlargement. However, IVUS depicted only 60% of all dissections identified by histology, mainly due to the limitations of IVUS in radial and axial resolution even under optimal ex-vivo settings. In almost every case the most severe damage of the vessel wall after PTCA was found at the narrowest spot of the vessel segment.

IVUS after PTCA in patients

In patients, various groups have reported findings obtained by IVUS after PTCA. These studies were in agreement concerning the feasibility and the relative safety of the procedure.[21–23] In order to obtain comparable data, the morphological findings after PTCA were classified concerning the presence or absence of calcification, dissections, and symmetry of the lesion. Furthermore, various mechanisms of luminal enlargement after PTCA were identified, such as plaque compression, overextension of the entire vessel segment, subintimal or submedial dissections, and stretching of the disease-free segment of the vessel wall. While initially the IVUS procedures were usually performed after PTCA, newer studies show the effect of PTCA before and after intervention.[24,25]

While some groups merely graded the effect of injury as 'superficial' and 'deep', others attempted more detailed classifications. Honye et al. proposed types A–E1/E2.[21] Initially surprising was the fact that even in angiographically successful cases the residual area stenosis after PTCA was in the order of 60%.

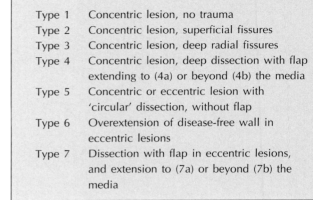

Classification proposed by Gerber et al.[22]

Type 1	Concentric lesion, no trauma
Type 2	Concentric lesion, superficial fissures
Type 3	Concentric lesion, deep radial fissures
Type 4	Concentric lesion, deep dissection with flap extending to (4a) or beyond (4b) the media
Type 5	Concentric or eccentric lesion with 'circular' dissection, without flap
Type 6	Overextension of disease-free wall in eccentric lesions
Type 7	Dissection with flap in eccentric lesions, and extension to (7a) or beyond (7b) the media

Based on the results of Waller,[8] Düber et al.[9] and Jungbluth et al.,[10] Gerber et al.[22] described the effects of IVUS after PTCA via a classification of seven subtypes. The majority of patients had eccentric lesions (Fig. 21.1) and dissections were found in approximately two-thirds of all patients after PTCA (Figs 21.2–21.5).

Thus post-PTCA IVUS examination proved to be effective in showing the effects of PTCA, not only on luminal diameters, but also on vessel wall morphology. However, these studies also showed the relative imperfection of current PTCA interventions in terms of residual area stenosis, leaving in many patients a large plaque burden.

Comparison of angiography and IVUS for morphology and luminal dimensions

In patients, after PTCA, comparison with quantitative coronary angiography (QCA) and with visually assessed angiography-based morphological classifications showed that the correlation of luminal dimensions between QCA and IVUS and detection of dissections is very poor.

Nakamura et al. showed that the differences between QCA and IVUS are more pronounced in deeper-injured vessels in comparison with vessels with only minor wall injuries detected by IVUS. Additionally, IVUS revealed more dissections than angiography, but probably less than expected from ex-vivo studies with histology as the gold-standard.[20,26]

Classification proposed by Honye et al.[21]

Type A	Radial fissure to intima
Type B	Radial fissure to media
Type C	Circular dissection beyond plaque < 180°
Type D	Circular dissection > 180°
Type E1	Concentric lesion, no fissures or flaps
Type E2	Eccentric lesion, no fissures or flaps

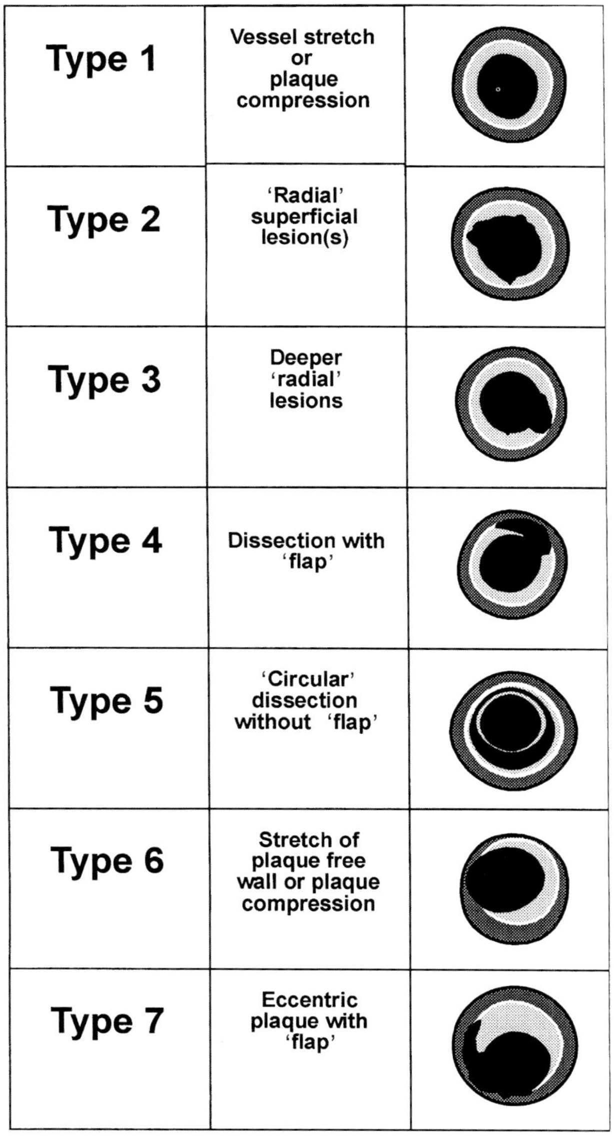

Type 1	Vessel stretch or plaque compression	
Type 2	'Radial' superficial lesion(s)	
Type 3	Deeper 'radial' lesions	
Type 4	Dissection with 'flap'	
Type 5	'Circular' dissection without 'flap'	
Type 6	Stretch of plaque free wall or plaque compression	
Type 7	Eccentric plaque with 'flap'	

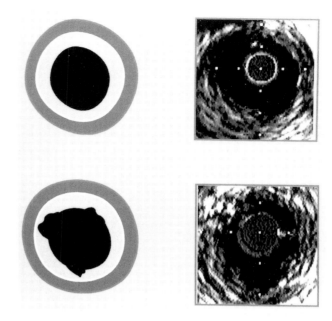

Figure 21.2 IVUS examples of Type 1 (top) and Type 2 (bottom) lesions after PTCA. In Type 1 segments, only plaque compression or stretch without apparent damage to the vessel wall or plaque is found. In Type 2, IVUS depicts only minor superficial fissures.

Figure 21.1 IVUS explains the acute effects of PTCA on the vessel wall and the underlying plaque. The classification proposed distinguishes between concentric (Types 1–4) and eccentric lesions (Types 6 and 7). Additionally, the amount of damage to the plaque or the stretch of the vessel wall can be categorized. In Type 1, only plaque compression, or stretch without apparent damage to the vessel wall or plaque in concentric lesions is found. In Type 2, found also in concentric lesions, IVUS depicts only minor superficial fissures, while in Type 3 these injuries increase in severity. The appearance of flaps is typical for Types 4a and b in concentric lesions. Type 4b lesions are lesions with injuries extending into the media. However, image quality does not always allow the distinction between Types 4a and b. Type 5 describes circular dissections after PTCA, found in either eccentric or concentric lesions. Type 6 defines the overextension of the plaque-free wall in eccentric lesions with or without plaque compression. Finally, Types 7a and b show dissections and flaps in eccentric lesions. Type 7b describes injuries extending to the media.

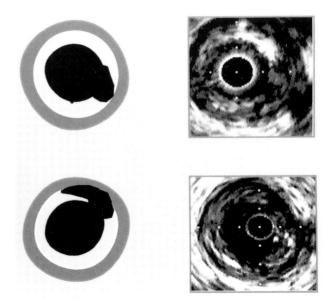

Figure 21.3 Type 3 lesions (top) after PTCA are defined by radial injuries not extenting to the media. In Type 4 lesions, clearly mobile flaps are visible by IVUS.

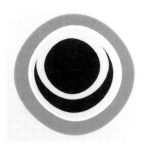
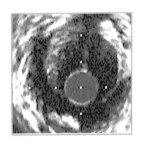

Figure 21.4 Circular dissections can be identified often by IVUS only. Type 5 lesions show circular dissections in either eccentric or concentric lesions. Long-term prognosis of patients with Type 5 lesions seems to be inferior to other lesions found after PTCA.

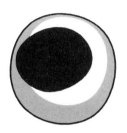
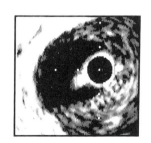

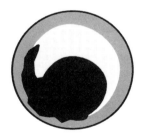
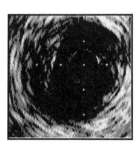

Figure 21.5 Type 6 lesions (top) show an overextension of the plaque-free wall in eccentric lesions. Eccentric lesions are found in over 70% of all lesions suitable for coronary interventions. In Type 7 lesions (bottom) clearly visible dissections with mobile flaps are found. Type 7 lesions are most commonly seen after PTCA. Despite their higher degree of damage in comparison to Type 6 lesions, complication or restenosis rate is not increased.

After PTCA

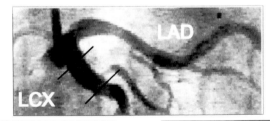

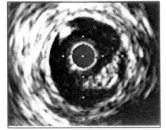
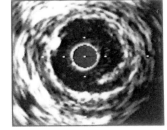

1 mm

proximal   distal

Figure 21.6 IVUS is more useful than angiography for the detection of vessel wall changes after PTCA. In this patient with PTCA of a high-grade LCX lesion, angiography revealed a good initial result. No filling defects or dissection membranes were seen. However, IVUS revealed two flaps. The proximal was very mobile, with an almost 'free-floating' appearance, while the distal lesion showed little motion. Residual plaque area was relatively small. Further PTCAs did not result in change of anatomy. Therefore it was decided to implant a stent (result shown in chapter 30).

Before PTCA

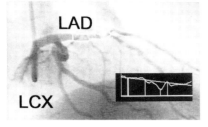
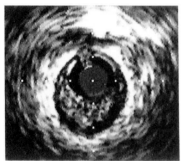

After PTCA

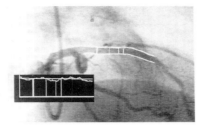
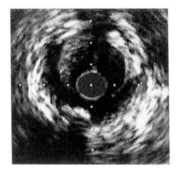

Figure 21.7 Example of a Type 5 'circular' dissection after PTCA of a proximal LAD lesion. The preinterventional IVUS shows an eccentric lesion with 'soft' plaque. After PTCA (3.5 mm balloon, 11 atm), a very satisfying angiographical appearance was found. Surprisingly, IVUS showed marked remodeling of the vessel with a circular dissection. The patient was kept in the catheterization laboratory for 15 minutes after PTCA. No signs of impaired contrast flow or depots outside the coronary artery were seen. The further clinical course of this patient was uneventful.

Serial IVUS studies before and after PTCA

Recently, studies assessing coronary artery lesions before and after PTCA brought even more insight into the mechanisms of PTCA (Fig. 21.6). Di Mario et al. and Baptista et al. showed that an increase in total vessel area accounted for over 40% of luminal enlargement.[24,25] Plaque compression was found more frequently in concentric than in eccentric lesions. Kimura et al., from the SURE trial (Serial Ultrasound Analysis of Restenosis), showed also that vessel area increases and plaque area decreases acutely after PTCA.[27] All studies addressing the question of post-PTCA IVUS showed that, even in angiographically successful interventions, the residual area stenosis is in the magnitude of 55–65%. The question remains as to whether IVUS-guided interventions can improve the outcome of PTCA by reducing the residual plaque burden (Fig. 21.7).

Hodgson et al., for the CLOUT study, reported an increase in post-PTCA luminal diameter by selecting PTCA balloon size from the mean value of the IVUS-estimated reference lumen and vessel measurements. This resulted in an upsizing of the balloon diameters in comparison with QCA-based selection of balloon dimensions. Complication rates were unchanged in proportion to other studies.[28]

Summary and outlook

In summary, IVUS allows for the first time the in-vivo assessment of the vessel wall response to PTCA. While pathology favored fissures, dissections, and plaque ruptures as main mechanisms of successful PTCA, IVUS confirmed these vessel wall responses but showed also that acute vessel enlargement is a significant component of angiographically successful PTCA. However, even in these cases, mean residual plaque burden is in the range of 60%. Further studies are needed to establish whether IVUS-guided PTCA will improve acute and long-term outcome.

References

1 Grüntzig A. Perkutane Dilatation von Koronarstenosen—Beschreibung eines neuen Kathetersystems. *Klin Wochenschr* 1976; **54**: 543–5.

2 Grüntzig A, Senning A, Siegenthaler WE. Nonoperative dilatation of coronary artery stenoses: percutaneous transluminal coronary angioplasty. *New Engl J Med* 1979; **301**: 61–8.

3 Waller BF. 'Crackers, breakers, stretchers, drillers, scrapers, shavers, burners, welders, and melders'—the future treatment of atherosclerotic coronary artery

disease? A clinical–morphological assessment. *J Am Coll Cardiol* 1989; **13**: 969–87.

4   Waller BF, Pinkerton CA, Slack JD. Intravascular ultrasound: a histological study of vessels during life. The new 'gold standard' for vascular imaging. *Circulation* 1992; **85**: 2305–10.

5   Tobis JM, Mahon DJ, Goldberg SL, Nakamura S, Colombo A. Lessons from intravascular ultrasonography: observations during interventional angioplasty procedures. *J Clin Ultrasound* 1993; **21**: 589–607.

6   Nishioka T, Luo H, Eigler NL et al. The evolving utility of intracoronary ultrasound. *Am J Cardiol* 1995; **75**: 539–41.

7   Dotter CT, Judkins MP. Transluminal treatment of arteriosclerotic obstruction: description of a new technique and a preliminary report on its application. *Circulation* 1964; **30**: 654–70.

8   Waller BF. Morphologic correlates of coronary angiographic patterns at the site of percutaneous transluminal coronary angioplasty. *Clin Cardiol* 1988; **11**: 817–22.

9   Düber C, Jungbluth A, Rumpelt H-J et al. Morphology of the coronary arteries after combined thrombolysis and percutaneous transluminal coronary angioplasty for acute myocardial infarction. *Am J Cardiol* 1986; **58**: 698–703.

10 Jungbluth A, Düber C, Rumpelt HJ, Erbel R, Meyer J. Morphologic changes in a coronary artery after cardiac tamponade following percutaneous transluminal coronary angioplasty (PTCA). *Z Kardiol* 1988; **77**: 125–9.

11 Serruys PW, Foley DP, Kirkeeide RL, King SB III. Restenosis revisited: insights provided by quantitative coronary angiography. *Am Heart J* 1993; **126**: 1243–67.

12 Weintraub WS, Ghazzal ZM, Douglas JS Jr et al. Long-term clinical follow-up in patients with angiographic restudy after successful angioplasty. *Circulation* 1993; **87**: 831–40.

13 Hirshfeld JW Jr, Schwartz JS, Jugo R et al. Restenosis after coronary angioplasty: a multivariate statistical model to relate lesion and procedure variables to restenosis. *J Am Coll Cardiol* 1991; **18**: 647–56.

14 Coy KM, Maurer G, Siegel RJ. Intravascular ultrasound imaging: a current perspective. *J Am Coll Cardiol* 1991; **18**: 1811–23.

15 Tobis JM, Mallery JA, Mahon D et al. Intravascular ultrasound imaging: a new method for guiding interventional vascular procedures. *Echocardiography* 1990; **7**: 415–24.

16 Yock PG, Johnson EL, Linker DT. Intravascular ultrasound: development and clinical potential. *Am J Card Imaging* 1988; **32**: 185–93.

17 The SH, Gussenhoven EJ, Zhong Y et al. Effect of balloon angioplasty on femoral artery evaluated with intravascular ultrasound imaging. *Circulation* 1992; **86**: 483–93.

18 van der Lugt A, Gussenhoven EJ, Stijnen T et al. Balloon angioplasty evaluated in vitro by intracoronary ultrasound: a validation with histology. *Eur Heart J* 1995; **16**: 203.

19 Gussenhoven EJ, Essed CE, Lancee CT et al. Arterial wall characteristics determined by intravascular ultrasound imaging: an in vitro study. *J Am Coll Cardiol* 1989; **14**: 947–52.

20 Di Marco C, The SH, Madretsma S et al. Detection and characterization of vascular lesions by intravascular ultrasound: an in vitro study correlated with histology. *J Am Soc Echocardiogr* 1992; **5**: 135–46.

21 Honye J, Mahon DJ, Jain A et al. Morphological effects of coronary balloon angioplasty in vivo assessed by intravascular ultrasound imaging. *Circulation* 1992; **85**: 1012–25.

22 Gerber TC, Erbel R, Görge G, Ge J, Rupprecht HJ, Meyer J. Classification of morphologic effects of percutaneous transluminal coronary angioplasty assessed by intra-vascular ultrasound. *Am J Cardiol* 1992; **70**: 1546–54.

23 Jain SP, Jain A, Collins TJ, Ramee SR, White CJ. Predictors of restenosis: a morphometric and quantitative evaluation by intravascular ultrasound. *Am Heart J* 1994; **128**: 664–73.

24 Di Mario C, Gil R, Camenzind E et al. Quantitative assessment with intracoronary ultrasound of the mechanisms of restenosis after percutaneous transluminal coronary angioplasty and directional coronary atherectomy. *Am J Cardiol* 1995; **75**: 772–7.

25 Baptista J, di Mario C, Ozaki Y et al. Impact of plaque morphology and composition on the mechanisms of lumen enlargement using intracoronary ultrasound and quantitative angiography after balloon angioplasty. *Am J Cardiol* 1996; **77**: 115–21.

26 Nakamura S, Mahon DJ, Maheswaran B et al. An explanation for discrepancy between angiographic and intravascular ultrasound measurements after percutaneous transluminal coronary angioplasty. *J Am Coll Cardiol* 1995; **25**: 633–9.

27 Kimura T, Kaburagi S, Tashima Y, Nobuyoshi M, Mintz GS, Popma JJ. Geometric remodeling and intimal growth as mechanisms of restenosis: observations from serial ultrasound analysis of restenosis (SURE) trial. *Circulation* 1995; **92(suppl)**: I76.

28 Hodgson JMcB, Stone GW, Linnemeier TJ, Sheehan HM, St Goar FG, Berry JL. Oversized balloons defined by intracoronary ultrasound results in dramatic improve-ments in angioplasty results: initial ultrasound analysis of the CLOUT pilot study. *Eur Heart J* 1995; **16**: 487.

22 Intravascular ultrasound after coronary laser angioplasty

Michael Haude

The major mechanism of luminal enlargement after percutaneous transluminal coronary balloon angioplasty (PTCA) is plaque disruption with creation of intimal and medial dissections.[1] These postangioplasty intimal and medial dissections were associated with the potential risk of acute vessel closure because of flow limitations and the potential exposure of thrombogenic parts of the disrupted vessel wall.[2] Plaque compression or reduction of plaque volume contributes marginally to the extent of luminal widening after PTCA.[1]

Different alternative interventional techniques from PTCA were developed to gain postinterventional luminal widening by reduction of the obstructive plaque volume. These techniques include directional coronary atherectomy, high-speed rotational angioplasty, the transluminal extraction catheter, and excimer laser angioplasty.

Excimer laser angioplasty is the preferred laser technique for application in coronary artery disease.[3,4] The name 'excimer' is an abbreviation for 'excited dimer'. Laser energy is produced when the active medium (for example, HCI gas) is excited by electrical energy and emits monochromatic, coherent light. Laser energy can be emitted as a continuous or pulsed wave. The excimer laser emits pulsed ultraviolet laser light at 308 nm. Excimer laser energy ablates inorganic material by photochemical mechanisms that involve the breaking of molecular bonds without generation of heat. In vivo, the exact mechanism of tissue ablation is unknown, but it probably consists of photochemical localized thermal and mechanical effects. Some intravascular ultrasound studies documented lumen enlargement due to atheroablation and vessel expansion,[5] while others demonstrate little or no plaque ablation.[6] Furthermore, laser angioplasty was thought to limit elastic recoil. This could not be demonstrated under clinical conditions.[5]

The excimer laser is a contact laser, which requires contact between the laser catheter and the coronary plaque. Blood or contrast medium avidly absorb ultraviolet laser energy, inducing significant acoustic effects resulting in tissue disruption and dissection. Intracoronary injection of saline solution during the period of laser activation with replacement of blood and contrast medium at the contact site of the laser has been shown to avoid these adverse mechanisms.[7]

Conventional excimer laser catheters are front-firing, concentric, and track over conventional coronary angioplasty guide wires. The current concentric designs use more than 200 individual fibers concentrically arranged around the guide wire lumen. Limitations of these concentric laser catheter designs include the inability to treat highly eccentric lesions on an inner curve of a severe bend. More recently, rapid exchange laser catheters have become available with an eccentric guide wire lumen better to treat eccentric lesions. Stand-alone laser angioplasty procedures are rare because catheter diameters range from 1.4 to 2.0 mm and usually leave substantial residual stenosis requiring adjunctive PTCA.[8,9] The overall laser success is reported to be greater than 80%. Peri- or postinterventional complications such as transient vessel closure, spasm or perforation are reported more frequently after laser angioplasty as compared with PTCA.[8,9] Angiographic restenosis was not reduced after excimer laser angioplasty compared with PTCA.[8–11]

Furthermore, a laser guide wire has been recently developed for crossing chronic total occlusions. This

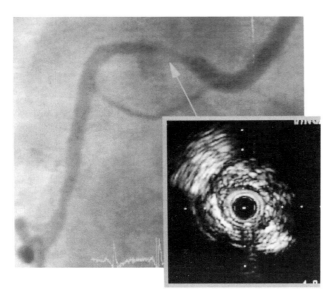

Figure 22.1. Angiogram and intravascular ultrasound image of a patient with an ostial stenosis of the right coronary artery before excimer laser angioplasty.

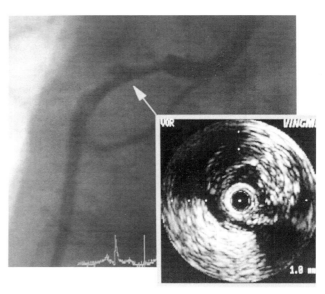

Figure 22.2. Angiogram and intravascular ultrasound image of the patient with ostial stenosis of the right coronary artery presented in Fig. 22.1 after excimer laser angioplasty with a 1.7 mm laser catheter.

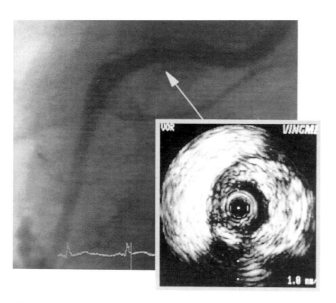

Figure 22.3. Angiogram and intravascular ultrasound image of the patient with ostial stenosis of the right coronary artery presented in Fig. 22.1 after excimer laser angioplasty with a 1.7 mm laser catheter and adjunct balloon angioplasty. 3.2 F, 30 MHz transducer, 1 mm calibration.

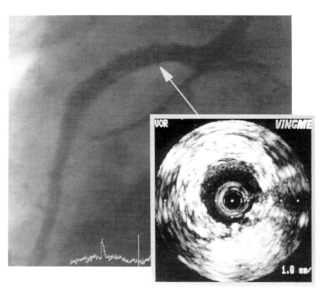

Figure 22.4. Angiogram and intravascular ultrasound image of the patient with ostial stenosis of the right coronary artery presented in Fig. 22.1 after excimer laser angioplasty with a 1.7 mm laser catheter, adjunct balloon angioplasty and stent implantation.

0.018 inch (0.46 mm) wire has a shapable tip and consists of 12 individual front-firing laser fibers of 45 micron in diameter.

The first case presented is a 53-year-old patient with an ostial lesion of the right coronary artery (Fig. 22.1). The corresponding intravascular ultrasound

image using a 3.2 F., 30 MHz CVIS catheter (Cardiovascular Imaging Systems, Sunnyvale CA, USA) documented sonolucent soft plaque material with some calcification, with echo shadowing from seven to nine o'clock. After passage of the lesion with a 0.014 inch (0.36 mm) floppy guide wire a 1.7 mm Vitesse excimer laser angioplasty rapid

before Intervention

after 1.4 mm Excimer laser

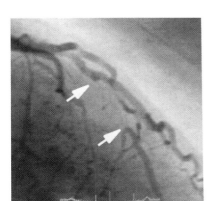
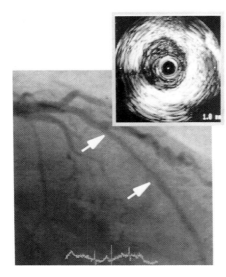

Figure 22.5. Angiograms and intravascular ultrasound image of a patient with chronic occlusion of the left anterior descending artery before (left) and after (right) successful recanalization with a laser guide wire and additional excimer laser angioplasty. White arrows indicate proximal and distal ends of the occlusion.

after PTCA
(3.0 mm balloon)

after stenting
(3.0 mm balloon)

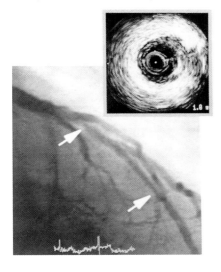
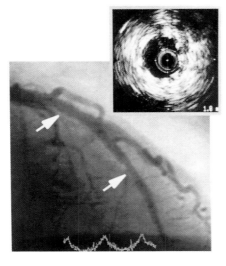

Figure 22.6. Angiograms and intravascular ultrasound images of the patient with chronic occlusion of the left anterior descending artery presented in Fig. 22.5 after successful recanalization with a laser guide wire, additional excimer laser angioplasty, adjunct balloon angioplasty (PTCA, left) and adjunct stent implantation (right) (3 mm balloon). White arrows indicate proximal and distal ends of the treated occlusion. 3.2 F, 30 MHz transducer, 1 mm calibration.

exchange catheter (Spectranetics, Colorado Springs CO, USA) was advanced through the target lesion with saline flushing during laser exposure. During the passage there was some resistance at the middle part of the lesion which was attributed to the calcification documented in the preprocedural intravascular ultrasound image. The angiogram after laser angioplasty documented some lumen widening with contrast-medium staining in a cave in the middle part of the slightly bent lesion (Fig. 22.2). The corresponding intravascular ultrasound image documented some eccentric lumen created in the plaque at one o'clock. To avoid potential vessel

perforation by using a larger laser angioplasty catheter, it was decided to perform adjunct balloon angioplasty with a 3.5 mm balloon catheter. Figure 22.3 shows the angiographic result after two inflations at 8 atm for 60 s. There was a marked improvement in lumen dimensions, and contrast staining in the cave was no longer present. Nevertheless, the corresponding intravascular ultrasound image still documented substantial plaque burden but no longer a cave in the plaque. To optimize the final result, a 16 mm NIR stent (Boston Scientific, Boston, MA) was implanted on a 4 mm balloon at 15 atm. Final angiographic and intravascular results documented the creation of a large lumen with complete stent strut apposition to the vessel wall (Fig. 22.4). This example supports the potential risk of vessel perforation by laser angioplasty even in slightly bent vessel segments.

The second case is a 73-year-old patient who had an anterior myocardial infarction nine months before the actual procedure. Coronary angiography was performed because of progressive angina pectoris during physical stress and documented a total occlusion of the left anterior descending coronary artery distal to the origin of the first diagonal branch with contrast filling of the distal vessel via collaterals from the diagonal branch (Fig. 22.5). Quantitative coronary angiography revealed an occlusion length of 30 mm. Recanalization with standard mechanical 0.014 inch guide wire systems, even with catheter back-up, failed. Therefore recanalization with a 0.018 inch Prima laser wire (Spectranetics) was attempted. After a total lasing time of 155 s the laser guide wire was advanced through the occlusion and entered the distal part of the left anterior descending artery. Then

a 1.4 mm Vitesse laser catheter was advanced over the laser guide wire through the occlusion. The angiographic result documented the creation of a smooth channel between the proximal and distal parts of the occlusion (Fig. 22.5). The corresponding intravascular ultrasound image (3.2 F., 30 MHz CVIS catheter) documented persisting soft tissue around the imaging catheter that obstructed the channel created by the 1.4 mm laser catheter. Adjunct PTCA with a 3.0 mm balloon (five inflations at 8 atm for a maximum of three minutes) was performed to improve lumen dimensions. The postinterventional angiogram and intravascular ultrasound image documented a clear improvement of the created lumen but some haziness and substantial residual stenosis in the proximal part (Fig. 22.6). Dissection membranes could not be documented by intravascular ultrasound. To optimize the interventional result, a 36 mm NIR stent (Scimed, USA) was implanted on a 3.0 mm balloon catheter at 15 atm. The final angiogram documented the creation of a reconstructed vessel conduit, while the intravascular ultrasound image documented complete stent strut apposition to the vessel wall (Fig. 22.6).

References

1 Waller BF. 'Crackers, breakers, stretchers, drillers, scrapers, shavers, burners, welders and melters'—the future treatment of atherosclerotic coronary artery disease? A clinical–morphologic assessment. *J Am Coll Cardiol* 1989; **13**: 969–87.

2 Tan K, Sulke N, Taube N, Sowton E. Clinical and lesion morphologic determinants of coronary angioplasty success and complications: current experience. *J Am Coll Cardiol* 1995; **25**: 855–65.

3 Litvack F. *Coronary Laser Angioplasty.* (Boston, MA: Blackwell Scientific Publications, 1992).

4 Parikh A, Eigler N, Litvack F. Excimer laser coronary angioplasty. In: Freed M, Crines C, Safian RD, eds. *The New Manual of Interventional Cardiology* (Birmingham, MI: Physicians Press, 1996): 573–81.

5 Mintz GS, Kovach JA, Javier SP et al. Mechanisms of lumen enlargement after excimer laser coronary angioplasty: an intravascular ultrasound study. *Circulation* 1995; **92**: 3408–14.

6 Honye J, Mahon DJ, Nakamura S et al. Intravascular ultrasound imaging after excimer laser angioplasty. *Cathet Cardiovasc Diagn* 1994; **32**: 213–22.

7 Deckelbaum LI, Natarjan MK, Bittl JA et al. for the percutaneous excimer laser coronary angioplasty (PELCA) investigators. Effect of intracoronary saline infusion on dissection during excimer laser coronary angioplasty: a randomized trial. *J Am Coll Cardiol* 1995; **26**: 1264–9.

8 Appleman YEA, Piek JJ, Strikwerda S et al. Randomized trial of excimer laser angioplasty versus balloon angioplasty for treatment of obstructive coronary artery disease. *Lancet* 1996; **347**: 79–84.

9 Strikwerda S, Montauban-van-Swijndregt E, Foley DP et al. Immediate and late outcome of excimer laser and balloon coronary angioplasty: a quantitative angiographic comparison based on matched lesions. *J Am Coll Cardiol* 1995; **26**: 939–46.

10 Ghazzal ZMB, Burton E, Weintraub WS et al. Predictors of restenosis after excimer laser coronary angioplasty. *Am J Cardiol* 1995; **75**: 1012–14.

11 Vandormael M, Reifart N, Preusler W et al. Six months follow-up results following excimer laser angioplasty, rotational atherectomy and balloon angioplasty for complex lesions: ERBAC study. *Circulation* 1994; **90**: I213.

23 Assessment of balloon angioplasty and directional atherectomy with three-dimensional intracoronary ultrasound

Clemens von Birgelen, Antonino Nicosia, Patrick W Serruys and Jos R T C Roelandt

Introduction

Intracoronary ultrasound (ICUS) permits the assessment of plaque eccentricity and composition before the intervention and the guidance of catheter-based interventional techniques.[1] Preintervention ICUS findings frequently give rise to a modification of the therapeutic concept.[2] One of the most frequent reasons for a change of therapeutic strategy or selecting a specific interventional device based on ICUS findings has been the calcification of the target lesion.

Detection of lesion calcification prior to the intervention

Using intracoronary ultrasound coherent deposits of calcium (Fig. 23.1) are found in about 80% of the patients undergoing coronary balloon angioplasty (BA).[3–5] Information on calcification of the target stenosis is clinically significant, since an increased incidence, depth, and circumferential extension of dissections have been observed post-BA in calcific plaques[6,7] and a higher incidence of complications with a smaller amount of retrievable material after directional coronary atherectomy has been found in the presence of diffuse subendothelial calcification.[8]

Three-dimensional (3D) ICUS[9] allows one to visualize and quantify the length of calcifications, thus permitting an estimation of the total extent of plaque calcification in an entire arterial segment.

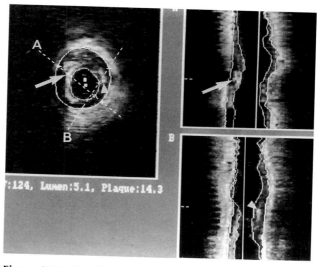

Figure 23.1. Calcified plaque in a right coronary artery before balloon angioplasty. The intimal leading edge and the external boundary of the vessel were detected by a custom-designed computerized three-dimensional intracoronary ultrasound analysis system developed at the Thoraxcenter, Rotterdam. Contour detection was performed in both the two perpendicular longitudinal sections (panels A and B) and the series of cross-sectional images (left panel). Arrowheads indicate calcium, visible in the longitudinal and cross-sectional view. (Reprinted, with permission, from ref. 35.)

Morphometric information on the plaque dimensions can generally be obtained with ICUS but cannot be gained in severely calcified arteries from two-dimensional cross-sectional ICUS images.

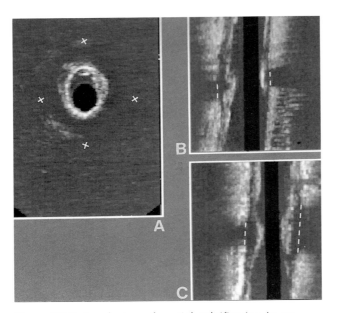

Figure 23.2. Focal circumferential calcification in an atherosclerotic mid-left anterior descending coronary artery. The whole vascular structures are hidden in the echo-shade of the superficial calcification. Using the cross-sectional view (panel A), no estimation of the vessel and plaque area is possible. However, the interpolation of the external vessel contour in two longitudinally reconstructed views (panels B and C) allows one to derive four edge-points (in panel A), which permit one to trace manually an (estimated) elliptical contour of the external vessel boundary.

Three-dimensional reconstruction techniques may permit a reliable estimation by manual tracing and thus a quantification of the vascular dimension even behind circumferential calcium (Fig. 23.2).

Guidance of directional coronary atherectomy

Directional coronary atherectomy (DCA) is particularly efficient when it is applied to 'soft', eccentric plaques without superficial calcium (Fig. 23.3) in proximal or midcoronary segments.[2,10–12] Furthermore, ICUS is clinically useful in guiding the device and provides reliable information on plaque eccentricity,[1,8,13] and permits one to minimize the damage of the nondiseased vessel wall.

Using 3D ICUS, the orientation of the atherectomy device in relation to side-branches is simplified (Fig. 23.4) and the detection of deep or spiral cuts is facilitated.[14] ICUS examinations before and after DCA suggest that the operative mechanism is mainly based on plaque removal, but also to a certain extent on vessel stretch.[15] Recently, 'plaque compression' was reported to account for 50% of the enlargement of lumen area by DCA;[16] however, this finding may reflect the problem of pre/post studies which consider only changes at the site of the minimal

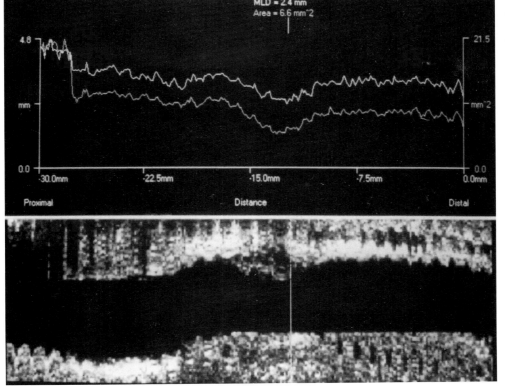

Figure 23.3. Short eccentric lesion in a proximal coronary artery. The longitudinal reconstruction (lower panel) and the on-line measurement of luminal area and minimal diameter are obtained from a three-dimensional reconstruction program (EchoQuant, Indec, Capitola, CA) which detects and subtracts the blood-pool based on acoustic quantification. The measurement of any site of the reconstructed vascular segment (vertical cursor in lower panel) can be displayed immediately (top of upper panel).

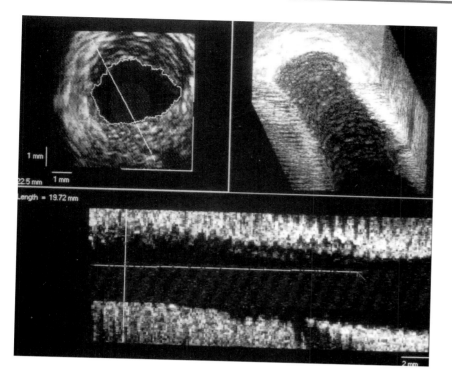

Figure 23.4. 'Soft' eccentric plaque and side-branch. The side-branch, distal to the eccentric plaque, is visible in both the reconstructed longitudinal view (bottom of lower panel) and the cylindrical display (dark side-spot in right upper panel). The longitudinal view can be rotated lengthwise by rotating a longitudinal cursor on the cross-sectional view (left upper panel). Measurement of distances can be performed. The horizontal measurement line in the longitudinal view is an example indicating a distance of 19.7 mm.

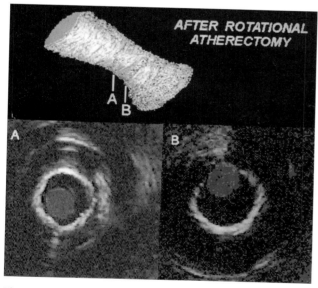

Figure 23.5. Circumferentially calcified proximal left anterior descending coronary artery after rotational atherectomy. The positions of the mid-stenotic (panel A) and proximal (panel B) ICUS cross-sections are indicated in a three-dimensionally reconstructed lumen cast (upper panel). In the cross-sectional images a relatively smooth and circular lumen can be observed. Computerized rotation of the reconstructed lumen cast allows one to evaluate rapidly the lumen shape of an entire vascular segment, demonstrating in this case a smooth shape with a residual luminal obstruction. (Reprinted, with permission, from ref. 20.)

luminal area, a limitation which can only be overcome by quantification with 3D ultrasound.[17,18] The applicability and benefit of 3D assessment of coronary plaque has been demonstrated in directional atherectomy.[19] A 3D lumen cast display may be used to facilitate the visual assessment of the luminal geometry (Fig. 23.5).

Balloon angioplasty and coronary dissections

The operative mechanism of interventional devices such as BA can be studied by use of quantitative angiography;[20] however, ICUS is superior since it directly visualizes the vessel wall.[21] ICUS detected that vessel wall stretching and dissection are the principal operative mechanisms and that dissections frequently occur adjacent to a calcific plaque portion (Fig. 23.6),[22] suggesting that localized calcium may play a significant role in promoting their incidence. Even in complex dissections, demonstrated by ICUS, filling defects are frequently not visualized in the angiogram.

Since dissections are important predictors of immediate outcome and adverse events,[23] information on the vessel trauma is of clinical interest.

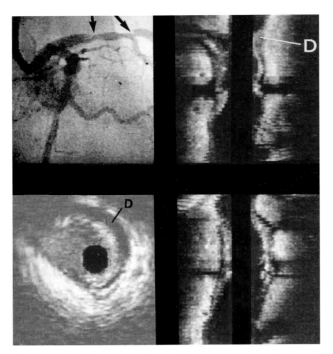

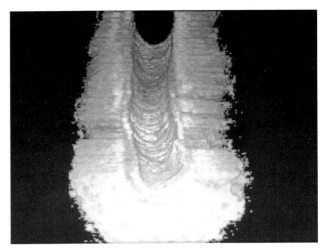

Figure 23.7. Cylindrical 3D reconstruction after balloon angioplasty. The spatial reconstruction demonstrates a good result after percutaneous transluminal coronary angioplasty of a focally calcified arterial segment. 'Gaps' in the reconstructed vessel represent the echo-shades behind the deposits of calcium.

Figure 23.6. Dissection after balloon angioplasty. In the angiogram (left upper panel) a dissection (smaller arrowhead) was found in a left anterior descending coronary artery (LAD) after dilatation of the severely calcified lesion. Also an unexplained obstruction of a large diagonal branch at its origin (larger arrowhead) was noticed, not observed on the preinterventional coronary angiogram. During a motorized pullback of the intracoronary ultrasound catheter through this diagonal branch and the LAD, the dissection could be demonstrated. Two perpendicular longitudinal views (right panels, blood signals removed) were derived from the three-dimensional image dataset, demonstrating the dissection which ranges from the almost circumferentially calcified lesion of the LAD (mid) to the large diagonal branch (top). The letter D in the longitudinal view indicates the spot where the dissection narrows the origin of the diagonal branch. This site corresponds with the cross-sectional intracoronary ultrasound image, displayed in the left lower panel. Note there the dissection (D) and the high echogenicity of the blood inside the lumen, indicating the impairment of blood flow.

Although the sensitivity of ICUS in detecting arterial dissections is high,[22] the longitudinal extent of complex flaps cannot reliably be determined by conventional two-dimensional ICUS imaging. Three-dimensional ICUS providing longitudinal reconstructions has been demonstrated to facilitate the analysis of dissections in peripheral and coronary arteries.[24–26] Excellent agreement between 3D reconstruction of ICUS images and pathologic

findings has been described in the evaluation of length and depth of dissections after balloon angioplasty.[27] During on-line studies with 3D ICUS, measurements of the target lesion and the reference segment can immediately be obtained in the reconstructed longitudinal view, thus facilitating the selection of the optimal type and size of interventional device. On-line reconstruction after BA is particularly valuable, since it permits the immediate assessment of the vessel wall changes (Fig. 23.7) after catheter-based interventions.[28,29] Thus, 3D ICUS may immediately prove the need for adjunctive therapy.

Benefit in the assessment of restenosis

Intracoronary ultrasound is able to help elucidate the vagueness surrounding the mechanisms underlying restenosis.[30] The authors' group studied the mechanism of restenosis separately in two populations of patients, treated by balloon angioplasty or directional coronary atherectomy.[31] It was found that increase in plaque area, representing intimal hyperplasia, was responsible for 92% of the late lumen loss after directional coronary atherectomy, whereas this mechanism accounts for 32% of the late lumen loss after balloon angioplasty. In the population treated by balloon angioplasty a decrease in the total

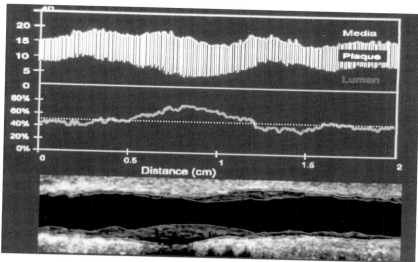

Figure 23.8. Quantitative 3D analysis of a restenotic lesion after directional coronary atherectomy. The detection of the intimal leading edge and the external vessel contour on a set of intracoronary ultrasound images, provided by the analysis system of the Thoraxcenter, Rotterdam,[17,18] allows one to quantify both lumen and plaque area and volume. In the upper panel the plaque area (white) is displayed with the free lumen below the plaque. A diagram of the area obstruction is displayed in the mid panel. The site of the maximum plaque burden and area obstruction corresponds well with the longitudinally reconstructed two-dimensional view (lower panel); however, the results displayed are derived from measurements in a volumetric image dataset. This approach allows the analysis of serial intracoronary ultrasound studies in a much more reliable way than by conventional approaches.

vessel area was the predominant mechanism of restenosis. These findings support the concept of a device-specific mechanism of restenosis, recently stated based on angiographic data.[32]

However, an important limitation of serial studies, using ICUS to compare initial findings with follow-up results,[30,31] is the fact that the sites of ultrasound measurement are not always identical. Longitudinal displays of the three-dimensionally reconstructed ICUS images (Fig. 23.8) allow one serially to evaluate identical sites of the coronary artery in a much more reliable way. Furthermore, measurements of plaque volume can be made which may be of particular interest in the evaluation of the effectiveness of DCA.

In summary, preintervention ICUS imaging is important for BA and DCA. Three-dimensional ICUS allows one to gain additional information and to guide the DCA procedure. Assessment by 3D ICUS after DCA helps to determine the procedural

endpoint. The main benefit after BA is the possibility of evaluating, in case of a threatening dissection or an ambiguous angiographic result, the need for further interventions such as coronary stenting, which is also facilitated by 3D ICUS.[33,34]

References

1 Yock PG, Fitzgerald PJ, Linker DT, Angelsen BAJ. Intravascular ultrasound guidance for catheter-based coronary interventions. *J Am Coll Cardiol* 1991; **17**: 39B–45B.

2 Mintz GS, Pichard AD, Kovach JA et al. Impact of preintervention intravascular ultrasound imaging on transcatheter treatment strategies in coronary artery disease. *Am J Cardiol* 1994; **73**: 423–30.

3 Mintz GA, Douek P, Pichard AD et al. Target lesion calcification in coronary artery disease: an intravascular ultrasound study. *J Am Coll Cardiol* 1992; **20**: 1149–55.

4   Honye J, Mahon DJ, Jain A et al. Morphological effects of coronary balloon angioplasty in vivo assessed by intravascular ultrasound imaging. *Circulation* 1992; **85**: 1012–25.

5   Mintz GS, Popma JJ, Pichard AD et al. Pattern of calcification in coronary artery disease: a statistical analysis of intravascular ultrasound and coronary angiography in 1155 lesions. *Circulation* 1995; **91**: 1959–65.

6   Fitzgerald PJ, Ports TA, Yock PG. Contribution of localized calcium deposits to dissection after angioplasty: an observational study using intravascular ultrasound. *Circulation* 1992; **86**: 64–70.

7   Potkin BN, Keren G, Mintz GS et al. Arterial responses to balloon coronary angioplasty: an intravascular ultrasound study. *J Am Coll Cardiol* 1992; **20**: 942–51.

8   Kimura BJ, Fitzgerald PJ, Sudhir K, Amidon TM, Strunk BL, Yock PG. Guidance of directional coronary atherectomy by intracoronary ultrasound imaging. *Am Heart J* 1992; **124**: 1365–9.

9   Roelandt JRTC, Di Mario C, Pandian NG et al. Three-dimensional reconstruction of intracoronary ultrasound images: rationale, approaches, problems and directions. *Circulation* 1994; **90**: 1044–55.

10 Ellis SG, De Cesare NB, Pinkerton CA et al. Relation of stenosis morphology and clinical presentation to the procedural results of directional coronary atherectomy. *Circulation* 1991; **84**: 644–53.

11 De Lezo JA, Romero M, Medina A et al. Intracoronary ultrasound assessment of directional coronary atherectomy: immediate and follow-up findings. *J Am Coll Cardiol* 1993; **21**: 298–307.

12 Popma JJ, Mintz GS, Satler LF et al. Clinical and angiographic outcome after directional coronary atherectomy: a qualitative and quantative analysis using coronary arteriography and intravascular ultrasound. *Am J Cardiol* 1993; **72**: 55E–64E.

13 Di Mario C, von Birgelen C, Prati F et al. Three-diemsional reconstruction of two-dimensional intracoronary ultrasound: clinical or research tool? *Br Heart J* 1995; **73**(suppl 2): 26–32.

14 Smucker ML, Kil D, Sarnat WS, Howard PF. Is three-dimensional reconstruction a gimmick or a useful clinical tool? Experience in coronary atherectomy. *J Am Coll Cardiol* 1992; **19**: 115A.

15 Braden GA, Herrington DM, Downes TR, Kutcher MA, Little WC. Qualitative and quantative contrasts in the mechanisms of lumen enlargement by coronary balloon angioplasty and directional coronary atherectomy. *J Am Coll Cardiol* 1994; **23**: 40–8.

16 Suneja R, Nair RN, Reddy KG, Rasheed Q, Sheehan HM, Hodgson J McB. Mechanisms of angiographically successful directional coronary atherectomy: evaluation by intracoronary ultrasound and comparison with transluminal coronary angioplasty. *Am Heart J* 1993; **126**: 507–14.

17 von Birgelen C, Di Mario C, Li W et al. Morphometric analysis in three-dimensional intracoronary ultrasound: an in-vitro and in-vivo study using a novel system for the contour detection of lumen and plaque. *Am Heart J* 1996; **132**: 516–17.

18 von Birgelen C, van der Lugt A, Nicosia A et al. Computerized assessment of coronary lumen and atherosclerotic plaque dimensions in three-dimensional intravascular ultrasound correlated with histomorphometry. *Am J Cardiol* 1996 (in press).

19 Dhawale PJ, Rasheed Q, Mecca W, Nair R, Hodgson J McB. Analysis of plaque volume during DCA using a volumetrically accurate three dimensional ultrasound technique. *Circulation* 1993; **88**: I550.

20 von Birgelen C, Umans V, Di Mario C et al. Mechanism of high-speed rotational atherectomy and ajunctive balloon angioplasty revisited by quantitative coronary angiography: edge detection versus videodensitometry. *Am Heart J* 1995; **130**: 405–12.

21 Wolfe CL, Klette MA, Trask RV et al. Assessment of the results of percutaneous transluminal coronary angioplasty using an integrated ultrasound imaging-angioplasty catheter. *Cathet Cardiovasc Diagn* 1994; **32**: 108–12.

22 Werner GS, Sold G, Buchwald A, Kreuzer H, Wiegand V. Intravascular ultrasound imaging of human coronary arteries after percutaneous transluminal angioplasty: morpholic and quantative assessment. *Am Heart J* 1991; **122**: 212–20.

23 Tenaglia AN, Buller CE, Kisslo KB, Phillips HR, Stack RS, Davidson CJ. Intracoronary ultrasound predictors of adverse outcomes after coronary artery interventions. *J Am Coll Cardiol* 1992; **20**: 1385–90.

24 Rosenfield K, Kaufman J, Pieczek A et al. Lumen cast analysis: a quantative format to expedite on-line analysis of 3D intravascular ultrasound images. *J Am Coll Cardiol* 1992; **19**: 115A.

25 Rosenfield K, Kaufman J, Pieczek A, Langevin RE, Razvi S, Isner JM. Real-time three-dimensional reconstruction of intravascular ultrasound images of iliac arteries. *Am J Cardiol* 1992; **70**: 412–15.

26 Schryver TE, Popma JJ, Kent KM, Leon MB, Eldredge S, Mintz GS. Use of intracoronary ultrasound to identify the true coronary lumen in chronic coronary dissection treated with intracoronary stenting. *Am J Cardiol* 1992; **69**: 1107–8.

27 Coy KM, Park JC, Fishbein MC et al. In vitro validation of three-diemsional intravascular ultrasound for the evaluation of arterial injury after balloon angioplasty. *J Am Coll Cardiol* 1992; **20**: 692–700.

28 Rosenfield K, Kaufman J, Pieczek AM et al. Human coronary and peripheral arteries: on-line three-dimensional reconstruction from two-dimensional intravascular US scans. *Radiology* 1992; **184**: 823–32.

29 Mintz GS, Leon MB, Satler LF et al. Clinical experience using a new three-dimensional intravascular ultrasound system before and after transcatheter coronary therapies. *J Am Coll Cardiol* 1992; **19**: 292A.

30 Mintz GS, Kovach JA, Pichard AD et al. Geometric remodeling is the predominant mechanism of clinical restenosis after coronary angioplasty. *J Am Coll Cardiol* 1994; **23**: 138A.

31 Di Mario C, Gil R, Camenzind E et al. Quantitative assessment with intracoronary ultrasound of the mechanisms of restenosis after percutaneous transluminal coronary angioplasty and directional coronary atherectomy. *Am J Cardiol* 1995; **75**: 772–7.

32 Serruys PW, Foley DP, Kirkeeide RL, King III SB. Restenosis revisited: insights provided by quantitative coronary angiography. *Am Heart J* 1993; **126**: 1243–67.

33 von Birgelen C, Kutryk MJB, Gil R et al. Quantification of the minimal luminal cross-sectional area after coronary stenting: two- and three-dimensional intravascular ultrasound versus edge detection and videodensitometry. *Am J Cardiol* 1996; **78**: 52–5.

34 von Birgelen C, Gil R, Ruygrok P et al. Optimized expansion of the Wallstent compared to the Palmaz-Schatz stent: online observations with two- and three-dimensional intracoronary ultrasound after angiographic guidance. *Am Heart J* 1996; **131**: 1067–75.

35 von Birgelen C, Di Mario C, van der Putten N et al. Quantification in three-dimensional intracoronary ultrasound: importance of image acquisition and segmentation. *Cardiologie* 1995; **2**: 67–72.

24 Intravascular ultrasound to predict and assess restenosis after coronary intervention

Günter Görge, Fengqi Liu, Junbo Ge, Michael Haude and Raimund Erbel

Introduction

Restenosis is defined as loss of lumen gained after an invasive coronary artery procedure.[1-5] Besides acute recoil, restenosis is the main drawback of percutaneous coronary angioplasty. It is a chronic event and after 6 months, the process does not usually progress.[3] In most cases, patients present with recurrence of symptoms such as angina or dyspnea, but a significant percentage will develop 'silent' restenosis.[6] Fortunately, restenotic lesions lead only occasionally to myocardial infarcts.[7] At present, from 20% to over 50% of patients will suffer from restenosis after coronary artery intervention, depending on procedural characteristics and the definition of restenosis.

The most commonly used definition of restenosis is dichotomous: it is defined as a >50% diameter stenosis at follow-up coronary angiography. This definition is best known as the 'Thoraxcenter I' definition. Because many patients are in the range of 30–60% diameter stenosis, other definitions are also in use. The 'Thoraxcenter II' definition is described as a loss of minimal luminal diameter >0.72 mm from the initial intervention to follow-up. This definition requires exact quantitative coronary angiography measurements. Besides these two definitions, other trials used other definitions, known as National Heart, Lung, and Blood Institute (NHLBI) definitions 1–4. NHLBI 1 is defined as a 30% increase in stenosis diameter between acute intervention and follow-up; NHLBI 2 is defined as an increase in stenosis diameter of <50% after intervention to >70% at control angiography; NHLBI 3 describes a <10%

difference of acute and follow-up luminal dimensions as restenosis. Finally, NHLBI 4 is characterized as a 50% loss of initial luminal gain.[1-3]

Theories to explain and interventions to prevent restenosis

Numerous efforts have been made to explain or prevent restenosis. To date, only a mechanical approach, the implantation of coronary artery stents, was able to reduce restenosis rate in de novo lesions.[8-11] Besides this, the results of attempts to predict the occurrence of restenosis in an individual patient on the basis of patient, lesion or interventional parameters have been puzzling.[12] Despite the identification of various predictive factors, these measures do not usually allow risk stratification in the individual patient with 100% predictability. The reasons lie in the complex mechanisms of restenosis. According to Haudenschild, the basic principles in the development of restenosis are the same as those for proper healing and remodeling of the vessel wall after the trauma of angioplasty, but different from the process of initial plaque formation and growth.[13] The difference between a clinically significant, that is, an hemodynamically relevant (re)stenosis and a 'physiologic' remodeling after percutaneous transluminal coronary angioplasty (PTCA) is in both the quantity and the timing of these processes. The majority of scientific knowledge favors local rather than systemic factors as largely determining the development of restenosis.

Potential role of intravascular ultrasound (IVUS)

In this context, what could be the potential role of IVUS in explaining restenosis? It is unlikely that IVUS will contribute to the cellular mechanisms of restenosis. But as a tomographic technique IVUS has the potential to

(a) assess the stenosis morphology before intervention to allow optimal device selection and to predict acute complications;

(b) identify the principles of luminal enlargement such as vessel stretch, plaque remodeling, and recoil;

(c) aid in finding the balance between the 'response to injury' theory for triggering restenosis and the 'bigger the better' dogma in interventional cardiology;

(d) describe the amount of intimal proliferation and vessel remodeling at follow-up angiography.

The acute success of therapeutic intervention is mainly determined by the acute gain in free lumen and avoidance of complications (Fig. 24.1). It is also known that an optimal, morphologic and functional initial result (or a 'stent-like' acute result after PTCA) lowers the chances of restenosis.[14–16] The questions are whether preinterventional IVUS can predict the outcome of the intervention, whether IVUS is superior to angiography in this respect, and whether postinterventional studies can optimize the

acute result or predict restenosis.[17–21] One principal problem is that preinterventional IVUS is only possible if the lesion can be passed over before the intervention. Even more time-consuming procedures like motorized pullbacks or ECG-triggered pullbacks to allow three-dimensional reconstruction are often not tolerated by patients or put them at an unacceptably high risk of ischemic complications. However, pre-PTCA IVUS of tight stenosis might be beneficial because of the Dotter effect of the IVUS catheter. Alfonso et al. showed an increase in diameter after IVUS, but before PTCA, from 0.84 to 1.16 mm in studies using 4.8 F. IVUS catheters.[22]

IVUS, device selection, and prediction of outcome

Theoretically, IVUS can help in choosing the optimal device for a given lesion. This could mean either to select the balloon dimensions and inflation pressures based on IVUS measurements of luminal and vessel dimensions, or to select an alternative technique, for example, rotablators in calcified lesions or atherectomy in lesions with a large plaque load. However, no prospective or randomized study has assessed the decision-making role of IVUS before intervention. Mintz et al. reported that preinterventional IVUS led to a different interventional strategy in 20% of cases. The same group reported in 1155 lesions on the presence and distribution of

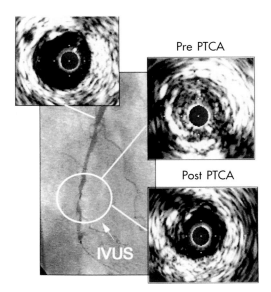

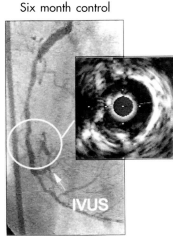

Figure 24.1. Example of a pre- and post-PTCA IVUS examination at six-month follow-up in a right coronary artery. The upper left image shows the proximal reference segment. The lesion is in the distal part of the right coronary artery. The 3.5 F. IVUS catheter leads to an occlusion distal to the stenosis (left angiogram). Pre-PTCA IVUS shows 180° deep calcification and superimposed plaque material with almost complete occlusion of the lumen. After PTCA, only very little residual stenosis is found and the formerly stenosed segment shows a smooth surface. The six-month follow-up (images on the right) is without angiographically visible restenosis. IVUS shows a large free lumen with no signs of intimal hyperplasia. 3.5 F, 20 MHz transducer, 1 mm calibration.

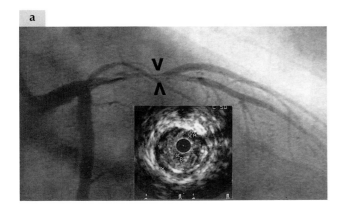

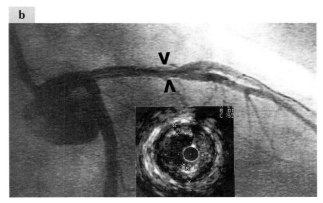

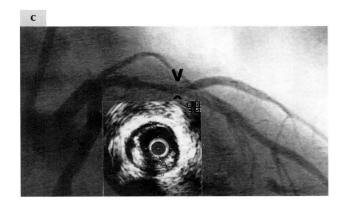

Figure 24.2. Serial angiographic and IVUS images in a 59-year-old patient with a proximal LAD lesion, shown in the 30° RAO view. Before PTCA (a), an eccentric stenosis was found, occlusive for the 3.5 French 30 MHz IVUS catheter (Hewlett and Packard Sonos system, distance between two dots equals 1 mm). After PTCA (b), a good angiographical result was found. However, IVUS revealed complex remodeling of the lesion, with an increase in total vessel diameter and a radial deep tear at 1 o'clock and residual plaque from 1 o'clock to 7 o'clock. The follow-up angiogram (c) in this asymptomatic patient revealed a decrease in total vessel area, but a large enough free lumen without apparent intimal hyperplasia.

calcium, where IVUS was superior to angiography in revealing the presence, length, and arc of calcification. The arc of calcification was predictive for the occurrence of dissections after PTCA.[21,23,24] Rotablation instead of PTCA or atherectomy might be superior in patients with heavy calcification discovered during preinterventional IVUS.

IVUS for mechanisms of PTCA

Several groups focused their interest on IVUS after PTCA better to understand the mechanisms of the procedure and to find predictors of restenosis.[25–29] The findings in post-PTCA IVUS studies led to various classifications of the effect of balloon angioplasty on the vessel wall. The most detailed classifications have been published by Honye et al. and by Gerber et al. (see chapter 23).[26,28] It could be shown that most lesions are eccentric in nature, and that tears and dissections are the main mechanisms leading to luminal enlargement, while stretching of the disease-free wall or plaque compression is found less frequently after PTCA. The implications of the postinterventional morphologic characteristics alone seem to be limited, and interest focuses at present on the definition of residual stenosis and residual

plaque load assessed by IVUS after angiographically 'optimal' (Fig. 24.2) PTCA.[30–32] Because of the limitations of angiography in revealing changes of the coronary artery wall, IVUS is at present the only method with which to measure exactly the residual area stenosis, or 'plaque load' in vivo. Different groups have shown an average residual stenosis of approximately 55–65% after PTCA (Fig. 24.3).[26,29,30,32] The question remains whether a reduction in the residual area stenosis could result in better long-term results.

Postinterventional IVUS for prognosis after PTCA

The PICTURE trial (Post Intra-Coronary Treatment Ultrasound Restenosis Evaluation) is the first larger trial to be completed looking at ultrasound markers for restenosis. The results were discouraging; in about 200 patients no correlation was found between the various morphologic and dimensional parameters and the outcome of the patients.[27] On the other hand, the GUIDE II trial showed a significant potential for residual plaque burden and luminal cross-sectional area to predict restenosis.[31]

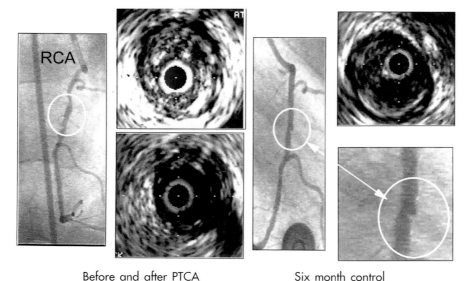

Before and after PTCA   Six month control

Figure 24.3. Development of restenosis after PTCA of a RCA lesion. Before PTCA an almost occlusive lesion with soft and fibrous parts was found (left angiogram and upper left IVUS image). After PTCA a good result with a 2.8 × 3 mm free lumen (distance between two white calibration spots = 1 mm) was achieved. After 3 months, the patient had exercise inducable angina and a positive bicycle stress test at 100 Watts. The follow-up angiography (right images) showed a short restenotic segment with half-moon shaped intimal hyperplasia at the distal stenosis.

Comparable results were published by Mintz et al. who found a >50% restenosis rate in patients with a >70% area stenosis after PTCA.[30] Reports of Görge et al. showed a significant prognostic effect for the development of restenosis for minimal luminal diameter and percentage residual area stenosis measured by IVUS. Additionally, patients with circular dissections had an inferior prognosis.[32]

IVUS-guided PTCA

In future IVUS should aid in identifying in particular patients with 'false-optimal' angiographic results. The cut-off point in percentage area stenosis predictive for an optimal long-term result has yet to be established. However, modifications of PTCA to provide a larger luminal gain post-PTCA are mainly limited to higher balloon inflation pressures and larger balloon diameters. A ratio of the reference segment to the expected balloon diameter of >1.1 assessed by angiography led to a higher complication rate without benefit in long-term outcome.[14] On the contrary, perliminary results of the CLOUT trial showed that balloon size selection based on IVUS instead of angiography improves acute PTCA results without an increase in complication rates.[33] Tobis et al. reported on 154 lesions treated with PTCA or atherectomy, randomized to IVUS-guided

or angiographically guided interventions. They found a higher restenosis rate in IVUS-guided interventions, explained by the fact that aggressive multiple interventions might further traumatize the vessel, leading to increased restenosis rates.[34] Therefore, given these conflicting yet preliminary results of various established groups, the role of IVUS-guided interventions and the impact on restenosis has yet to be evaluated.

IVUS for understanding restenosis

Intravascular ultrasound has already contributed to the explanation of the morphology of restenosis in patients.[35–37] Di Mario et al. studied 18 patients treated with PTCA before, immediately after, and 6 months after coronary interventions by angiography and IVUS. The increase in lumen area was the result of a combination of plaque reduction (52% of luminal increase) and increase in total lumen area (48%). This last mechanism was prevalent in the lesions showing wall fracture or dissection after treatment and in the lesions with a mixed or calcific composition. Concentric lesions showed a greater plaque compression than eccentric lesions. Plaque increase was responsible for 32% of the late lumen

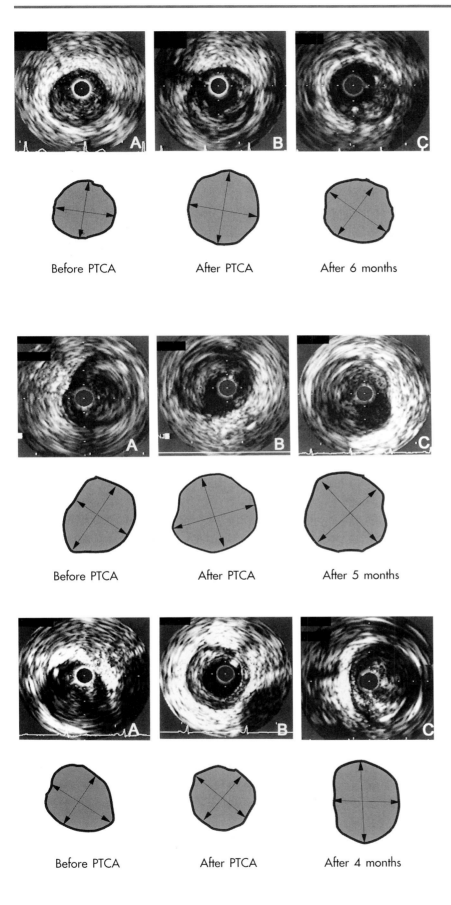

Before PTCA   After PTCA   After 6 months

Before PTCA   After PTCA   After 5 months

Before PTCA   After PTCA   After 4 months

Figure 24.4. Effect of PTCA on lumen and total vessel dimensions. Before PTCA (left), IVUS depicts an eccentric plaque and a narrow residual lumen. After PTCA, a Type 7 dissection with flap is found. Luminal dimensions also increased and the angiographical appearance was normal. The total vessel area had increased significantly, as illustrated by the drawings below the IVUS images. For 6 months, the clinical course had been uneventful. Follow-up IVUS showed a decrease in total vessel area. However, the flap had disappeared and the luminal dimensions were almost the same. 3.5 F, 20 MHz transducer, 1 mm calibration.

Figure 24.5. Example of a patient with unstable angina. Before PTCA, a very narrow free lumen with a large plaque load was found during IVUS. The plaque showed signs of 'layering'. PTCA resulted in a limited increase in total vessel area, but a significant increase in luminal area and inhomogenous composition of the plaque (see echolucent area from 10 o'clock–11.30 within plaque). At follow-up, the total vessel and plaque area had increased, but the luminal dimensions were unchanged. 3.5 F, 20 MHz transducer, 1 mm calibration.

Figure 24.6. Example of restenosis most likely due to intimal hyperplasia, despite adaptive plaque growth and vessel remodeling. Before PTCA, an eccentric plaque with a 'hazy' surface was found. Surprisingly, PTCA resulted in a complete redistribution and compression of the plaque material and its increased echodensity. Exact orientation within the vessel was possible due to the side-branch imaged in image A (2 o'clock to 5 o'clock) and image B (4 o'clock to 6 o'clock). The patient developed angina CCS class II after three months. Despite an increase in total vessel area, the authors found an almost complete narrowing of the lumen due to a very 'soft' plaque formation.

loss after PTCA. In PTCA patients, a chronic reduction in total vessel area was the main operative mechanism of lumen reduction (67%) and was mainly prevalent in lesions with a mixed or calcific composition. Additionally, Kimura et al. from the SURE trial described the results of serial IVUS examinations in 25 patients before and after balloon angioplasty, at 24 hours after angioplasty, at 1 month after PTCA and at 6 months. They also identified geometric remodeling as the main cause of late lumen loss in 83% of patients, where intimal hyperplasia alone had only an additional effect. The main argument for the role of geometric remodeling was the occurrence of 63% of total plaque increase within 24 hours after PTCA, excluding intimal hyperplasia as a main cause of restenosis (Figs 24.4–24.6).[38]

Summary and outlook

Post-PTCA IVUS examination enables one to assess the effects of the invasive procedure on luminal dimensions and the amount of residual plaque. The latter is a unique feature of IVUS in comparison with angiography. These values seem to be related to the occurrence of restenosis, although the prognostic significance in an individual patient is still unclear. IVUS has contributed significantly to the understanding of restenosis in humans. Serial IVUS studies have underlined the role of geometric remodeling. This explains the beneficial effects seen by stenting after PTCA and the failure of most therapeutic interventions to reduce restenosis that aimed at the reduction of intimal hyperplasia alone.[39]

References

1　Gershlick A, Brack MJ, More RS, Syndercombe-Court D, Balcon R. Angiographic restenosis after angioplasty: comparison of definitions and correlation with clinical outcome. *Coron Artery Dis* 1993; **4**: 73–81.

2　Kelsey SF, James M, Holubkov AL, Holubkov R, Cowley MJ, Detre KM. Results of percutaneous transluminal coronary angioplasty in women. 1985–1986 National Heart, Lung, and Blood Institute's Coronary Angioplasty Registry. *Circulation* 1993; **87**: 720–7.

3　Serruys PW, Luijten HE, Beatt KJ et al. Incidence of restenosis after successful coronary angioplasty: a time-related phenomenon. A quantitative angiographic study in 342 consecutive patients at 1, 2, 3, and 4 months. *Circulation* 1988; **77**: 361–71.

4　Rensing BJ, Hermans WRM, Vos J et al. Angiographic risk factors of luminal narrowing after coronary balloon angioplasty using balloon measurements to reflect stretch and elastic recoil at the dilatation site. *Am J Cardiol* 1992; **69**: 584–91.

5　Rozenman Y, Gilon D, Welber S, Sapoznikov D, Gotsman MS. Clinical and angiographic predictors of immediate recoil after successful coronary angioplasty and relation to late restenosis. *Am J Cardiol* 1993; **72**: 1020–5.

6　Rupprecht HJ, Brennecke R, Kottmeyer M et al. Short- and long-term outcome after PTCA in patients with stable and unstable angina. *Eur Heart J* 1990; **11**: 964–73.

7　Weintraub WS, Ghazzal ZM, Douglas JS Jr et al. Long-term clinical follow-up in patients with angiographic restudy after successful angioplasty. *Circulation* 1993; **87**: 831–40.

8　Bourassa MG, Lesperance J, Eastwood C et al. Clinical, physiologic, anatomic and procedural factors predictive of restenosis after percutaneous transluminal coronary angioplasty. *J Am Coll Cardiol* 1991; **18**: 368–76.

9　Califf RM, Fortin DF, Frid DJ et al. Restenosis after coronary angioplasty: an overview. *J Am Coll Cardiol* 1991; **17(Suppl B)**: 2B–13B.

10　Fischman DL, Leon MB, Baim DS et al. A randomized comparison of coronary-stent placement and balloon angioplasty in the treatment of coronary artery disease. Stent Restenosis Study Investigators. *N Engl J Med* 1994; **331**: 496–501.

11　Serruys PW, de Jaeger P, Kiemeneij F et al. For the Benestent study group. A comparison of balloon-expandable-stent implantation with balloon angioplasty in patients with coronary heart disease. *N Engl J Med* 1994; **331**: 489–95.

12　Hirshfeld JW Jr, Schwartz JS, Jugo R et al. Restenosis after coronary angioplasty: a multivariate statistical model to relate lesion and procedure variables to restenosis. *J Am Coll Cardiol* 1991; **18**: 647–56.

13　Haudenschild CC. Restenosis: pathophysiologic considerations. In: Topol EJ, ed. *Textbook of Interventional Cardiology*, Volume 1, second edition (Philadelphia, PA: WB Saunders Company, 1994): 382–98.

14　Roubin GS, Douglas JS Jr, King SB III et al. Influence of balloon size on initial success, acute complications, and restenosis after percutaneous transluminal coronary angioplasty. A prospective randomized study. *Circulation* 1988; **78**: 557–65.

15　Zijlstra F, Den-Boer A, Reiber JHC, Van-Es GA, Lubsen J, Serruys PW. Assessment of immediate and long-term functional results of percutaneous transluminal coronary angioplasty. *Circulation* 1988; **78**: 15–24.

16 De Feyter PJ, Van den Brand M, Jaarman G, Van Domburg R, Serruys PW, Suryapranata H. Acute coronary artery occlusion during and after percutaneous transluminal coronary angioplasty. Frequency, prediction, clinical course, management, and follow-up. *Circulation* 1991; **83**: 927–36.

17 Coy KM, Meurer G, Siegel RJ. Intravascular ultrasound imaging: a current perspective. *J Am Coll Cardiol* 1991; **18**: 1811–23.

18 Fitzgerald PJ, Yock PG. Mechanisms and outcomes of angioplasty and atherectomy assessed by intravascular ultrasound imaging. *J Clin Ultrasound* 1993; **21**: 579–88.

19 Görge G, Erbel R, Gerber TC, Ge J, Trauth B, Meyer J. Morphologic findings by intravascular ultrasound and clinical outcome after PTCA. *Circulation* 1992; **84**: 518 (abst).

20 Hodgson JM, Reddy KG, Suneja R, Nair RN, Lesnefsky EJ, Sheehan HM. Intracoronary ultrasound imaging: correlation of plaque morphology with angiography, clinical syndrome and procedural results in patients undergoing coronary angioplasty. *J Am Coll Cardiol* 1993; **21**: 35–44.

21 Mintz GS, Pichard AD, Kovach JA et al. Impact of preintervention intravascular ultrasound imaging on transcatheter treatment strategies in coronary artery disease. *Am J Cardiol* 1994; **73**: 423–30.

22 Alfonso F, Macaya C, Goicolea J et al. Angiographic changes (Dotter effect) produced by intravascular ultrasound imaging before coronary angioplasty. *Am Heart J* 1994; **128**: 244–51.

23 Mintz GS, Douek P, Pichard AD et al. Target lesion calcification in coronary artery disease: an intravascular ultrasound study. *J Am Coll Cardiol* 1992; **20**: 1149–55.

24 Mintz GS, Popma JJ, Pichard AD et al. Patterns of calcification in coronary artery disease. A statistical analysis of intravascular ultrasound and coronary angiography in 1155 lesions. *Circulation* 1995; **91**: 1959–65.

25 Tenaglia AN, Buller CE, Kisslo KB, Stack RS, Davidson CJ. Mechanisms of balloon angioplasty and directional coronary atherectomy as assessed by intracoronary ultrasound. *J Am Coll Cardiol* 1992; **20**: 685–91.

26 Honye J, Mahon DJ, Jain A et al. Morphological effects of coronary balloon angioplasty in vivo assessed by intravascular ultrasound imaging. *Circulation* 1992; **85**: 1012–25.

27 Peters RJG for the PICTURE study group. Prediction of risk of angiographic restenosis by intracoronary ultrasound imaging after coronary balloon angioplasty. *J Am Coll Cardiol* 1995; **35A**: 701.

28 Gerber TC, Erbel R, Görge G, Ge J, Rupprecht HJ, Meyer J. Classification of morphologic effects of percutaneous transluminal coronary angioplasty assessed by intravascular ultrasound. *Am J Cardiol* 1992; **70**: 1546–54.

29 Jain SP, Jain A, Collins TJ, Ramee SR, White CJ. Predictors of restenosis: a morphometric and quantitative evaluation by intravascular ultrasound. *Am Heart J* 1994; **128**: 664–73.

30 Mintz GS, Pichard AD, Satler LF, Bucher TA, Griffin C, Leon M. The final percent cross-sectional narrowing (residual plaque burden) is the strongest intravascular ultrasound predictor of angiographic restenosis. *J Am Coll Cardiol* 1995; **35A**: 701.

31 The GUIDE Trial investigators. IVUS-determined predictors of restenosis in PTCA and DCA: an interim report from the GUIDE trial, phase II. *Circulation* 1994; **90**: I23.

32 Görge G, Liu F, Ge J, Haude M, Baumgart D, Caspari G. Intravascular ultrasound variables predict restenosis after PTCA. *Circulation* 1995; **92**: I148.

33 Hodgson JMcB, Stone GW, Linnemeier TJ, Sheehan HM, St Goar FG, Berry JL. Oversized balloons defined by intracoronary ultrasound result in dramatic improvements in angioplasty results: initial ultrasound analysis of the CLOUT pilot study. *Eur Heart J* 1995; **16**: 487.

34 Tobis J, Colombo A, Almagor Y et al. Intravascular ultrasound guidance of multiple interventions does not reduce restenosis. *Circulation* 1995; **92**: I148.

35 Mintz GS, Pichard AD, Kent KM, Satler LF, Popma JJ, Leon MB. Intravascular ultrasound comparison of restenotic and de novo coronary artery narrowings. *Am J Cardiol* 1994; **74**: 1278–80.

36 Baptista J, Di Mario C, Ozaki Y et al. Impact of plaque morphology and composition on the mechanisms of lumen enlargement using intracoronary ultrasound and quantitative angiography after balloon angioplasty. *Am J Cardiol* 1996; **77**: 115–21.

37 Di Mario C, Gil R, Camenzind E et al. Quantitative assessment with intracoronary ultrasound of the mechanisms of restenosis after percutaneous transluminal coronary angioplasty and directional coronary atherectomy. *Am J Cardiol* 1995; **75**: 772–7.

38 Kimura T, Kaburagi S, Tashima Y, Nobuyoshi M, Mintz GS, Popma JJ. Geometric remodeling and intimal growth as mechanisms of restenosis: observations from serial ultrasound analysis of restenosis (SURE) trial. *Circulation* 1995; **92(suppl)**: I76.

39 Haude M, Erbel R, Issa H, Meyer J. Quantitative analysis of elastic recoil after balloon angioplasty and after intracoronary implantation of balloon-expandable Palmaz–Schatz stents. *J Am Coll Cardiol* 1993; **21**:26–34.

25 Functional assessment of intracoronary Doppler: the Doppler Endpoints Balloon Angioplasty Trial Europe (DEBATE) study: preliminary results

Madoka Sunamura, Carlo Di Mario, Jan Piek, Erwin Schroeder, Olivier Gurné, Christian Vrints, Peter Probst, Gerold Porenta, Bernard de Bruyne, Guy Heyndrickx, Claude Hanet, Eckart Fleck, Ernst Wellnhofer, Raimund Erbel, Michael Haude, Dietrich Baumgart, Vasilis Voudris, Eduardo Verna, Herbert J Geschwind, Hakan Emanuelsson, Volker Mühlberger, Luigi Campolo, Gan Bapptistta Danzi, Joj Peels, Robert Gil and Patrick W Serruys

Introduction

The limitations of angiography have prompted investigators to use alternative methods for the functional assessment of angioplasty results. Various digital angiographic techniques[1] and Doppler catheters were introduced and tested.[2–6] However, only with the introduction of a Doppler angioplasty guide wire has the continuous measurement of blood flow velocity during a routine angioplasty procedure become possible.[7–10] The main advantage of this system is the possibility of positioning the guide wire distal to the stenosis and reliably assessing the flow impairment induced by the stenosis under treatment. The velocity measurements can be repeated after angioplasty leaving the guide wire in place, distal to the stenosis, during dilatation. A normalization of flow velocity parameters after successful angioplasty will indicate that an adequate lumen enlargement has been achieved and a normal vascular conductance restored. The results of small-sized single-center studies have shown an improvement of the flow velocity indices in most cases after percutaneous transluminal coronary angioplasty (PTCA).[6–9] Up to now, however, no appropriately sized prospective studies have assessed the value of flow velocity indices in predicting immediate complications and recurrence of symptoms after PTCA.

The aim of the DEBATE study (Doppler Endpoints Balloon Angioplasty Trial Europe) was to identify Doppler flow velocity indices predictive of the short-term and long-term clinical outcome after angioplasty. This chapter reports the preliminary results of the correlation between functional status one month after angioplasty and flow velocity measurements immediately after angioplasty.

Methods

Patient selection

The study population consisted of 297 patients undergoing balloon angioplasty because of chest pain at rest or with exertion. All patients gave witnessed, written, informed consent and the study protocol was approved by the institutional review boards of all participating hospitals. Patients with stable and unstable angina, undergoing a PTCA of a single lesion in a major native coronary artery were eligible for inclusion.

Exclusion criteria were: multivessel disease; previous transmural myocardial infarction in the territory of the vessel to be dilated; acute myocardial infarction less than one week prior to PTCA; total coronary occlusion; presence of left bundle-branch block or second- or third-degree atrioventricular block; open bypass graft distal to the lesion to be treated; extreme tortuosity of the vessel to be dilatated; application of alternative or additional interventional treatment (directional or rotational atherectomy, stent implantation, etc.).

Documentation of electrocardiographic, scintigraphic or echocardiographic changes (spontaneously or during provocative tests) was required.

Angioplasty procedure

Before angioplasty all patients were treated with heparin and acetyl salicylic acid. A 0.014-inch Doppler-tipped guide wire was used as primary angioplasty guide wire. The guide wire has a 15 MHz piezoelectric transducer mounted at the tip, while maintaining a floppy shapable distal end (FloWire, Cardiometrics, Mountain View, CA).[11] The Doppler guide wire was introduced into the proximal segment of the artery to be dilatated and baseline and hyperemic flow velocity measurements were obtained in an angiographically normal segment of the artery. Afterwards, the Doppler guide wire was advanced distal to the lesion after recording of the velocity of the stenotic jet, if present, and new velocity recordings were obtained in basal and hyperemic conditions. For both proximal and distal measurements a distance greater than three times the vessel diameter was maintained in order to avoid prestenotic acceleration of flow or poststenotic turbulent flow.

Maximal hyperemia was induced by intracoronary bolus injection of adenosine, 12 µg for the right coronary artery (RCA) and 18 µg for the left coronary artery (LCA) (Fig. 25.1).[12] The Doppler guide wire

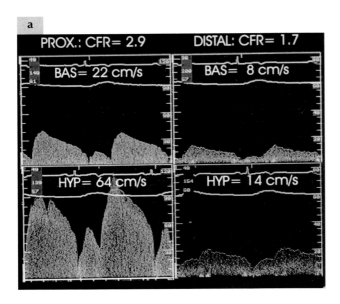
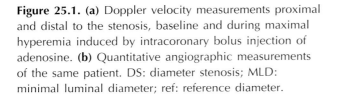
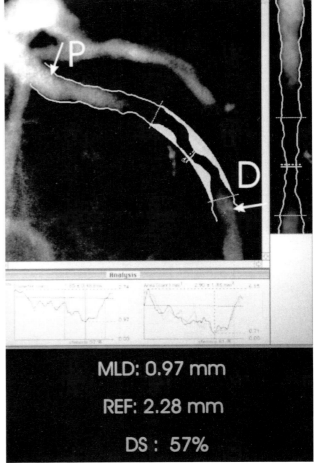

Figure 25.1. (a) Doppler velocity measurements proximal and distal to the stenosis, baseline and during maximal hyperemia induced by intracoronary bolus injection of adenosine. **(b)** Quantitative angiographic measurements of the same patient. DS: diameter stenosis; MLD: minimal luminal diameter; ref: reference diameter.

was left in place and flow velocity was continuously monitored during balloon inflation and deflation and for 15 minutes after documentation of an angiographically successful result. During this trend recording interventions which could interfere with the stability of the velocity signal were avoided (for example, injection through the guiding catheter or repositioning of the Doppler guide wire). Afterwards, baseline and hyperemic flow velocity recordings were obtained in the same position as before dilatation (Fig. 25.2). During pullback, high velocities in the treated segment were recorded, if present, and new baseline and hyperemic flow velocity measurements were obtained proximal to the stenosis.

Follow-up procedures

Two to four weeks after the initial angioplasty procedure the patient was examined and possible anginal complaints, classified according to the Canadian Cardiovascular Society (CCS) Angina Classification, were recorded. A bicycle stress test was performed after withdrawal of all antianginal medication when possible.

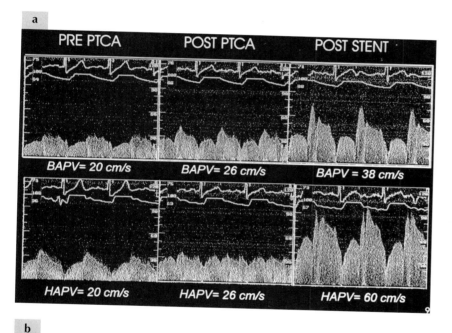

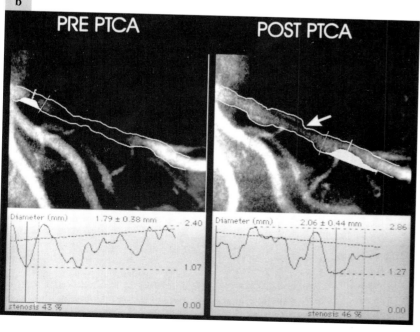

Figure 25.2. Example of coronary flow reserve for the assessment of the result after PTCA. **(a)** Basal and hyperemic flow velocity measurements distal to the stenosis before and after PTCA. Note the persistent impaired flow reserve after PTCA and the significant increase in flow velocity after final stent implantation. **(b)** Quantitative angiographic measurements of the same patient before and after PTCA. Bas: baseline; hyper: hyperemic; DS: diameter stenosis; MLD: minimal luminal diameter.

Quantitative angiographic measurement

At least two cineangiograms, in orthogonal projections, were performed before coronary angioplasty and repeated after angioplasty in the same projections. Nitroglycerin 0.1–0.3 mg or isosorbide dinitrate 1–3 mg was administered intracoronarily to achieve maximal coronary vasodilatation. All films were sent to an independent Core Laboratory, unaware of the clinical results and of the Doppler measurements, and matched views and frames were selected appropriately for off-line quantitative analysis. A computer-assisted analysis system was used (CAAS system, Pie Medical data, Maastricht, The Netherlands)[13] which performs an automatic detection of the vessel centerline, applying a weighted first- and second-derivative function to the brightness profile on each scanline perpendicular to the vessel centerline. By using the guiding catheter diameter (filmed without contrast) as a scaling device, minimal luminal diameter, reference diameter and percentage diameter stenosis were calculated. For the videodensitometric analysis, the brightness profile of each scanline perpendicular to the lumen centerline was transformed into an absorption profile by means of a logarithmic transfer function to correct for the Lambert–Beer law. The background contribution was estimated by computing the linear regression line through background points directly left and right of the detected contours. Subtraction of this background portion from the absorption profile yielded the net cross-sectional absorption profile. By repeating this procedure for all scanlines, the cross-sectional area function was obtained.[14]

Flow velocity measurement

During the angioplasty procedure, the Doppler flow velocity spectra were recorded continuously on videotape.

A real-time fast Fourier transform algorithm was used to process the quadrature audio signal. The Doppler ultrasound instrument (FloMap, Cardiometrics, Mountain View, CA) calculates and displays on-line several spectral variables, including: the time-averaged peak velocity (normalized to the cardiac cycle); the maximum peak velocity; the average diastolic peak velocity; the average systolic peak velocity; the ratio of the average diastolic to average systolic peak velocities (DSVR); and the integral versions for each of these parameters.[11] The accuracy of these flow velocity measurements has been validated in vitro and in an animal model using simultaneous electromagnetic flow measurements for comparison.[11] The following quotients were also computed: coronary flow reserve (CFR),

calculated as the ratio between maximal flow velocity during the peak effect of the adenosine injection and the basal flow velocity; and the proximal-to-distal (P/D) ratio, calculated as the ratio of the flow velocity proximal and distal to the lesion. Correction and manual tracing of the Doppler signals were performed when necessary during the off-line review of the videotapes.

Statistical analysis

Continuous variables are expressed as mean ± standard deviation. Group differences were tested using Student's t-test. P-values less than 0.05 are considered to be statistically significant.

Results

At this stage of the trial 224 analysable patients were left of the total number of 297 patients: on 33 patients data was not yet available; three patients

Table 25.1 **Patient clinical and angiographic characteristics**

No. of patients	224
Age (years)	59 ± 9
Sex (male)	175 (78%)
Hypertension[a]	77 (14%)
Hypercholesterolemia[b]	116 (52%)
Previous myocardial infarction	42 (19%)
Previous PTCA	26 (12%)
Unstable angina	113 (50%)
Treated vessel:	
LAD	108 (48%)
LCX	61 (27%)
RCA	55 (25%)
Type of lesion[c]:	
Type A	31 (14%)
Type B	191 (85%)
Type C	2 (1%)
Type of lesion[d]:	
Eccentric	175 (78%)
Length of lesion ≥ 10 mm	39 (17%)

[a]blood pressure ≥ 150/95 in repeated measurements.
[b]Total cholesterol ≥ 6.5 mmol/l.
[c]Type of lesion, as defined by the ACC/AHA Task Force.
[d]Type of lesion, according to the Ambrose classification.
LAD: left anterior descending artery; LCX: left circumflex artery; RCA: right coronary artery.

were excluded because of protocol violations; in one patient it was impossible to cross the lesion with the FloWire or other wires; in 10 patients there were no distal velocity measurements available post-PTCA. Coronary angioplasty was successful in 224 cases; of the remaining 26 cases (10%), 24 patients required stent implantation and two emergency coronary artery bypass graftings (CABGs) because of acute or threatened occlusion. All complications occurred after balloon dilatation and were not related to the use of the Doppler guide wire.

Clinical and angiographic characteristics of the study patients are shown in Table 25.1.

Angiographic and Doppler measurements

Minimal luminal diameter (MLD) increased from 1.05 ± 0.27 mm before PTCA to 1.78 ± 0.34 mm after PTCA (Fig. 25.3). Diameter stenosis (DS) decreased from 62% to $37 \pm 8\%$ (both $P<0.0001$), while percentage cross-sectional area stenosis (CSA-St) measured independently with videodensitometry, decreased from $82 \pm 11\%$ to $48 \pm 14\%$ ($P<0.0001$) and minimal luminal cross-sectional area (CSA) increased from 1.11 ± 0.76 mm^2 to 3.35 ± 1.39 mm^2 ($P <0.0001$). Reference diameter was unchanged from before to after PTCA (2.82 ± 0.47 mm versus 2.84 ± 0.46 mm).

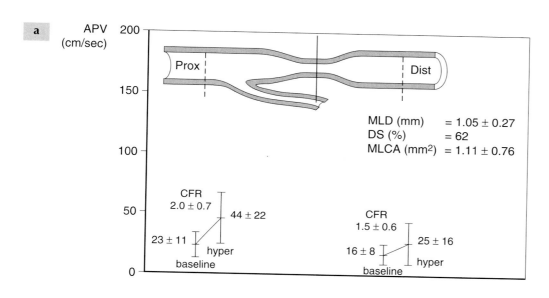

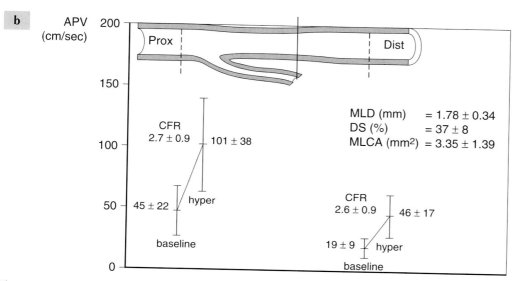

Figure 25.3. Flow velocity (**a**) and angiographic measurements (**b**) before and after angioplasty.

The flow velocity measurements in baseline and hyperemic conditions, proximal and distal to the stenosis, before and after PTCA, are summarized in Fig 25.3.

Distal CFR increased from 1.5 ± 0.6 before PTCA to 2.6 ± 0.9 after PTCA, $P<0.0001$. The distal DSVR increased from 1.68 ± 0.68 to 2.12 ± 0.97 ($P<0.0001$).

Flow velocity measurements and early recurrence of ischemic events

Two in-hospital complications occurred in the group of patients with successful PTCA. At the date of data analysis, 224 patients had undergone a clinical evaluation and a bicycle stress test 2–4 weeks after PTCA; 189 patients (84%) were free of ischemic events, whereas 35 patients (16%) either complained of typical chest pain (11 patients) or had an electrocardiographically positive exercise test (16 patients). Six patients had both typical angina and a positive stress test.

Patients with or without ischemic events one month after PTCA had similar angiographic measurements (Fig. 25.4(a)). Distal CFR after angioplasty was significantly lower in the patients with recurrence of ischemia than in the patients asymptomatic after PTCA ($P<0.02$) (Fig 25.4(b)).

For the left coronary system (left anterior descending or circumflex artery) an even larger difference between the two groups was observed. Despite a similar trend, the difference in CFR between patients with and without recurrence of ischemia did not reach statistical significance for the right coronary artery (Fig. 25.4(c)). The other indices based on flow velocity measurements (DSVR, proximal-to-distal velocity ratio) showed similar values in both groups.

Percentage correct classification of recurrence of ischemia (sensitivity) and percentage correct classification of absence of ischemia (specificity) at early follow-up as a function of cut-off points for quantitative angiographic and flow velocity measurements for the whole group (left and right coronary artery system) are given in Fig 25.5. The point of intersection of the sensitivity and specificity curves represents the cut-off point for which diagnostic

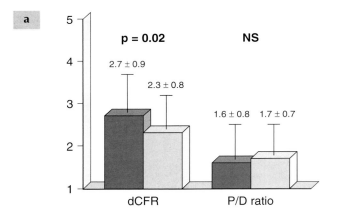

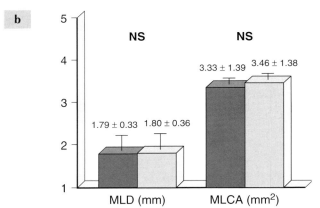

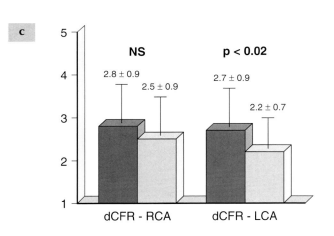

Figure 25.4. Correlation between flow velocity measurements, angiographic measurements and recurrence of ischemia at early follow-up. Flow velocity measurements distal to the lesion immediately after PTCA (a) and (c) but not angiographic measurements (b) were predictive of early ischemic events. dCFR: distal coronary flow reserve; P/D ratio: proximal-to-distal flow velocity ratio; LCA: left coronary artery system; RCA: right coronary artery system; MLD (mm): minimal luminal diameter; MLCA (mm²): minimal luminal cross-sectional area.

accuracy was optimal. Coronary flow reserve had a sensitivity and specificity of 59% at a cut-off point of 2.34, whereas minimal luminal diameter had a sensitivity and specificity of 41% at a cut-off point of 1.80 mm.

Discussion

Qualitative and quantitative angiographic parameters are poor predictors of recurrence of symptoms or restenosis after PTCA.[15–17]

The use of other techniques for morphologic assessment of the stenosis after PTCA (intracoronary ultrasound, angioscopy) has shown that angiography is unable to detect presence and severity of dissections and thrombosis after PTCA.[18–21]

Intracoronary ultrasound, in particular, has shown that a severe atherosclerotic burden is present in most cases after PTCA and that the angiographic appearance of lumen enlargement is mainly correlated with the presence of circumferential dissections, while a small central lumen for blood passage is available.[18–20,22,23] The complexity and high costs of these imaging techniques, however, make them unsuitable for routine assessment of the results of coronary interventions. Intracoronary Doppler can be easily incorporated into an interventional procedure, such as coronary angioplasty, since the

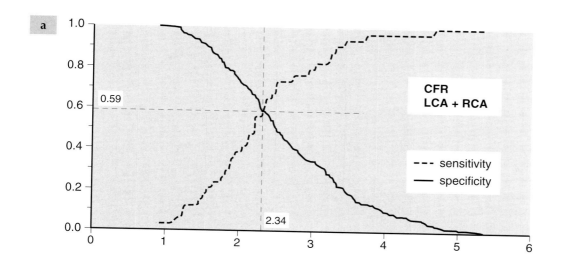

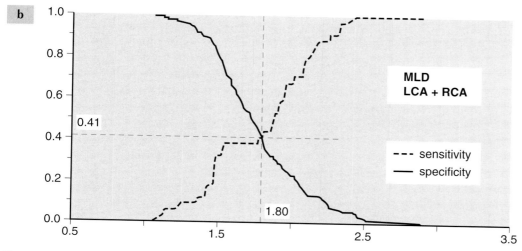

Figure 25.5. Percentage correct classification of recurrence of ischemia (sensitivity) and percentage correct classification of no recurrence of ischemia (specificity) at early follow-up as a function of cut-off points for CFR and MLD. The point of intersection of the two curves denotes the cut-off point with the highest diagnostic accuracy. **(a)** Curves for coronary flow reserve; **(b)** curves for minimal luminal diameter.

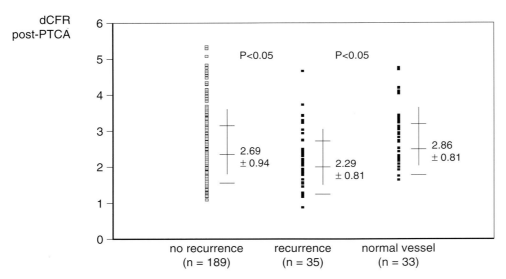

Figure 25.6. Coronary flow reserve (CFR) immediately after PTCA in patients with recurrence and without recurrence of angina at one-month follow-up. Note the presence of a subgroup of asymptomatic patients with abnormal measurements after PTCA. A group of 38 angiographically normal arteries is shown for comparison. Note the similar average measurement of CFR and the presence of a subgroup with abnormal measurements.

Doppler guide wire can safely be used as an alternative to a conventional angioplasty guide wire.[24]

A persisting impairment of flow velocity indices after PTCA may detect the inability of the dilatation procedure to restore a normal vascular conductance. Up to now, however, the correlation between flow velocity measurements and functional and clinical results of PTCA has not been established. In this study, a low CFR was significantly correlated with recurrence of symptoms after PTCA, confirming that the flow velocity measurements can provide a reliable assessment of the physiologic significance of residual stenosis.

A cut-off criterion of CFR equal to 2.34 can be used to predict whether a patient with an angiographically 'successful' PTCA will display symptoms of recurrence of ischemia at one month after PTCA and for whom additional intervention at the time of the PTCA may be warranted.

As shown in Fig 25.5, the specificity and sensitivity of the flow velocity measurements after PTCA remain limited. In particular, a subgroup of patients without recurrence of ischemia presents low values of coronary flow reserve (Fig 25.6). Explanation of this phenomenon already described in previous Doppler studies,[4–7] can be the presence of acute disturbance of flow regulation after angioplasty by release of endothelin, thrombin or microemboli,[25–27] modifications in the hemodynamic conditions after

PTCA, alterations of smooth muscle vasomotor tone due to mechanical trauma after PTCA and chronic impairment of microvascular response. Figure 25.6 shows that also in normal arteries, a subgroup of patients presents values of CFR lower than 2.0.[27]

Since flow velocity measurements are available at the time of the procedure, additional interventions can be immediately performed after PTCA to prevent the recurrence of symptoms.

Coronary stenting has been shown to be associated with a larger lumen gain immediately after stenting and a reduced long-term restenosis.[28] Since stent implantation remains a technically demanding and expensive procedure, the use of flow velocity measurements can represent a useful way of selecting the patients who can benefit most from this intervention (Fig 25.2).

Conclusion

Flow velocity measurements distal to the lesion immediately after PTCA, but not quantitative angiographic measurements, are predictive of early ischemic events suggesting that intracoronary Doppler can reveal the presence of a critical residual impairment of lumen conductance which remains undetected by angiography.

References

1 Zijlstra F, Reiber JC, Juillière Y, Serruys PW. Normalization of coronary flow reserve by percutaneous transluminal angioplasty. *Am J Cardiol* 1988; **61**: 55–60.

2 Donohue TJ. Clinical application of intracoronary Doppler. In: de Feyter PJ, di Mario C, Serruys PW, eds. *Quantitative Coronary Imaging* (Delft: Barjesteh, Meeuwes & Co., 1995) 251–66.

3 Wilson RF, Johnson MR, Marcus ML et al. The effect of coronary angioplasty on coronary blood flow reserve. *Circulation* 1988; **71**: 873–5.

4 Serruys PW, Juillière Y, Zijlstra et al. Coronary blood flow velocity during percutaneous transluminal coronary angioplasty as a guide for assessment of the functional result. *Am J Cardiol* 1988; **61**: 253–9.

5 Kern MJ, Deligonul U, Vandormael M et al. Impaired coronary vasodilator reserve in the immediate postcoronary angioplasty period: analysis of coronary artery flow velocity indexes and regional cardiac venous reflux. *J Am Coll Cardiol* 1989; **13**: 860–72.

6 Segal J, Kern MJ, Scott NA et al. Alterations of phasic coronary artery flow velocity in humans during percutaneous transluminal coronary angioplasty. *J Am Coll Cardiol* 1992; **20**: 276–86.

7 Ofili EO, Kern MJ, Labovitz AJ et al. Analysis of coronary blood flow velocity dynamics in angiographically normal and stenosed arteries before and after endoluminal enlargement by angioplasty. *J Am Coll Cardiol* 1993; **21**: 308–16.

8 Segal J. Applications of coronary flow velocity during angioplasty and other coronary interventional procedures. *Am J Cardiol* 1993; **71**: 17D–25D.

9 Serruys PW, Di Mario C, Meneveau N et al. Intracoronary pressure and flow velocity with sensor-tip guidewires: a new methodologic approach for assessment of coronary hemodynamics before and after coronary interventions. *Am J Cardiol* 1993; **71**: 41D–53D.

10 di Mario C, Gil R, Sunamura M, Serruys PW. New concepts for interpretation of intracoronary velocity and pressure tracings. *Br Heart J* 1995; **74**: 485–92.

11 Doucette JW, Douglas CP, Payne HP et al. Validation of a Doppler guide wire for intravascular measurement of coronary artery flow velocity. *Circulation* 1992; **85**: 1899–911.

12 Wilson RF, Wyche K, Christensen BV, Laxson DD. Effects of adenosine on human coronary arterial circulation. *Circulation* 1990; **82**: 1595–1606.

13 Keane D, Haase J, Slager CJ. Comparative validation of quantitative coronary angiography systems. Results and implications from a multicenter study using a standardized approach. *Circulation* 1995; **91**: 2174–83.

14 Di Mario C, Haase J, de Feyter PJ et al. Videodensitometry versus edge detection for the assessment of in vivo intracoronary phantoms. *Am Heart J* 1992; **124**: 1181–9.

15 Rensing BJ, Hermans WRM, Deckers JW et al. Which angiographic parameter best describes functional status 6 months after successful single vessel coronary balloon angioplasty? *J Am Coll Cardiol* 1993; **21**: 317–24.

16 Rensing BJ, Hermans WRM, Vos J et al. Luminal narrowing after PTCA. A study of clinical, procedural and lesional factors related to long term angiographic outcome. Coronary Artery Restenosis Prevention on Repeated Thromboxane Antagonism (CARPORT) Study Group. *Circulation* 1993; **88**: 975–85.

17 Hermans WR, Rensing BJ, Foley DP et al. Therapeutic dissection after successful coronary balloon angioplasty: no influence on restenosis or on clinical outcome in 693 patients. The MERCATOR study group (Multicenter European Research Trial with Cilazapril after Angioplasty to prevent Transluminal Coronary Obstruction and Restenosis). *J Am Coll Cardiol* 1992; **20**: 767–80.

18 Nakamura S, Mahon DJ, Colombo A et al. An explanation for discrepancy between angiographic and intravascular ultrasound measurements after PTCA. *J Am Coll Cardiol* 1995; **25**: 633–9.

19 Di Mario C, Escaned J, Baptista J et al. Advantages and limitations of intravascular ultrasound for the assessment of vascular dimensions. *J Intervent Cardiol* 1994; **7**: 43–56.

20 Hodgson JM, Reddy KG, Suneja R et al. Intravascular ultrasound imaging: correlation of plaque morphology with angiography, clinical syndrome and procedural results in patients undergoing coronary angioplasty. *J Am Coll Cardiol* 1993; **21**: 35–44.

21 Den Heijer P, Van Dijk RB, Pentinga ML et al. Serial angioscopy during the first hour after successful PTCA. *Circulation* 1992; **86**: 458–62.

22 Tenaglia AN, Buller CE, Kisslo KB et al. Intracoronary ultrasound predictors of adverse outcomes after coronary artery interventions. *J Am Coll Cardiol* 1992; **20**: 1385–90.

23 Di Mario C, Gil R, Camenzind E et al. Quantitative assessment with intracoronary ultrasound of the mechanisms of restenosis after PTCA and DCA. *Am J Cardiol* 1995; **75**: 772–7.

24 Serruys PW, Di Mario C, Kern MJ. Intracoronary Doppler. In: Topol EJ, ed. *Textbook of Interventional Cardiology* (Philadelphia: Saunders, 1994): 1069–121.

25 Marmur JD, Merlini PA, Sharma SK et al. Thrombin generation in human coronary arteries after percutaneous transluminal balloon angioplasty. *J Am Coll Cardiol* 1995; **24**: 1484–91.

26 Uren NG, Crake T, Lefory DC et al. Delayed recovery of coronary resistive vessel function after coronary angioplasty. *J Am Coll Cardiol* 1993; **21**: 612–21.

27 Di Mario C, Gil R, Serruys PW et al. Long-term reproducibility of coronary flow velocity measurements in patients with coronary artery disease. *Am J Cardiol* 1995; **75**: 1177–80.

28 Serruys PW, De Jaegere PJ, Kiemeneij F et al. A comparison of balloon-expandable-stent implantation with balloon angioplasty in patients with coronary artery disease. *New Engl J Med* 1994; **331**: 489–95.

Appendix

The following institutions and investigators participated in the DEBATE study: Academical Medical Center, Amsterdam, The Netherlands: J Piek, K Koch; Clinique Universitaire de Mont-Godinne, Yvoir, France: E Schroeder, O Gurné; Universitair Ziekenhuis Antwerp, Belgium: C Vrints; Thoraxcenter, Rotterdam, The Netherlands: C di Mario, R Gil, P Nierop, PW Serruys; Kardiologische Universitatsklinik Wien, Vienna, Austria: P Probst, G Porenta; Onze Lieve Vrouwe Kliniek, Aalst, Belgium: G Heyndrickx, B de Bruyne, W Wijns; Clinique Universitaire St Luc, Brussels, Belgium: C Hanet; Deutsches Herzzentrum, Berlin, Germany: E Fleck, E Wellnhofer, H Sauer; Universität Essen, Essen, Germany: R Erbel, M Haude, F Baumgart; Ospedale di Circolo, Varese, Italy: E Verna; Onassis Cardiac Surgery Center, Athens, Greece: V Voudris; CHU Henri Mondor, La Creteil, France: H Geschwind; Universitätsklinik fur Innere Medizin, Innsbruck, Austria: V. Mühlberger, N Moes, G Friedrich; Sahlgrenska Hospital, Göteborg, Sweden: H Emanuelsson; Ospedale Niguarda Ca'Granda, Milan, Italy: L Campolo, G Danzi; Academisch Ziekenhuis, Groningen, The Netherlands: H Peels.

26 Assessment of high-frequency rotational angioplasty with intravascular ultrasound

Junbo Ge and Raimund Erbel

High-frequency rotational angioplasty (HFRA), also known as high-speed rotational atherectomy, ablates and pulverizes noncompliant coronary plaque material by high-frequency rotation of a diamond-coated burr. It is usually used for coronary recanalization in total or subtotal occlusion and subsequently combined with other interventional procedures to achieve optimal results, as the maximal burr size used is 2.5 mm in diameter; this is sometimes not large enough for proximal epicardial coronary arteries. Recently, it has been generally used for debulking of plaque material with subsequent percutaneous transluminal coronary angioplasty (PTCA) and stenting. Studies have shown that the mechanism of PTCA is mainly via plaque breaks or dissections, especially in calcified plaques, thus creating a wider lumen.[1-3] HFRA,

however, functions by pulverizing plaque material to create a wider lumen.[4]

Morphological observations

Coronary angiography is usually unable to detect the effect of coronary interventions on the vessel wall. The authors compared a group of patients who underwent PTCA and HFRA using intravascular ultrasound (IVUS) with those who underwent angiography and found that patients with HFRA only seldom have intimal dissection. The postintervention consequences of the plaques are closely related to their character.[5] Intravascular ultrasound studies have shown that the vessel lumen after

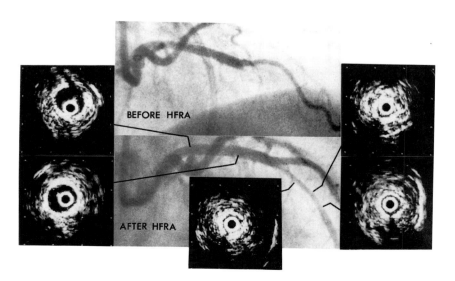

Figure 26.1. A patient with total occlusion of the LAD (upper panel). High-frequency rotational angioplasty was carried out using 1.25 mm, 1.75 mm, and 2.25 mm burrs. IVUS shows a good result, with a circular, symmetrical lumen with a smooth surface. 4.8 F catheter, 20 MHz transducer.

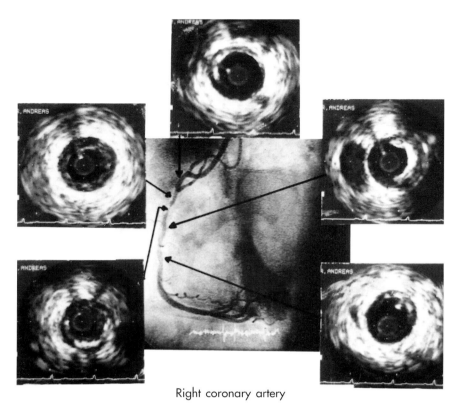

Right coronary artery

Figure 26.2. Coronary angiogram and IVUS images of a right coronary artery after HFRA. Superficial calcification can be seen on ultrasound images. No intimal dissection was found. 4.8 F catheter, 20 MHz transducer.

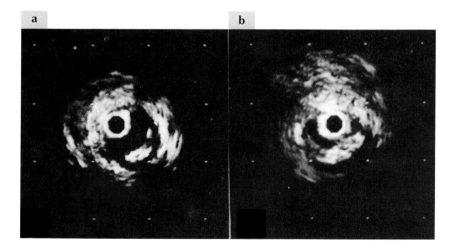

Figure 26.3. IVUS images of two patients with superficial calcification of the plaques. Dissection is seen at the edge of the calcified plaque after PTCA. 4.8 F catheter, 20 MHz transducer.

HFRA is usually circular and symmetrical with a smooth surface without intimal dissection.[5,6] Figures 26.1 and 26.2 show examples of patients after HFRA. In severe calcified lesions PTCA normally results in intimal dissection at the junction of calcium and fibrotic plaque as described by Fitzgerald et al.[7] Figure 26.3 shows typical examples of post-PTCA dissection in calcified plaques. Even in severe superficial calcified plaque, PTCA creates only small breaks of the plaque surface to increase the lumen, which normally presents an appearance of angiographic haziness. In patients with HFRA, after subsequent PTCA the incidence of intimal dissection increases. One possible reason might be the damage to the integrity of the intima by HFRA. Therefore PTCA should be used at a lower pressure post-HFRA. Figure 26.4 shows a patient after HFRA and subsequent PTCA. A large intimal dissection is seen by IVUS, which is not detected by coronary angiography. Figure 26.5 shows another patient with HFRA and subsequent PTCA. Coronary angiography shows haziness in the intervention segment. IVUS demonstrated plaque breaks (tears) in the intervention segment.

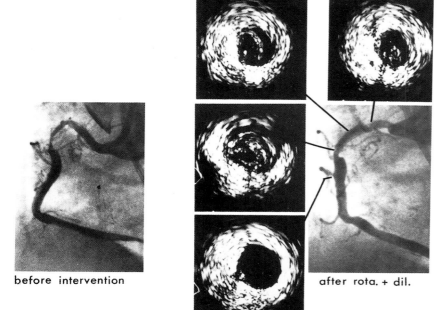

Figure 26.4. Coronary angiograms before (left) and after (right) interventions. After HFRA and subsequent PTCA, a large intimal dissection is seen on IVUS (upper left and middle part) which is not detected by coronary angiography. 4.8 F catheter, 20 MHz transducer.

before intervention

after rota. + dil.

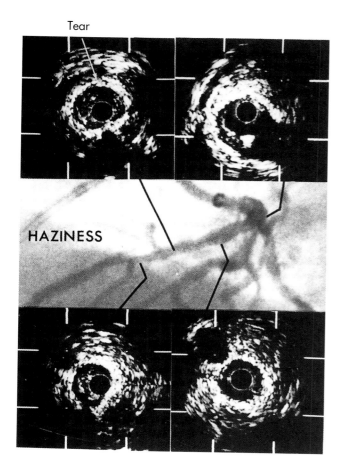

Tear

HAZINESS

Figure 26.5. Angiographic haziness in a patient after HFRA and subsequent PTCA. IVUS visualized multiple tears of the plaque which explains the angiographic haziness. 4.8 F catheter, 20 MHz transducer.

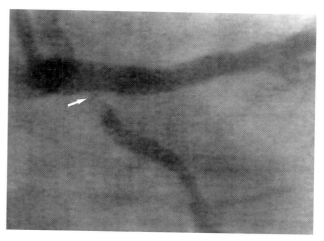

Figure 26.6. A patient with unstable angina for diagnostic angiography. Coronary angiography shows a subtotal occlusion of the ostium of the left circumflex coronary artery which required intervention.

Decision-making

Coronary angiography, a contour technique, provides only the silhouette of the lumen with little information on the lumen wall or the plaque characteristics. It is not a sensible method to use in the detection of calcium deposits and is unable to detect superficial or deep calcification. Figure 26.6 shows a patient with unstable angina who attended for

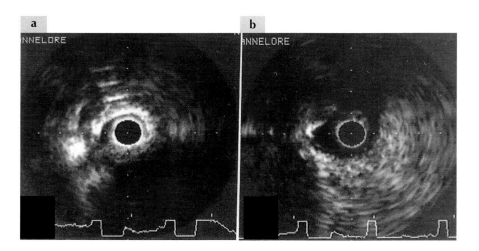

Figure 26.7. IVUS images of the patient shown in Fig. 28.6 before (A) and after (B) HFRA. Severe superficial calcification of the plaque was found. Based on the IVUS finding, HFRA was performed using 1.25 mm and 1.75 mm burrs. (B) An optimal plaque debulking after HFRA. 3.5 F catheter, 20 MHz transducer, 1 mm calibration.

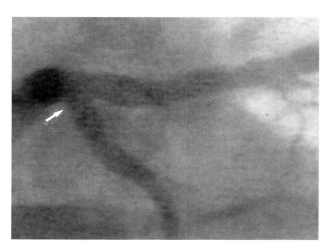

Figure 26.8. The same patient as shown in Figs 28.6 and 28.7. After HFRA, subsequent stenting was performed with an excellent result.

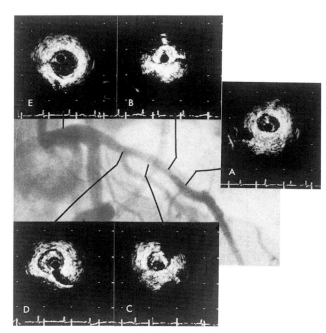

Figure 26.9. A severely calcified stenosis of the LAD. After PTCA, IVUS shows that only two small cracks (B) were made by the balloon. No proper improvement of the vessel lumen. HFRA would have been more appropriate in this situation. 4.8 F catheter, 20 MHz transducer, 1 mm calibration.

coronary intervention. Contrast coronary angiography shows a subtotal stenosis of the ostium of the left circumflex artery on which it was intended to carry out directional coronary atherectomy. IVUS was performed before coronary intervention. A circular severely calcified plaque with severe stenosis is visualized (Fig. 26.7(a)). The patient developed severe chest pain during IVUS examination because of the severe stenosis. Based on the IVUS images, HFRA was selected for debulking the plaque. After rotablation with 1.25 mm and 1.75 mm burrs, IVUS showed that the superficial calcium was partly ablated with a good lumen but still a significant stenosis (Fig. 26.7(b)). Excellent results were achieved with subsequent PTCA and stenting (Fig. 26.8). When based only on coronary angiography, directional coronary atherectomy could not have obtained optimal results because of the severe superficial calcification.

Figure 26.9 shows a patient after PTCA with a poor result. IVUS was performed after intervention and shows that only a small crack occurred in the middle of the severely calcified plaque. The superficial calcium deposit has not changed. The widened lumen was created via small cracks with little improvement of the vessel lumen. In the case of deep calcification with a covering of soft plaque (Fig. 26.10), HFRA might be of little help. An optimal result was achieved with PTCA alone (Fig. 26.10). It is important therefore, to carry out IVUS

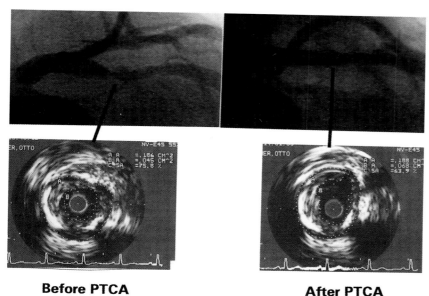

Before PTCA   **After PTCA**

Deep Calcification

Figure 26.10. Coronary angiograms and IVUS images of a patient with severe LAD stenosis. IVUS shows only deep calcification. Conventional PTCA was performed with a good result. 3.5 F catheter, 20 MHz transducer, 1 mm calibration.

not only after intervention in order to evaluate the results of coronary intervention but also prior to intervention to guide in the selection of proper interventional procedures.

Summary

Because IVUS offers a new tool for visualizing the vessel wall and plaque characteristics which conventional coronary angiography cannot provide, it is helpful if it is performed before coronary interventions in order to select correct interventional procedures. As calcium deposits occur frequently in coronary atherosclerosis, it is necessary to know whether there is superficial or deep calcification of the plaque in order to select proper interventional devices. For superficial calcification, HFRA is suitable. For soft plaque or deep calcified plaque, HFRA may be of little help.

References

1   Block PC, Myler RK, Stertzer S, Fallon JT. Morphology after transluminal angioplasty in human beings. *New Engl J Med* 1981; **305**: 382–5.

2   Mizuno K, Kurita A, Imazeki N. Pathological findings after percutaneous transluminal coronary angioplasty. *Br Heart J* 1984; **52**: 588–90.

3   Honye J, Mahon DJ, Jain A et al. Morphological effects of coronary balloon angioplasty in vivo assessed by intravascular ultrasound imaging. *Circulation* 1992; **85**: 1012–25.

4   Erbel R, Zotz R, Stähr P, Dietz U, Rupprecht HJ, Meyer J. Percutaneous transluminal coronary rotational angioplasty. In: Topo EJ, Serruys PW eds. *Current Review of Interventional Cardiology*, (Philadelphia, PA: Current Medicine, 1994): 10.2–10.25.

5   Ge J, Erbel R, Rupprecht HJ et al. Differentiation of the effects of balloon and high-frequency rotational coronary angioplasty by intravascular ultrasound and angiography. *J Am Coll Cardiol* 1992; **19**: 333A.

6   von Birgelen C, Umans VA, Di Mario C et al. Mechanisms of high-speed rotational atherectomy and adjunctive balloon angioplasty revisited by quantitative coronary angiography: edge detection versus videodensitometry. *Am Heart J* 1995; **130**: 405–12.

7   Fitzgerald PJ, Portss TA, Yoc PG. Contribution of localized calcium deposits to dissection after angioplasty: an observational study using intravascular ultrasound. *Circulation* 1992; **86**: 64–70.

27 Intravascular ultrasound after directional coronary atherectomy

Michael Haude

Percutaneous transluminal coronary balloon angioplasty (PTCA) has proven to be an effective treatment for obstructive coronary artery disease. The mechanism behind luminal enlargement by PTCA was first thought to be compression of the plaque.[1] However, in vitro histology examinations after balloon dilatation and, more recently, in vivo intravascular ultrasound imaging have shown that plastic deformation of the obstructive plaque during PTCA with the creation of intimal and medial dissections is the major reason for luminal enlargement.[2–9] Thereby, no significant change in plaque volume could be detected after PTCA. Postangioplasty intimal and medial dissections were associated with the potential risk of acute vessel closure because of flow limitations and the potential exposure of thrombogenic parts of the disrupted vessel wall.[9]

Different alternative interventional devices were developed to achieve luminal enlargement by reducing plaque volume instead of disrupting the plaque. Directional coronary atherectomy, as developed by Simpson and co-workers, is a percutaneous, over-the-wire cutting system, which allows retrieval of plaque specimens.[10,11] The device consists of a metal housing at the distal end of the catheter with an affixed balloon, a nose-cone collection chamber, and a hollow torque tube, which accommodates a 0.014-inch (0.36-mm) guide wire. A cup-shaped cutter inside the housing is attached to a flexible driveshaft, and is activated by a hand-held, battery-operated motor drive unit. The device is advanced into the lesion over a 0.014-inch (0.36-mm) guide wire with the cutting window oriented toward the atheroma. The balloon is inflated, pushing the plaque into the cutting window and holding the

housing in place. A lever on the motor drive unit allows the operator to activate and slowly advance the cutter through the lesion as it rotates at 2000 rpm. Excised atheroma is stored in the distal nose-cone collection chamber. After balloon deflation the chamber can be rotated and reoriented and further cuts can be performed. Finally the system is retrieved and the excised particles can be examined. The directional coronary atherectomy technique especially targets eccentric noncalcified lesions in the proximal part of large coronary vessels or bypass grafts.

The concept of plaque excision versus plaque rupture has been evaluated clinically by the Coronary Atherectomy versus Angioplasty (CAVEAT) I and II and CCAT trials which compared directional coronary atherectomy and PTCA for the treatment of coronary or saphenous bypass graft stenoses.[12–14] All these trials failed to document a clear reduction of long-term restenosis after directional atherectomy.[12–15] Furthermore, procedure-associated complications tend to be similar to those after PTCA, while non-Q-wave myocardial infarction and perforation were reported to occur more frequently.[12] These somewhat disappointing results are now re-evaluated in the Balloon versus Optimal Atherectomy (BOAT) and Optimal Atherectomy Restenosis Study (OARS) trials applying optimal atherectomy with the creation of a maximum postatherectomy final lumen diameter.

The angiographic and intravascular ultrasound appearance after directional coronary atherectomy is described by two examples. Figure 27.1 shows the angiogram of a patient with an eccentric proximal stenosis of the left anterior descending artery, who

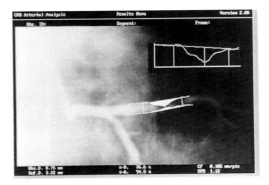 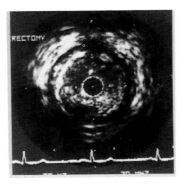

Figure 27.1 Angiogram and intravascular ultrasound image of a patient with stenosis of the left anterior descending artery before directional coronary atherectomy. 3.5 F catheter, 20 MHz transducer, 1 mm calibration.

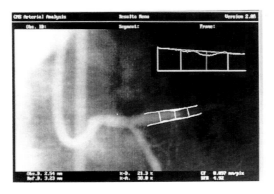 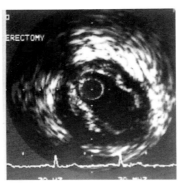

Figure 27.2 Angiogram and intravascular ultrasound image of the patient with stenosis of the left anterior descending artery presented in Fig. 27.1 after directional coronary atherectomy.

presented with unstable angina. Quantitative coronary angiography documented a minimal lumen diameter of 0.75 mm and a reference vessel diameter of 3.22 mm. The corresponding intravascular ultrasound image showed a soft, echolucent plaque formation and the imaging catheter obstructed the residual lumen. No substantial calcification could be documented at the lesion site.

Figure 27.2 illustrates the final postinterventional results. A total of 18 cuts were performed during three attempts with a 7 F. Atherocath SCA-EX (Devices for Vascular Intervention, Inc., Redwood City, CA). After each attempt the nose-cone collection chamber was filled with soft material. Angiographically, minimal lumen diameter increased to 2.54 mm with a 21.3% residual diameter stenosis. The corresponding intravascular ultrasound image documented the creation of an elliptical lumen without dissections to the vessel wall. Almost all echolucent material was removed. Histopathologic examination of the retrieved tissue documented fresh thrombus plus lipid-rich plaque formation including medial cells and lamina elastica interna.

Figure 27.3 illustrates the angiogram of a patient with a circumscript eccentric restenosis in the mid-

part of the left anterior descending artery six months after a PTCA procedure. Quantitative coronary angiography documented a minimal lumen diameter of 1.21 mm and a 69.2% diameter stenosis. The corresponding intravascular ultrasound image showed some echolucent material around the imaging catheter with some more echodense parts within the plaque. A circumscript calcification with echo shadowing was detected at ten o'clock.

Figure 27.4 summarizes the postinterventional angiographic and intravascular ultrasound results. In this patient 15 cuts were performed during five attempts with a 7 F. Atherocath GTO (Devices for Vascular Intervention, Inc., Redwood City, CA). Only after the first three attempts could tissue be retrieved from the nose-cone collection chamber, while after the final attempt no tissue was found in the chamber. The retrieved tissue had a gray and yellow color. Control angiography documented a minimal lumen diameter of 3.04 mm with a 21.2% residual diameter stenosis. In contrast to the angiographic appearance, intravascular ultrasound documented three deep cuts into the plaque and vessel wall with small slaps between. Compared with the result of the previous patient, postinterventional lumen surface at the treated vessel site is not so smooth. A calcification could not be documented at the treated vessel site after directional

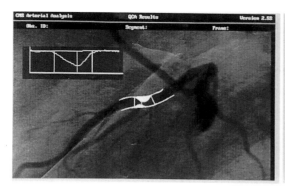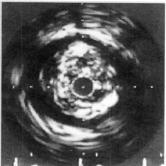

Figure 27.3 Angiogram and intravascular ultrasound image of a patient with restenosis of the left anterior descending artery before directional coronary atherectomy. The concentric plaque contains deep calcification with shadowing.

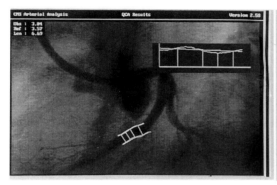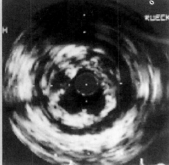

Figure 27.4 Angiogram and intravascular ultrasound image of the patient with restenosis of the left anterior descending artery presented in Fig. 27.3 after directional coronary atherectomy.

coronary atherectomy. Histopathologic examination of the retrieved tissue documented proliferative tissue consisting of cells of smooth muscle cell origin. In addition, a small amount of calcified tissue could be documented microscopically in the retrieved tissue.

References

1 Waller BF. 'Crackers, breakers, stretchers, drillers, scrapers, shavers, burners, welders and melters'–the future treatment of atherosclerotic coronary artery disease? A clinical-morphologic assessment. *J Am Coll Cardiol* 1989; **13**: 969–87.

2 Vlodaver Z, Edwards JE. Pathology of coronary atherosclerosis. *Prog Cardiovasc Dis* 1971; **14**: 256–74.

3 Düber C, Jungbluth A, Rumpelt HJ, Erbel R, Meyer J, Thoenes W. Morphology of the coronary arteries after combined thrombolysis and percutaneous transluminal coronary angioplasty for acute myocardial infarction. *Am J Cardiol* 1986; **58**: 698–703.

4 Jungbluth A, Düber C, Rumpelt HJ, Erbel R, Meyer J. Koronararterienmorphologie nach transluminaler Koronarangioplastie (PTCA) mit Hämoperikard. *Z Kardiol* 1988; **77**: 125–9.

5 Block PC, Baughman KI, Pasternak RC, Fallon JT. Transluminal angioplasty: correlation of morphologic and angiographic findings in an experimental model. *Circulation* 1980; **61**: 778–85.

6 Faxon DP, Weber VJ, Haudenschild C, Gottsman SB, McGovern WA, Ryan TJ. Acute effects of transluminal angioplasty in three experimental models of atherosclerosis. *Arteriosclerosis* 1982; **2**: 152–63.

7 Block PC, Myler RK, Sterzer S, Fallon JT. Morphology after transluminal angioplasty in human beings. *N Engl J Med* 1981; **305**: 382–5.

8 Castaneda-Zuniga WR, Formarck A, Todavarthy M, Edwards JE. The mechanism of balloon angioplasty. *Radiology* 1980; **135**: 565–9.

9 Tan K, Sulke N, Taub N, Sowton E. Clinical and lesion morphologic determinants of coronary angioplasty

success and complications: current experience. *J Am Coll Cardiol* 1995; **25**: 855–65.

10   Simpson JB, Johnson DE, Thapliyal HV, Marks DM, Braden LJ. Transluminal atherectomy: a new approach to the treatment of atherosclerotic vascular disease. *Circulation* 1985; **72(suppl III)**: 146 (abst).

11   Hinohara T, Robertson GC, Simpson JB. Directional coronary atherectomy. In: Topol EJ, ed. *Textbook of Interventional Cardiology* (Philadelphia, PA: WB Saunders Company, 1994), **1**: 641–58.

12   Topol EJ, Leya F, Pinkerton CA et al. A comparison of directional atherectomy with coronary angioplasty in patients with coronary artery disease. *N Engl J Med* 1993; **329**: 221–7.

13   Adelman A, Cohen E, Kimball B et al. A comparison of directional coronary atherectomy with balloon angioplasty for lesions of the left anterior descending coronary artery. *N Engl J Med* 1993; **329**: 228–33.

14   Holmes D, Topol E, Califf R et al. A multicenter, randomized trial of coronary angioplasty versus directional atherectomy for patients with saphenous vein bypass graft lesions. *Circulation* 1995; **91**: 1966–74.

15   Hinohara T, Robertson GC, Selmon MR et al. Restenosis after directional coronary atherectomy. *J Am Coll Cardiol* 1992; **20**: 623–32.

28 Ultrasound angioplasty

Dietrich Baumgart and Michael Haude

Ultrasound angioplasty has been introduced as a new, alternative treatment in interventional cardiology. Basically, there are three major indications for the application of ultrasound angioplasty. The first indication is for the treatment of heavily calcified and fibrous lesions. Ultrasound angioplasty is said to soften heavily calcified lesions using this device as an 'intracoronary lithotryptor'. A number of these complicated and tight lesions are sometimes impassable by conventional balloons, thus reducing the overall acute success rate. The softening mechanism of ultrasound angioplasty is said to enhance the passage of balloons in heavily calcified and tight lesions. Secondly, by this softening mechanism, balloon angioplasty should be applicable at lower inflation pressures. Furthermore, large and complicated dissections should be avoided during subsequent balloon angioplasty.

Safety studies in canine coronary arteries revealed that ultrasound angioplasty can be conducted with few side-effects with respect to endothelial denudation or changes in laboratory values, for example, serum creatinine kinase (CK) levels or coagulation parameters.[1]

Initial clinical experience was gained in peripheral arteries.[2] Eighty-six per cent of the occluded segments could be recanalized. From these experiences in 50 patients the restenosis rate in peripheral arterial stenosis was around 20% in the first 6–12 months. Dissections and perforations occurred in 8% of cases, respectively. As a positive side-effect, vessel vasodilation was noted, which may result in enhanced arterial run-off and could potentially reduce the risk of ischemia.[3] One of the major drawbacks of this technique is the fact that it can seldom be used as a stand-alone technique. In over 90% of cases additional balloon angioplasty or stenting had to be used to optimize the result.

Initial experience with intracoronary ultrasound angioplasty was also reported by Siegel and co-workers.[4] All lesions were treated with additional balloon angioplasty. Coronary artery stenosis fell from 80 ± 12% to 60 ± 18% after ultrasound angioplasty and to 26 ± 11% after additional balloon

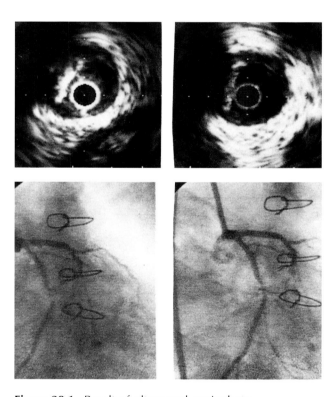

Figure 28.1. Result of ultrasound angioplasty demonstrated in intravascular ultrasound and conventional angiography. Left (before): highly significant stenosis in the left circumflex coronary artery (LCX) following aortocoronary bypass grafting and closure of the bypass to the LCX. Intravascular ultrasound reveals a coronary stenosis with superficial as well as deep calcifications (acoustic shadowing). Right (after): following a stepwise passage with a 1.2 and a 1.7 mm ultrasound angioplasty catheter, the lumen has widened and the calcification is no longer as dense. IVUS as well as angiographic findings indicate only a suboptimal result. 3.5 F, 30 MHz transducer, 1 mm calibration.

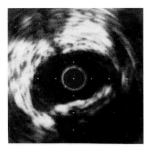
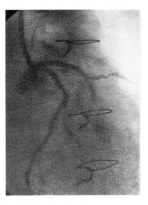

Figure 28.2. Same case as in Fig. 28.1. Angioplasty result following ultrasound angioplasty as well as additional 3.0 mm balloon angioplasty. In intravascular ultrasound findings, minimal luminal diameter has increased significantly. No major dissection can be detected; however, the lumen is rather elliptically shaped. Also the angiographic finding has improved. Some irregularities of the proximal part of the stenosis remain.

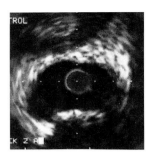
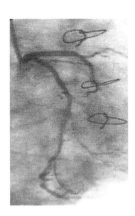

Figure 28.4. Same case as in Fig. 28.1. Angioplasty result following ultrasound angioplasty as well as additional 3.5 mm balloon angioplasty. The vessel lumen now appears more circular with a sufficient minimal luminal diameter. Also, following this intervention, no major dissection can be visualized. Angiography shows a satisfying angioplasty result with no major residual stenosis.

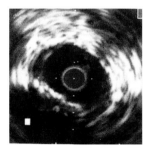
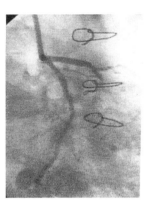

Figure 28.3. Same case as in Fig. 28.1. Follow-up on the next day still demonstrates a very good angioplasty result. Minimal luminal diameter has remained without major elastic recoil. Functional results based on the international study on Thrombolysis in Myocardial Infarction (TIMI) flow as well as morphologic results in intravascular ultrasound and angiography demonstrate the effectiveness of this alternative angioplastic technique.

angioplasty. No ultrasound-related complications were encountered. It was concluded that intracoronary ultrasound angioplasty appears to be safe. In addition, the technique was found to be useful for debulking and enhancing arterial distensibility, allowing balloon angioplasty to be carried out at low pressures.

The second indication is seen for chronic subtotal and total occlusions. Again, the basic principle of

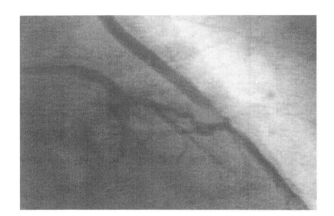
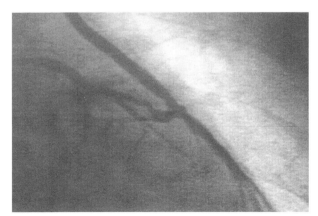

Figure 28.5. Venous bypass to the LAD with significant stenosis just proximal to the anostomosis.

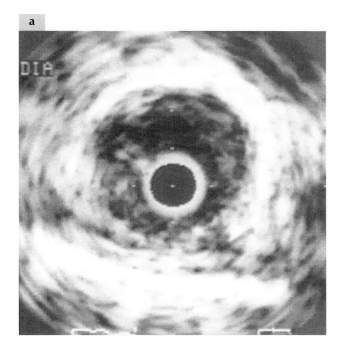

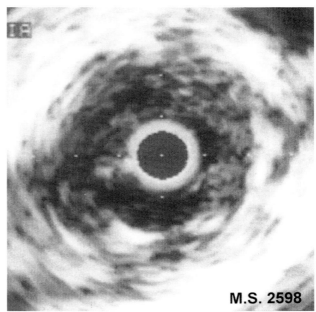

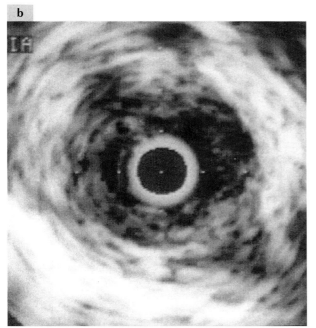

Figure 28.6. Same case as in Fig. 28.5. (a) IVUS images following successful ultrasound angioplasty drawn back from distal to proximal. Both images show remnants of significant plaque material in the bypass graft. There is an irregular borderline between lumen and plaque. (b) Parts of plaque material seem to protrude into the lumen. Most likely this demonstrates old organized thrombus and plaque material. Ultrasound angioplasty was unable to eliminate these organized structures probably composed of fibroblasts and interconnective matrix. 3.5 F catheter, 30 MHz transducer, 1 mm calibration.

ultrasound angioplasty for this type of lesion was to prepare the lesion in such a way that it would be passable by a conventional angioplasty balloon. For subtotal occlusions, this normally required at least the passage of a guide wire distal to the lesion as the ultrasound angioplasty technique is guide-wire-based. Once the guide wire had been passed, it was generally simple to advance the ultrasound probe using sonification times of 2–5 minutes. For chronic total occlusions it was also advisable to use ultrasound angioplasty without the guidance of a guide wire. As for shorter total occlusions with a lesion length of less than or equal to 1 cm, this can be a manageable approach without the risk of major perforations. However, in the authors' experience not every lesion could be successfully treated (Fig. 28.1). Longer chronic total occlusions with a lesion length of > 1 cm were not approached with this

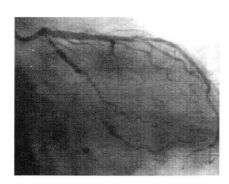

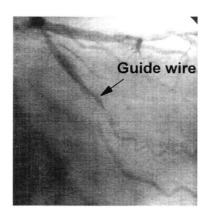

Figure 28.7. Before (left) and after (right) unsuccessful ultrasound angioplasty. The guide wire should be advanced into the distal LCX branch. Instead, it is reaching only the marginal branch. As the technique is guide-wire-based, the inability to advance the guide wire across the lesion limits the approach technically. Attempts to advance the ultrasonic probe without the guide wire resulted in failure or major dissections of the coronary artery and cannot be recommended.

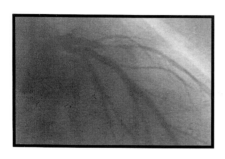

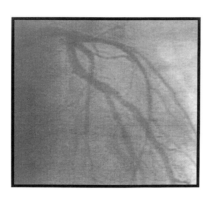

Figure 28.8. Angiographic images before (left) and after (right) ultrasound angioplasty of a subtotal LAD occlusion. This demonstrates one of the few cases where no additional balloon angioplasty was performed. The initial result can be classified as fair.

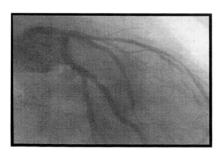

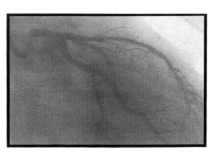

Figure 28.9. Same case as in Fig. 28.8. Result on day 1 (left) and after 6 months (right). Overall a good result with no sign of restenosis.

technique at the authors' institution. Alternative techniques, such as the laser wire, are more promising technologies associated with a lesser risk of major complications.

A third indication is seen for the treatment of total acute thrombotic occlusions, as in acute myocardial infarctions, where the ultrasound is said to dissolve the thrombotic material. The mechanism is mainly due to a physical dissolution of fibrin bonds. Initial experiences of Rosenschein and co-workers have been very promising[1,5,6] and will be further investigated in forthcoming prospective multicenter trials.

The present authors' own experience with ultrasound angioplasty in the clinical setting is based on participation in the Coronary Revascularization Ultrasound Angioplasty Device (CRUSADE) trial which was conducted in multiple centers in Europe. The main indication for ultrasound angioplasty in this trial concentrated on complicated type C lesions and chronic subtotal occlusions.

In over 90% of cases the ultrasound probe could be advanced, operating at a sonification frequency of about 20 kHz. Probes of 1.2 and 1.7 mm were used which were provided by Baxter Healthcare

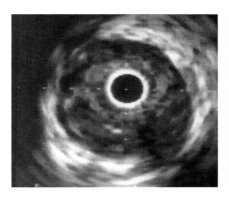 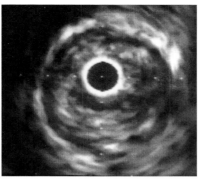

Figure 28.10. IVUS examination of an ultrasound angioplasty in a subtotal LCX occlusion. Before intervention (left) a concentric plaque with multiple layering is shown, indicating the presence of an organized thrombus. After sonification (right) the luminal gain is rather minimal. The plaque burden and morphology have not changed greatly. 3.5 F catheter, 30 MHz transducer, 1 mm calibration.

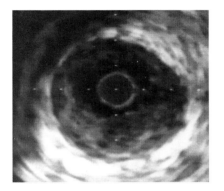 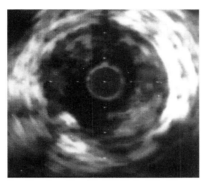

Figure 28.11. Same case as in Fig. 28.10. Balloon angioplasty with a 3.0 mm compliant balloon (left) achieves only a small additional lumen gain. A 3.5 mm balloon (right) improves the result although a satisfactory result is not obtained. The plaque burden has not decreased significantly.

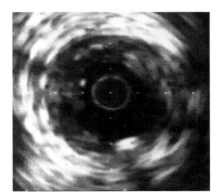 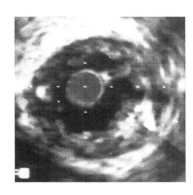

Figure 28.12. Same case as in Figs 28.10 and 28.11. Only after use of a 3.5 mm perfusion balloon is a satisfactory result obtained (left). The plaque has been condensed. Again ultrasound angioplasty has made subsequent balloon angioplasty possible at low inflation pressures; however, organized material of plaque and/or thrombus was not eliminated. The result on day one is acceptable (right). Elastic recoil has occurred to a certain extent. However, stent placement was not indicated as the luminal size was more than 2.5 × 2.5 mm.

Corporation (Cedex, France). A light pressure had generally to be applied to the probe to enable proper advancement. As shown in the illustrations, the initial lumen gain following the passage of the probe was rather small. More insights into the ablation process and its limitations were only gained from additional intravascular ultrasound (IVUS) examination. With the chronic subtotal occlusions in particular, the lumen gain seldom exceeded the diameter of the ultrasound probe. The IVUS image showed a significant plaque burden of soft, noncalcified tissue with a layering phenomenon typically encountered with organized thrombus formation.[7] Subsequent passages of angioplasty balloons were easily made; however, even upsizing the balloons did not improve the lumen gain significantly. The soft or softened plaque showed a significant elastic recoil. Additional stent implantation did finally improve the result; however, the plaque material was so soft that parts of it protruded through the stent struts into the vessel lumen. Similar phenomena were observed with different types of lesions where ultrasound angioplasty was not capable of ablating organized thrombus or plaque material. The inability of ultrasound angioplasty to debulk these structures might be attributed to their histologic nature. Both organized

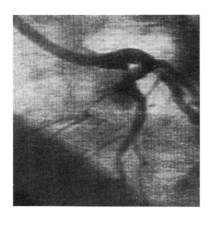
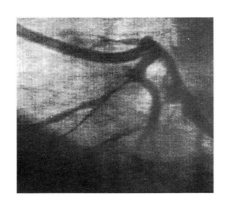

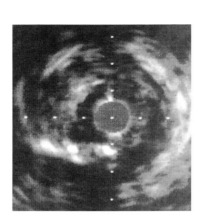

Figure 28.13. Angiograms (top) and IVUS images (bottom) before (left) and after (right) ultrasound angioplasty. Both imaging modalities indicate that the luminal gain was rather small with ultrasound angioplasty alone. From the IVUS image, with signs of multiple layering and the absence of calcification, it can be concluded that the plaque consists mainly of organized thrombus material at this subtotal LAD occlusion. 3.5 F catheter, 30 MHz transducer, 1 mm calibration.

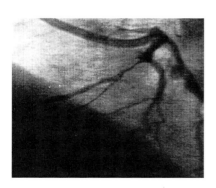
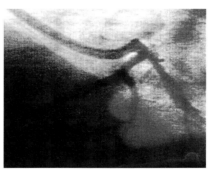

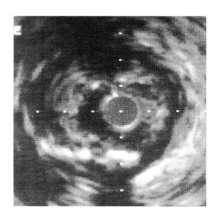
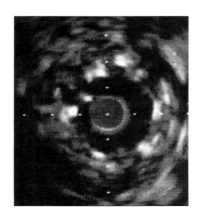

Figure 28.14. Angiograms (top) and IVUS images (bottom) after balloon (left) and after stenting (right) in the same lesion as in Fig. 28.13. Also in this case, additional balloon angioplasty is possible at low inflation pressures; however, plaque burden and area stenosis are not significantly reduced. Only after adjunctive stenting can a satisfactory lumen size be obtained. Of note, however, is that the soft plaque or thrombus material seems to protrude through the stent struts into the lumen. The edges of the stent are not outlined as clearly as in normal cases without previous ultrasound angioplasty. Thus the softening effect of ultrasound angioplasty may have additional adverse effects when adjunctive stenting is performed.

thrombi and plaque consist of fibroblasts and inter-connective tissue. Although ultrasound angioplasty is able to soften and dissolve calcified structures, it is apparently not able to dissolve cellular structures of fibroblasts and connective matrix. In contrast, acute thrombi consist mainly of cellular structures, for example, mainly erythrocytes and thrombocytes and fibrin bonds that can easily be dissolved by sonification. Subsequently erythrocytes and thrombocytes are fragmented and washed away with the bloodstream.

From the experience to date, which is still very limited, it can be stated that ultrasound angioplasty is a supplementary angioplastic technique for complicated lesions and special indications. From additional IVUS examination it has to be stated that the ablation of plaque burden in chronic lesions does not occur, or only to a minor extent. In contrast, early experiences with acute disorganized thrombi demonstrate that these thrombi can be effectively dissolved with ultrasound waves.

References

1 Rosenschein U, Rozenszajn LA, Bernheim J et al. Safety of coronary ultrasound angioplasty: effects of sonication on intact canine coronary arteries. *Cathet Cardiovasc Diagn* 1995; **35**: 64–71.

2 Siegel RJ, Gaines P, Crew JR, Cumberland DC. Clinical trial of percutaneous peripheral ultrasound angioplasty. *J Am Coll Cardiol* 1993; **22**: 480–8.

3 Steffen W, Cumberland D, Gaines P et al. Catheter-delivered high intensity, low frequency ultrasound induces vasodilation in vivo. *Eur Heart J* 1994; **15**: 369–76.

4 Siegel RJ, Gunn J, Ahsan A et al. Use of therapeutic ultrasound in percutaneous coronary angioplasty: experimental in vitro studies and initial clinical experience. *Circulation* 1994; **89**: 1587–92.

5 Rosenschein U, Bernstein JJ, DiSegni E, Kaplinsky E, Bernheim J, Rozenzsajn LA. Experimental ultrasonic angioplasty: disruption of atherosclerotic plaques and thrombi in vitro and arterial recanalization in vivo. *J Am Coll Cardiol* 1990; **15**: 711–17.

6 Rosenschein U, Frimerman A, Laniado S, Miller HI. Study of the mechanism of ultrasound angioplasty from human thrombi and bovine aorta. *Am J Cardiol* 1994; **74**: 1263–6.

7 Kearney P, Erbel R, Ge J, Zamorano J, Koch L, Görge G, Meyer J. Assessment of spontaneous coronary artery dissection by intravascular ultrasound in a patient with unstable angina. *Cathet Cardiovasc Diagn* 1994; **31**: 58–61.

29 Intravascular ultrasound in coronary artery stents

Günter Görge, Michael Haude, Junbo Ge and Raimund Erbel

Introduction

Coronary artery stents are a very effective method for the management of complications during interventions, to prevent recoil after percutaneous transluminal coronary angioplasty (PTCA), and to increase minimal luminal diameter in elective procedures.[1–3] Stenting as an adjunct to recanalization or dilatation of vessels was first suggested by Dotter in 1969.[4] Puel in Lille implanted the first coronary artery stent in a patient and Sigwart was the first to report on a larger series of patients with coronary artery stents.[1] But the acceptance of coronary artery stenting other than for bail-out indications in patients with symptomatic dissections was questionable, because patients suffered from a high subacute stent thrombosis rate.[5,6] To limit subacute thrombotic events, patients were treated with elaborate regimens of heparin, warfarin, and asprin, which resulted in high rates of bleeding complications and prolonged hospitalization.[7]

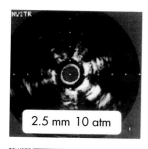
2.5 mm 10 atm

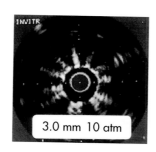
3.0 mm 10 atm

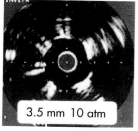
3.5 mm 10 atm

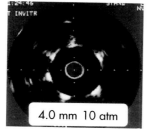
4.0 mm 10 atm

Figure 29.1. IVUS is ideal for the imaging of coronary artery stents. Clearly, the radial echoes of the stent struts (Palmaz–Schatz stents by Johnson and Johnson) are visible by IVUS. However, this example shows also that IVUS in coronary stents produces artefacts such as echo shadowing, reverberation and the echoes are wider than the actual size of the stent struts.

RCA
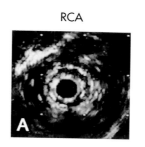

LAD
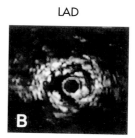

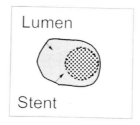
Lumen
Stent

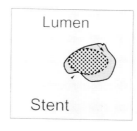
Lumen
Stent

Figure 29.2. Two examples of incomplete stent expansion (Palmaz–Schatz stents). In image A a large, almost circumferential echo-free space between stent and inner luminal border is shown by IVUS. Image B shows incomplete asymmetric stent expansion and 'oblique' stent struts. The shaded area depicts the stent area, the light grey area shows the inner vessel borders.

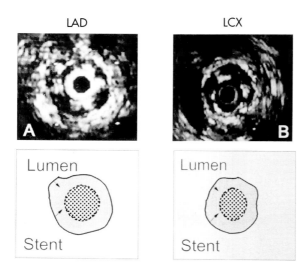

LAD   LCX

Figure 29.3. Two examples of incomplete stent expansion (Palmaz–Schatz stent). Image A: after implantation with 8 atm, a large, almost circular echo-free space was found. Motion picture in image B showed that the echo dense structure at 6 o'clock was mobile and not completely adherent to the stent or vessel wall. This patient developed subacute stent thrombosis after eight days.

The role of intravascular ultrasound (IVUS) in stenting

The reason for these complications was generally incomplete stent expansion (Fig. 29.1). Because most stents are not radiolucent, complete stent expansion cannot be assessed in high detail by angiographic techniques (Figs 29.2 and 29.3).[8] Therefore, IVUS seems to be the ideal adjunct to angiography in patients after stenting, and the first studies were carried out mainly in the peripheral circulation.[9,10] Although many studies documented incomplete stent expansion and asymmetric stent geometry,[11] no negative consequences were reported for patients with stents in their peripheral circulation (Fig. 29.4).[12] It was Colombo from Milan who drew the logical conclusion from incomplete stent expansion imaged by IVUS in the coronary circulation. He inaugurated high-pressure coronary artery stent deployment and proved its effectiveness.[13–15] As a consequence, high-pressure coronary artery stent deployment is now the standard procedure and has been a breakthrough in coronary artery stenting

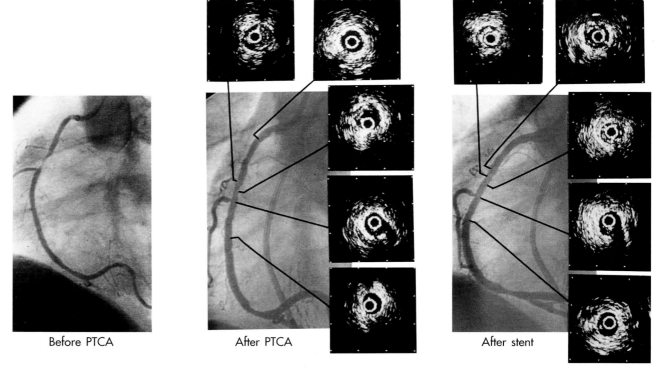

Before PTCA   After PTCA   After stent

Figure 29.4. After PTCA of an RCA restenostic lesion, IVUS revealed a satisfactory increase in free lumen (all images obtained by a 4.8 F, 20 MHz catheter, Diasonics imaging system). After stent implantation (Palmaz–Schatz by Johnson and Johnson), the angiographical appearance improved. However, IVUS depicted incomplete stent expansion (two upper right IVUS images). No acute consequences were drawn in this patient studied in 1992. This patient suffered from subacute stent thrombosis ten days after implantation.

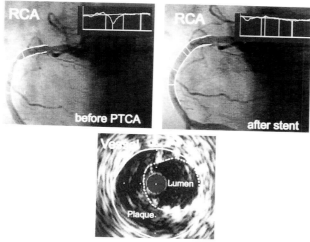

Figure 29.5. De novo stent implantation (Palmaz–Schatz stent by Johnson and Johnson) in a high-grade right coronary artery lesion. The quantitative coronary artery angiography images before and after stent implantation are shown on top. Angiography gave the appearance of a concentric lesion and showed a perfect acute result. IVUS after high-pressure PTCA with a 4.25 mm balloon at 17 atm revealed perfect stent expansion and geometry. However, the gain in free lumen was almost completely due to overextension of the plaque-free wall, leaving a high residual plaque area.

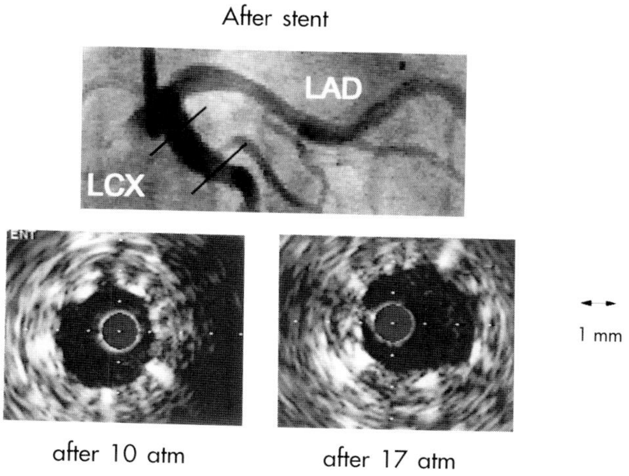

Figure 29.6. Effect of PTCA and a 'step-up' approach in balloon size and inflation pressure on stent size, luminal dimensions, and stent geometry. In a patient with a bail-out situation after PTCA of a proximal LCX stenosis, a 3.5 mm Palmaz–Schatz stent was implanted with 8 atm. (left lower image). A high-pressure PTCA with a 4.0 mm balloon at 18 atm resulted in a clearly visible further increase in stent luminal area. However, in this case no perfect 'circular' geometry of the stent could be achieved.

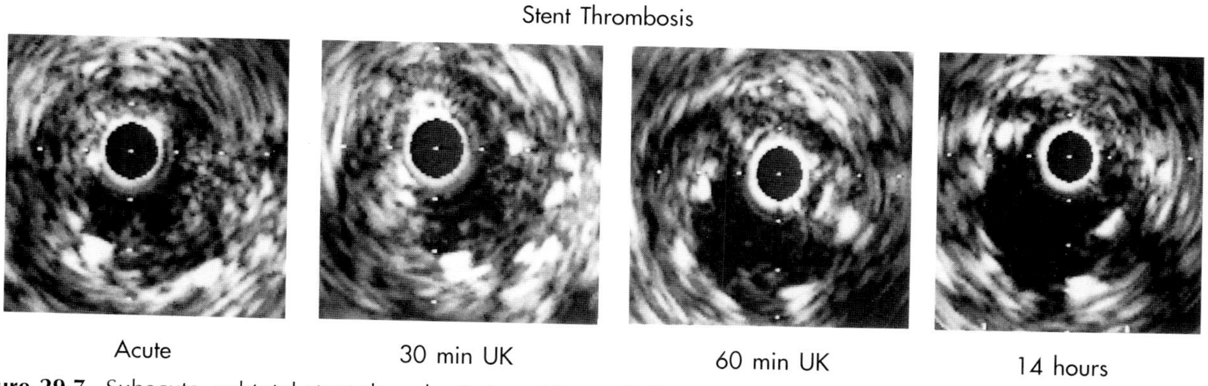

Figure 29.7. Subacute, subtotal stent thrombosis in a 47-year-old patient. Two days after stent implantation in the proximal LAD, the patient reported chest pain. The ECG showed only minor T-wave abnormalities in the precordial leads. Angiography showed TIMI III flow, but a haziness within the stent (not reproduced). IVUS showed soft, mobile structures throughout the entire stent ('Acute' left image). Additional inflations with PTCA balloons were ineffective. Therefore, it was decided to give 2 million units of urokinase (UK) intracoronarily. After 30 minutes, no apparent clinical or morphological effect was found. However, after 60 minutes, the angina resolved and IVUS showed less thrombotic tissue. The next day, the angiographic and IVUS image were normal (14 hours, right). The further course of the patient was uneventful.

(Fig. 29.5). In conjunction with ticlopidine, subacute thrombosis and bleeding complications are now in the range of 1% or even less.[16,17]

Serial IVUS images during stent implantation confirmed the value of high-pressure stent deployment, requiring sometimes 20 atm or more to achieve complete stent expansion (Fig. 29.6).[14,16–18] In comparison with standard techniques, this approach led to an almost 100% increases of the postprocedural coronary minimal luminal areas.[19] The overestimation of luminal dimensions by quantitative coronary angiography, found after low-pressure coronary artery stent deployment, was

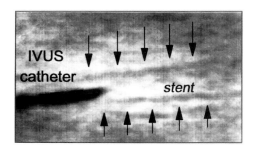

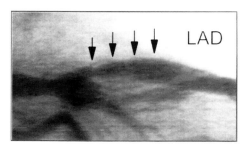

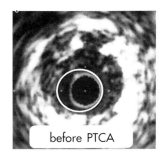

before PTCA

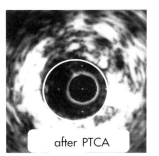

after PTCA

Figure 29.8. In comparison to PTCA, coronary artery stents reduce the restenosis rate. However, a certain proportion of patients develop restenosis even after stent implantation. The cause is mainly intimal hyperplasia. The images show an example of a stent restenosis in the proximal LAD. The upper left image shows the position of the 3.5 F IVUS catheter within the stent. IVUS reveals mainly intimal hyperplasia as cause of restenosis. After PTCA with a 3.5 mm balloon at 6 atm, a significant increase in luminal area without increase in stent area could be achieved.

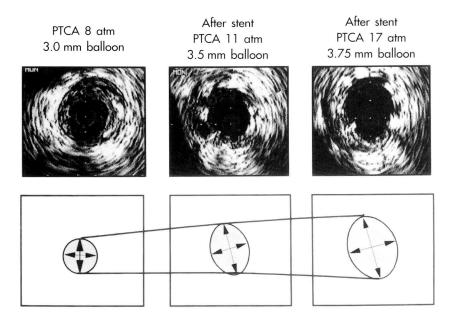

PTCA 8 atm
3.0 mm balloon

After stent
PTCA 11 atm
3.5 mm balloon

After stent
PTCA 17 atm
3.75 mm balloon

Figure 29.9. Effect of increasing balloon pressures and diameters on stent geometry in a proximal, restenotic LAD lesion. Already satisfactory result after PTCA (left), further increase in luminal dimensions after 3.5 mm balloon at 3.5 atm. The high-pressure PTCA with a 3.75 mm balloon resulted in a further increase in luminal area, but also asymmetric stent expansion.

caused by contrast filling of gaps between the outer stent border and the inner luminal margin. With high-pressure stent deployment, this systematic overestimation can be avoided.[20]

IVUS can reveal more precisely than angiography the action of coronary artery stents in attaching dissection membranes and insure that the entire length of dissection is covered by the stent. In a recent study, IVUS revealed incomplete or suboptimal stent expansion in 80% of cases, and even after the application of high-pressure stent deployment 40% of patients still had abnormal IVUS findings.[21]

It is unclear whether the prognosis for these patients is different from those with symmetrical stent expansion.

Beneficial results with high-pressure stent deployment, but without IVUS, have been reported; nevertheless, IVUS-guided implantation results in larger luminal diameters in comparison with angiographically guided stent implantation.[16,17,22]

The consequences of IVUS-guided stent deployment on long-term prognosis are not clear and will be addressed in ongoing trials (Fig. 29.7). IVUS will most likely have a place in the future in all complicated stent deployments (long lesions, diffuse disease, inconclusive angiographical results, very proximal or side-branch implantation) and during follow-up studies to reveal the amount of intimal hyperplasia within the stent.

IVUS and in-stent restenosis

Stent restenosis and the assessment of PTCA for in-stent restenosis can be best evaluated by IVUS. The main process of stent restenosis is intimal hyperplasia within the stent and in the adjacent coronary artery segments. Stent recoil plays no significant role, at least not in stents of the Palmaz–Schatz type (Fig. 29.8).[23,24]

Preliminary results show that PTCA of in-stent restenosis does not achieve the initial luminal dimensions in all patients.[25–27] In these cases, IVUS may help to guide other interventions instead of or as an adjunct to PTCA.

Summary and outlook

In summary, IVUS revolutionized the implantation technique for coronary artery stents. High-pressure coronary artery stent deployment is the present gold-standard. Whether IVUS-guided interventions are superior to angiographically guided procedures alone needs to be evaluated in prospective trials. In the patients who develop in-stent restenosis, IVUS will help in selecting the optimal intervention to restore endoluminal dimensions.

References

1 Sigwart U, Puel J, Mirkovitch V, Joffre F, Kappenberger L. Intravascular stents to prevent occlusion and restenosis after transluminal angioplasty. *N Engl J Med* 1987; **316**: 701–6.

2 Fischman DL, Leon MB, Baim DS et al. (Stent Restenosis Study Investigators). A randomized comparison of coronary-stent placement and balloon angioplasty in the treatment of coronary artery disease. *N Engl J Med* 1994; **331**: 496–501.

3 Serruys PW, de Jaegere P, Kiemeneij F et al. (Benestent Study Group). A comparison of balloon-expandable-stent implantation with balloon angioplasty in patients with coronary artery disease. *N Engl J Med* 1994; **331**: 489–95.

4 Dotter TC. Transluminally placed coilspring endarterial tube grafts: longterm patency in canine popliteal artery. *Invest Radiol* 1969; **4**: 329–32.

5 Haude M, Erbel R, Straub U, Dietz U, Meyer J. Short- and long-term results after intracoronary stenting in human coronary arteries: monocentre experience with the balloon-expandable Palmaz–Schatz stent. *Br Heart J* 1991; **66**: 337–45.

6 Haude M, Erbel R, Straub U, Dietz U, Schatz R, Meyer J. Results of intracoronary stents for management of coronary dissection after balloon angioplasty. *Am J Cardiol* 1991; **67**: 691–6.

7 Haude M, Hafner G, Jablonka A et al. Guidance of anticoagulation after intracoronary implantation of Palmaz–Schatz stents by monitoring prothrombin and prothrombin fragment 1 + 2. *Am Heart J* 1995; **130**: 228–38.

8 Schatz RA. A view of vascular stents. *Circulation* 1989; **79**: 445–7.

9 Cavaye DM, Tabbara MR, Kopchok GE, Termin P, White RA. Intraluminal ultrasound assessment of vascular stent deployment. *Ann Vasc Surg* 1991; **5**: 241–6.

10 Isner JM, Rosenfield K, Losordo DW et al. Percutaneous intravascular US as adjunct to catheter-based interventions: preliminary experience in patients with peripheral vascular disease. *Radiology* 1990; **175**: 61–70.

11 Keren G, Bartorelli AL, Bonner RF, Douek PC, Leon MB. Intravascular ultrasound examination of coronary stents. In: Tobis JM, Yock JM, eds. *Intravascular Ultrasound Imaging*, first edition. Edinburgh: Churchill Livingstone, 1992: 219–30.

12 Görge G, Erbel R, Ge J et al. Intravascular ultrasound after stent implantation. Can stent compression or recoil occur? *Eur Heart J* 1992; **13**: 308.

13 Goldberg SL, Colombo A, Nakamura S, Almagor Y, Maiello L, Tobis JM. Benefit of intracoronary ultrasound in the deployment of Palmaz–Schatz stents. *J Am Coll Cardiol* 1994; **24**: 996–1003.

14 Colombo A, Hall P, Nakamura S et al. Intracoronary stenting without anticoagulation accomplished with intravascular ultrasound guidance. *Circulation* 1995; **91**: 1676–88.

15 Nakamura S, Colombo A, Gaglione A et al. Intracoronary ultrasound observations during stent implantation. *Circulation* 1994; **89**: 2026–34.

16 Morice MC, Zemour G, Benveniste E et al. Intracoronary stenting without coumadin: one-month results of a French multicenter study. *Cathet Cardiovasc Diagn* 1995; **35**: 1–7.

17 Morice MC, Breton C, Bunouf P et al. Coronary stenting without anticoagulation, without intravascular ultrasound. Results of the French registry. *Circulation* 1995; **92**: I796.

18 Mudra H, Klauss V, Blasini R et al. Ultrasound guidance of Palmaz–Schatz intracoronary stenting with a combined intravascular ultrasound balloon catheter. *Circulation* 1994; **90**: 1252–61.

19 Görge G, Haude M, Ge J et al. Intravascular ultrasound after low and high inflation pressure coronary artery stent implantation. *J Am Coll Cardiol* 1995; **26**: 725–30.

20 Blasini R, Schühlen H, Mudra H et al. Angiographic overestimation of lumen size after coronary stent placement: impact of high pressure dilatation. *Circulation* 1995; **92**: I223.

21 Serruys PW, di Mario C. Who was the thrombogenic: the stent or the doctor? *Circulation* 1995; **91**: 1676–88.

22 Nunez BD, Foster-Smith K, Berger PB et al. Benefit of intravascular ultrasound guided high pressure inflations in patients with a 'perfect' angiographic result: the Mayo Clinic experience. *Circulation* 1995; **92**: I545.

23 Ellis SG, Savage M, Fischman D et al. Restenosis after placement of Palmaz–Schatz stents in native coronary arteries: initial results of a multicenter experience. *Circulation* 1992; **86**: 1836–44.

24 Painter JA, Mintz GS, Wong SC et al. Serial intravascular ultrasound studies fail to show evidence of chronic Palmaz–Schatz stent recoil. *Am J Cardiol* 1995; **75**: 398–400.

25 Baim DS, Levine MJ, Leon MB, Levine S, Ellis SG, Schatz RA. Management of restenosis within the Palmaz–Schatz coronary stent (the US multicenter experience). *Am J Cardiol* 1993; **71**: 364–6.

26 Ikari Y, Yamaguchi T, Tamura T, Isshiki T, Saeki F, Hara K. Transluminal extraction atherectomy and adjunctive balloon angioplasty for restenosis after Palmaz–Schatz coronary stent implantation. *Cathet Cardiovasc Diagn* 1993; **30**: 127–30.

27 Ikari Y, Hara K, Tamura T, Saeki F, Yamaguchi T. Luminal loss and site of restenosis after Palmaz–Schatz coronary stent implantation. *Am J Cardiol* 1995; **76**: 117–20.

30 Stenting: functional assessment using Doppler flow velocimetry

Michael Haude

Coronary stent implantation has gained wide acceptance as an adjunct to balloon angioplasty by minimizing postinterventional residual stenosis and by scaffolding the treated arterial conduit.[1] Thereby, peri-interventional flow-limiting dissections can be tacked against the vessel wall, thus preventing acute vessel closure.[2–13] Furthermore, it has been shown that long-term restenosis can be limited by intracoronary implantation of stents in patients with selected de novo and restenotic coronary stenoses.[13–16]

Beside morphologic improvements after stent implantation there might also be a beneficial impact on coronary flow and flow reserve by the minimization of residual stenosis and the creation of a more circular conduit without flaps protruding into the lumen, and a smoother surface.

In contrast to formerly applied Doppler catheters,[17–19] which merely allowed the measurement of coronary flow velocity proximal to stenoses, the Doppler FloWire is a 0.014- or 0.018-inch (0.36 or 0.46 mm) flexible guide wire of 175 cm in length, which has a 12 or 15 MHz Doppler crystal mounted at its distal end which spreads ultrasound at a 20° angle.[20] With the FloWire, coronary flow velocity can be also measured distal to coronary stenoses without having a clear obstructive influence on flow velocity at the stenotic site.[21,22] Doppler spectra are analyzed by fast Fourier transformation and flow velocity can be quantified. Coronary flow velocity ratio can be calculated as the ratio of hyperemic average peak velocity (after intracoronary injection of 12–18 µg adenosine) divided by baseline average peak velocity.[21] The FloWire can also be used as a guide wire for coronary interventions.[23]

Several attempts have been made to use coronary Doppler flow velocimetry for physiology-guided coronary interventions.[24,25] It has been shown that an angiographically successful angioplasty procedure improves coronary flow velocity ratio.[24–27] The DEBATE (Doppler Endpoints Balloon Angioplasty Trial Europe) trial, which tried to identify Doppler flow velocity parameters that are predictive for the outcome after coronary balloon angioplasty with respect to anginal status, recurrent ischemia, major adverse cardiac events and late restenosis or target lesion revascularization, showed that a postinterventional coronary flow velocity reserve ≥ 2.5 (coronary flow velocity ratio) and a residual stenosis ≤ 35% discriminated an angioplasty patient population that had a beneficial long-term outcome compared with the patients in the stent arm of the BENESTENT trial. Nevertheless, a majority of cases is reported to have persisting pathological ratios below 3.0 immediately after the angioplasty procedure, which was identified as the cut-off level in patients without coronary artery disease and other diseases that have an impact on microvascular capacity such as arterial hypertension, diabetes, left ventricular hypertrophy or myocardial infarction. Potential explanations for these findings are several. First, quantitative coronary angiography is known to overestimate postangioplasty lumen dimensions, especially in the presence of dissections. As a result, potential local flow-limiting flaps cannot be identified. Second, postangioplasty residual diameter stenosis is about 30% on average, which could additionally influence flow and flow reserve. Third, changes in baseline flow velocity during the measurement sequence can have an impact on subsequently calculated coronary flow velocity ratios. Fourth, metabolic and humoral disorders can

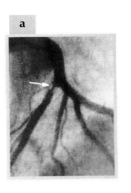
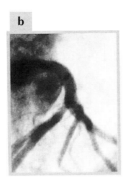
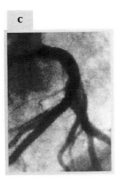

Figure 30.1. Angiograms (**a**) before and (**b**) after coronary balloon angioplasty (PTCA) and (**c**) after stent implantation in a patient with a proximal LAD stenosis (3.5 mm balloon). Reference vessel diameter: (a) 3.45 mm; (b) 3.54 mm; (c) 3.51 mm.

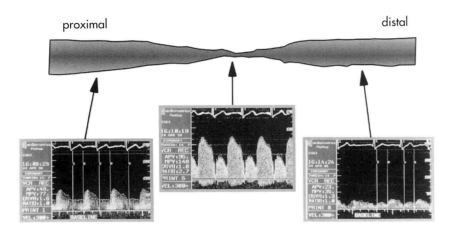

Figure 30.2. Doppler flow velocity spectra while advancing the Doppler FloWire through a coronary stenosis.

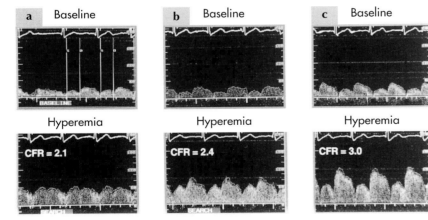

Figure 30.3. Doppler recordings (**a**) before and (**b**) after coronary balloon angioplasty (PTCA) and (**c**) after stent implantation distal to the treated site both at baseline (top row) and during hyperemia (bottom row) induced by intracoronary injection of adenosine.

influence coronary flow and microvascular capacity, especially in complicated angioplasty procedures with prolonged ischemia. Fifth, chronic changes in microvascular capacity might not be reversible immediately after a successful angioplasty procedure.

Since coronary stents can eliminate some of the potential explanations, such as residual stenosis and flow-limiting dissections, the subsequent improve-ment of coronary flow velocity and coronary flow velocity ratio may improve in comparison with balloon angioplasty.[28–32]

As an example, Fig. 30.1 illustrates the angiograms of a patient with proximal stenosis of the left anterior descending artery (LAD). Minimal stenosis diameter was 0.95 before intervention, 2.25 mm after percutaneous transluminal coronary angioplasty (PTCA) and 3.28 mm after stent implantation. The

proximal   distal

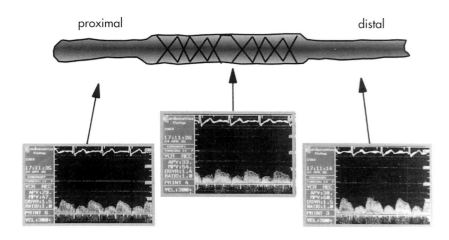

Figure 30.4. Doppler flow velocity spectra during pullback of the Doppler FloWire through the stented vessel segment.

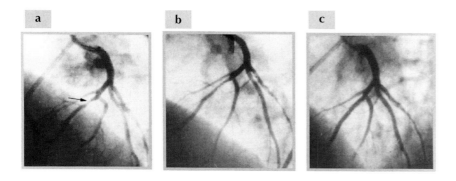

Figure 30.5. Angiograms (**a**) before and (**b**) after coronary balloon angioplasty (PTCA) and (**c**) after stent implantation in a patient with a mid-LAD restenosis (3 mm balloon). Minimal lumen diameter: (a) 0.86 mm; (b) 1.78 mm; (c) 2.88 mm. Reference vessel diameter: (a) 3.02 mm; (b) 3.08 mm; (c) 3.10 mm.

baseline   hyperemia

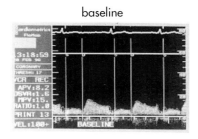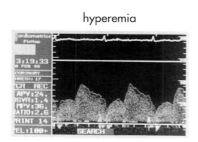

Figure 30.6. Doppler spectra at baseline (left) and during hyperemia (right) before intervention of the patient presented in Fig. 34.5.

patient had no history of myocardial infarction, arterial hypertension, diabetes, hypercholesterolemia, or left ventricular hypertrophy.

When advancing the Doppler FloWire through the stenosis, a significant jetting effect could be documented with acceleration of coronary flow velocity (Fig. 30.2). Distal coronary flow velocity ratio was 2.1 before intervention, which increased to 2.4 after balloon angioplasty and to 3.0 after stent implantation (Fig. 30.3). Remarkably, there was almost no change in baseline flow velocity, while there was a subsequent increase in hyperemic flow velocity being responsible for the improvement of coronary flow velocity ratio. Finally, during pullback of the stent segment there was no longer a jetting effect to be documented (Fig. 30.4).

Thus coronary stent implantation was associated with a morphologic and functional improvement in

baseline

hyperemia

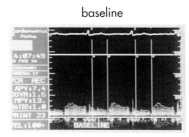
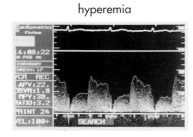

Figure 30.7. Doppler spectra at baseline (left) and during hyperemia (right) after PTCA of the patient presented in Fig. 34.5.

baseline

hyperemia

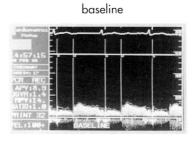
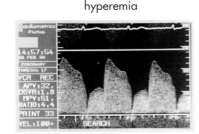

Figure 30.8. Doppler spectra at baseline (left) and during hyperemia (right) after stent implantation of the patient presented in Fig. 34.5.

before intervention

after PTCA

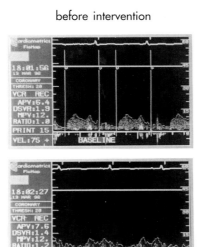
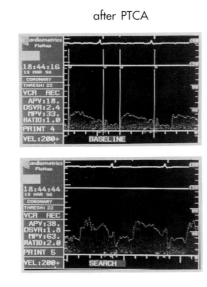

Figure 30.9. Doppler spectra at baseline (above) and during hyperemia (below) before (left) intervention and after (right) PTCA in a patient with LCX stenosis.

comparison with PTCA in this patient, in whom maximal balloon sizes for both procedures were identical. This raises the question whether similar results can be obtained even when the preinterventional coronary flow velocity reserve is only slightly reduced.

Figure 30.5 illustrates the angiograms before and after PTCA and after stent implantation of a patient with an intermediate LAD restenosis six months after an angioplasty procedure. The patient presented with angina class II according to the Canadian Cardiovascular Society and a pathological stress test. The post-PTCA angiogram documented substantial residual stenosis primarily due to elastic recoil. Therefore stenting was attempted to inhibit elastic recoil. The final angiogram after stent implantation documented a clearly improved angiographic appearance of the treated vessel site.

Distal Doppler flow velocity measurements documented a coronary flow velocity ratio of 2.6, which increased to 3.2 after PTCA and to 4.4 after stent implantation (Figs 30.6, 30.7 and 30.8). Similarly to the previously presented case, there was no change in baseline flow velocity, while

after stent implantation

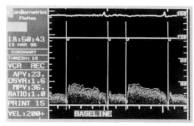

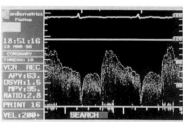

reference vessel

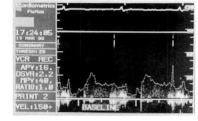

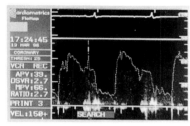

Figure 30.10. Doppler spectra at baseline (above) and during hyperemia (below) after stent implantation (left) and in the reference vessel (LAD) (right) in a patient with LCX stenosis.

hyperemic flow velocity also did not change after PTCA but increased by 25% after stenting.

This raises the issue of the target value of coronary flow velocity ratio which should be aimed for during an angioplasty procedure. At least in patients with single vessel disease the coronary flow velocity ratio of a nonstenotic vessel can be used as an intraindividual reference. The additional impact of other parameters which contribute to microvascular capacity, such as myocardial infarction, hypertension or diabetes, can be ruled out by measuring an intraindividual reference coronary flow velocity reserve.

An example is presented in Figs 30.9 and 30.10. Coronary flow velocity ratio distal to a stenosis in the LCX increased from 1.2 before intervention to 2.0 after PTCA. After stent implantation distal coronary flow velocity reserve was 2.8 and thus was almost identical to the coronary flow velocity ratio in the reference vessel (LAD) with a value of 2.7 (Fig. 30.10).

This concept of measurement of coronary flow velocity ratio in a nonstenotic vessel for intraindividual reference has been applied to Doppler flow velocity measurements in a small patient group with stenoses in the LAD, in whom PTCA and stent implantation were performed.[33] Results showed that only distal coronary flow velocity after stent implantation, but not after PTCA, reached the reference level.

References

1   Haude M, Erbel R, Issa H, Meyer J. Quantitative analysis of elastic recoil after balloon angioplasty and after intracoronary implantation of balloon-expandable Palmaz-Schatz stents. *J Am Coll Cardiol* 1993; **21**: 26–34.

2   Erbel R, Schatz R, Dietz U et al. Ballondilatation und koronare Gefäßstützenimplantation. *Z Kardiol* 1989; **78**: 71–7.

3   Haude M, Erbel R, Straub U, Dietz U, Meyer J. Short- and long-term results after intracoronary stenting in human coronary arteries: monocenter experience with the balloon-expandable Palmaz–Schatz stent. *Br Heart J* 1991; **66**: 337–45.

4   Sigwart U, Urban P, Golf S et al. Emergency stenting for acute occlusion after coronary balloon angioplasty. *Circulation* 1988; **78**: 1121–7.

5   Sigwart U, Puel J, Mirkovitch V, Joffre F, Kappenberger L. Intravsacular stents to prevent occlusion and restenosis after transluminal angioplasty. *N Engl J Med* 1987; **316**: 701–706.

6   de Feyter PJ, de Scheerder I, van den Brand M et al. Emergency stenting for refractory acute coronary artery occlusion. *Am J Cardiol* 1990; **66**: 1147–50.

7   Haude M, Erbel R, Straub U et al. Results of intracoronary stents for management of coronary dissection after balloon angioplasty. *Am J Cardiol* 1991; **67**: 691–6.

8   Maiello L, Colombo A, Gianrossi R, McCanny R, Finci L. Coronary stenting for treatment of acute or threatened closure following dissection after coronary balloon angioplasty. *Am Heart J* 1993; **125**: 1570–5.

9   Lincoff AM, Topol EJ, Chapekis AT et al. Intracoronary stenting compared with conventional therapy for abrupt vessel closure complicating coronary angioplasty: a matched case–control study. *J Am Coll Cardiol* 1993; **21**: 866–75.

10 Schömig A, Kastrati A, Mudra H et al. Four-year experience with Palmaz–Schatz stenting in coronary angioplasty complicated by dissection with threatened or present vessel closure. *Circulation* 1994; **90**: 2716–24.

11 Herrmann HC, Buchbinder M, Clemen MW et al. Emergent use of balloon-expandable coronary artery stenting for failed percutaneous transluminal coronary angioplasty. *Circulation* 1992; **86**: 812–19.

12 Vrolix M, Piessens J. Usefulness of the Wiktor stent for treatment of threatened or acute closure complicating coronary angioplasty. *Am J Cardiol* 1994; **73**: 737–41.

13 Haude M, Erbel R, Hafner G et al. Multicenter results after intracoronary implanation of balloon-expandable Palmaz–Schatz stents. *Z Kardoil* 1993; **82**: 77–86.

14 Fischman DI, Leon MB, Baim DS et al. A randomized comparison of coronary stent placement and balloon angioplasty in the treatment of coronary artery disease. *N Engl J Med* 1994; **331**: 496–501.

15 Serruys PW, de Jaegere P, Kiemeneij F et al. A comparison of balloon-expandable stent implantation with balloon angioplasty in patients with coronary artery disease. *N Engl J Med* 1994; **331**: 489–95.

16 Erbel R, Haude M, Höpp HW et al. on behalf of the REST Study Group. REstenosis STent (REST) study: randomized trial comparing stenting and balloon angioplasty for treatment of restenosis after balloon angioplasty. *J Am Coll Cardiol* 1996; **27(suppl A)**: 732–4 (abst).

17 Cole JS, Hartely CJ. The Doppler coronary artery catheter: preliminary report of a new technique for measuring rapid changes in coronary artery flow velocity in man. *Circulation* 1977; **56**: 18–25.

18 Hartely CJ, Cole JS. An ultrasonic pulsed Doppler system for measuring blood flow in small vessels. *Appl Physiol* 1974; **37**: 626–30.

19 Kern MF, Courtois M, Ludbrook P. A simplified method to measure coronary blood flow velocity in patients: validation and application of a new Judkins style Doppler tipped angiographic catheter. *Am Heart J* 1990; **120**: 1202–8.

20 Doucette JW, Coral TD, Payne HM et al. Validations of a Doppler guidewire for intravascular measurement of coronary artery flow velocity. *Circulation* 1992; **85**: 1899–911.

21 Wilson RF, Laughlin DE, Ackell PH et al. Transluminal subselective measurement of coronary artery blood flow velocity and vasodilator reserve in man. *Circulation* 1985; **72**: 82–92.

22 Ofili EO, Labovitz AJ, Kern MJ. Coronary flow dynamics in normal and diseased arteries. *Am J Cardiol* 1993; **71**: 3D–9D.

23 The DEBATE Study Group. Doppler guide wire as a primary guide wire for PTCA. Feasibility, safety, and continuous monitoring of the results. *Circulation* 1995; **92**: I263.

24 Ofili EO, Labovitz AJ, St Vrain JA et al. Analysis of coronary blood flow dynamics in angiographically normal and stenosed arteries before and after endoluminal enlargement by angioplasty. *J Am Coll Cardiol* 1993; **21**: 308–16.

25 Segal J, Kern MJ, Scott NA et al. Alterations of phasic coronary artery flow velocity in man during percutaneous coronary angioplasty. *J Am Coll Cardiol* 1992; **20**: 276–86.

26 The DEBATE Study Group. Cyclic flow variations after PTCA are predictive of immediate complications. *Circulation* 1995; **92**: I725.

27 The DEBATE Study Group. Are flow velocity measurements after PTCA predictive of recurrence of angina or of a positive exercise stress test early after balloon angioplasty? *Circulation* 1995; **92**: I547.

28 Rupprecht HJ, Erbel R, Kooymann C, Schmitz A, Görge G. Stent implantation: cosmetics or functional improvement? *Circulation* 1991; **84**: I196A.

29 Haude M, Lang M, Issa H, Renneisen U, Brennecke R. Additional improvement of stenosis dimensions and coronary flow after intracoronary implantation of Palmaz–Schatz stents. *Circulation* 1991; **84**: II196 (abst).

30 Ge J, Erbel R, Zamorano J et al. Improvement of coronary morphology and blood flow after stenting: assessment by intravascular ultrasound and intracoronary Doppler. *Int J Card Imaging* 1995; **11**: 81–7.

31 Haude M, Caspari G, Baumgart D et al. Normalisierung der myokardialen Perfusionsreserve nach koronarer Stentimplantation im Gegensatz zur alleinigen Ballonangioplastie. *Z Kardiol* 1996; **85**: 260–72.

32 Haude M, Caspari G, Baumgart D, Brennecke R, Meyer J, Erbel R. Comparison of myocardial perfusion reserve before and after coronary ballon angioplasty and after stent implantation in patients with post-angioplasty restenosis. *Circulation* 1996 (in press).

33 Haude M, Baumgart D, Caspari G, Erbel R. Does adjunct coronary stenting in comparison to balloon angioplasty have an impact on Doppler flow velocity parameters? *Circulation* 1995; **92**: 547.

31 Three-dimensional intravascular ultrasound for stenting

Francesco Prati, Carlo Di Mario, Robert Gil, Clemens von Birgelen, Nico Bruining, Patrick W Serruys and Jos R T C Roelandt

Introduction

Conventional two-dimensional intravascular ultrasound assessment of stent deployment

The use of intravascular ultrasound (IVUS) has exerted a strong influence in the strategy of stent positioning. The Colombo group documented with IVUS incomplete stent apposition to the vessel wall and residual narrowings within the stented segments in a high percentage of cases, despite the achievement of optimal angiographic results.[1–4] The attainment of a substantial increase of lumen dimensions and the elimination of residual narrowing in the stented segment obtained with IVUS translate into two major clinical benefits: a large reduction of the incidence of subacute stent thrombosis and a decrease in the restenosis rate.[5–9]

Rationale for the use of three-dimensional reconstruction of intravascular ultrasound for guidance of stent deployment

The current assessment of proper stent expansion by two-dimensional IVUS requires a cumbersome and subjective review of the examination at each step of the procedure, selecting and measuring the minimal cross-sectional area within the stented segment and two appropriate reference cross-sectional areas proximal and distal to the stent. These limitations can be overcome by a recently developed, fully automated, on-line, three-dimensional reconstruction system that facilitates stenting guidance by providing a proper definition of longitudinal vessel architecture before and after stent positioning.

This chapter reports the authors' experience with the use of an on-line 3D IVUS system, capable of automated vessel lumen identification, for guidance of interventional procedures.

Three-dimensional reconstruction techniques

The acquisition, digitization and segmentation of two-dimensional ultrasound cross-sectional images, and the final display, are the sequential steps required to obtain a three-dimensional reconstruction.[10,11] Different modalities of 2D IVUS image acquisition, digitization and segmentation have been used for on-line and off-line applications of 3D reconstruction. The acoustic quantification system has been used at the Thoraxcenter, Rotterdam, for guidance of interventional procedures. The system is based on rapid acquisition and segmentation steps that allow an automated lumen volume assessment of the reconstructed segment and which is therefore suitable for on-line applications.

Acoustic quantification system

Acquisition

IVUS images are obtained with a mechanical 2.9 F. (diameter 0.96 mm) ultrasound catheter (Micro-View 30 MHz, CVIS, Sunnyvale, CA). Ultrasound catheters are equipped with a transparent distal sleeve that can accept alternatively a guide wire for intracoronary insertion or a flexible ultrasound imaging rotating cable.

IVUS assessment is performed by pulling back the guide wire to a radio-opaque marker and positioning the imaging probe distal to the lesion. Image acquisition is then performed using a continuous pullback device. In the authors' experience a 1 mm/s pullback speed is an adequate compromise between resolution of longitudinal reconstruction and avoidance of excessive duration of examination. Ultrasound catheter design facilitates image acquisition since the presence of the transparent sleeve avoids direct contact of imaging core and vessel wall and therefore reduces the risk of a nonuniform pullback.

Digitization and image segmentation

The system operates on a dedicated Intel Pentium 60 MHz personal computer using the OS/2 operating system, digitizing the analog video image on-line at a digitization frame rate of 8.5 images per second. A maximum of 255 basic IVUS images can be used for 3D reconstruction. Since the image acquisition rate is fixed, using a 1.0 mm/s pullback speed, a vessel segment with a maximal length of 30 mm can be reconstructed.

IVUS images are processed on-line with a blood speckle identification method that is able to detect the blood–intima interface by distinguishing between the vessel wall backscatter and the backscatter pattern of blood cells that exhibits more variation in time than the former (EchoQuant, Indec

Systems Inc., Capitola, CA). Segmentation is then performed by removing the blood pool, identified in all the images.

This method has been previously validated in an animal model[12] and has been already described.[10,11]

On-line reconstruction and quantification

After acquisition, the cross-sectional images are rapidly processed and the system can display the reconstructed 3D image and the quantitative analysis of the selected segment. The short time required for acquisition and segmentation (155 seconds for a segment 30 mm in length) allows the system to be used on-line in the catheterization laboratory for clinical decision making.

The longitudinal view of the analyzed segment and a diagram showing measurements of minimal lumen diameter and of minimal lumen area over the segment itself are displayed. By scrolling the longitudinal view and the measurement diagram with a cursor, automatically contoured lumen cross-sectional areas can be selected. With this approach the minimal lumen cross-sectional area within the stent is automatically detected and a reference proximal and distal frame can be easily selected 3–5 mm on either side of the stented segment. The residual stent stenosis is automatically calculated as the ratio of the minimal stent lumen area to the reference lumen area. The contours of the stent

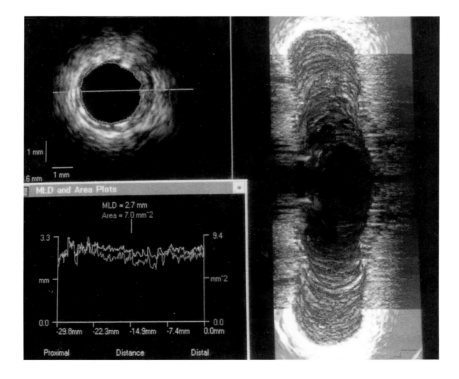

Figure 31.1. A well deployed Cordis stent is shown. The measurement diagram with measurements of lumen area and diameter (lower panel) facilitated the selection of the transverse view of the stented segment with the minimal lumen area (left upper panel). A moderate residual plaque burden and a minimal residual percentage area stenosis are present. In the right panel the 3D cylindrical format is displayed as a 'clam shell' view, with the vessel open longitudinally and both halves tilted back 30°, showing the inner surface of the vessel.

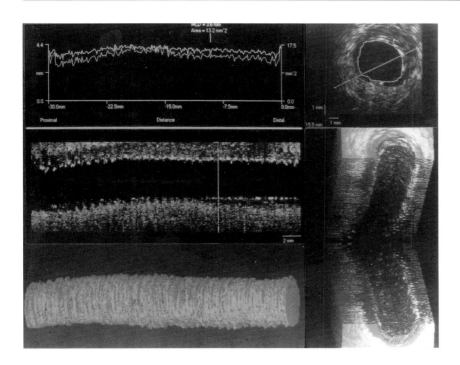

Figure 31.2 A 3D reconstruction of the proximal mid-right coronary artery after implantation of two sequential Wallstents. The longitudinal display of the vessel (mid-left panel), the measurement diagram (upper left panel) and the lumen cast format (lower left panel) demonstrate that a regular lumen was achieved after high-pressure balloon dilatations of the stented segment. A moderate residual plaque is present in the transverse view (right upper panel). The cylindrical reconstruction of the artery ('clam shell' view) confirms the adequacy of stent expansion (lower right panel).

lumen area and of the reference segments can be manually corrected in case of failure of the automated detection. Furthermore, the external contour of the total vessel area, defined as the area inside the interface between plaque–media complex and adventitia (area inside the external elastic membrane), can be traced manually.

Lengths of segments of interest or distances between anatomic landmarks can be measured on the 3D longitudinal display.

A 3D cylindrical format is also available and is displayed as a 'clam shell' view, with the vessel open longitudinally and both halves tilted back 30°, showing the inner surface of the vessel (Figs 31.1, 31.2).

Thoraxcenter experience on feasibility and clinical usefulness of on-line 3D IVUS for stent deployment

Methods

Population

Between June, 1994 and February, 1995 the authors assessed the feasibility and clinical usefulness of on-line 3D IVUS in 49 patients undergoing stent deployment. A reliable 3D reconstruction could be obtained in 41 patients (80%) which represent the study population.

In total 70 stents were imaged with 3D IVUS. Table 31.1 reports patient clinical profile and procedural characteristics. No complications occurred due to 3D IVUS use. All patients were put on oral anticoagulants for at least three months at a dosage sufficient to maintain the thrombin time between 5 and 10%.

Procedure

Stents were deployed with an aggressive approach consisting of high-pressure inflations exerted with balloons 0.5 mm greater than the interpolated reference diameter. After a negative percentage diameter stenosis was obtained by on-line quantitative coronary angiography (QCA) (minimal lumen diameter within the stent larger than the reference diameter), 3D IVUS was carried out.

The treatment strategies planned before and after 3D IVUS were compared to assess the impact of 3D IVUS on subsequent revascularization strategy.

In a group of 10 patients (30%) 3D IVUS was also successfully carried out before stenting and its results could then be used to plan the subsequent stent selection.

Table 31.1. Clinical, angiographic and procedural data.

	N
No. of patients	49
Age (years)	58.9±6.8
Sex (male)	36 (73%)
Treated vessel:	
LAD	23 (47%)
RCA	16 (33%)
LCX	3 (6%)
SVBG	7 (14%)
De Novo lesion	34 (69%)
Restenosis	15 (31%)
Elective procedure	38 (78%)
Bail-out procedure	11 (22%)
Single stent	35 (72%)
Multiple stent	14 (28%)
Inflation pressure (atm)	14.2±3.3
Balloon diameter (mm)	3.6±0.7
Balloon–artery ratio	1.3±0.2
No. of stents	70
Stents/patient	1.4
Stent type:	
Palmaz–Schatz[a]	31 (44%)
Wallstent[b]	22 (31%)
Cordis[c]	7 (10%)
Microstent[d]	6 (9%)
Gianturco–Roubin[e]	2 (3%)
Multilink[f]	2 (3%)

[a]Johnson & Johnson Interventional Systems, Warren, NJ.
[b]Schneider, Zurich, Switzerland.
[c]Cordis Corporation, Miami, FL.
[d]Applied Vascular Engineering, Edmonton, Canada.
[e]Cook Inc., Bloomington, IN.
[f]Advanced Cardiovascular Systems Inc., Temecula, CA.
LAD: left anterior descending artery; RCA: right coronary artery; LCX: left circumflex artery; SVBG: saphenous venous by-pass graft.

The 3D IVUS criteria indicative of optimal stent expansion were (a) complete apposition of stent struts to the vessel wall and (b) a symmetry index (minimum divided by maximum lumen ratio) greater than 0.7. Furthermore, an attempt was made to maximize the intrastent lumen area to match the lumen area of the reference segment and to cover with stents all the segments with residual significant lesions (plaque burden > 50%).

Results

Feasibility of on-line 3D reconstruction

A reliable 3D reconstruction of target lesions before stenting was obtained in eight cases (80%). After interventional procedures 3D IVUS reconstruction was successfully performed in 41 out of 49 cases (80%).

Three-dimensional IVUS for assessment of stent positioning

In two out of 10 patients who underwent 3D IVUS assessment before stent implantation an additional significant lesion (plaque burden more than 50%) was revealed by 3D IVUS. The stent minimal lumen diameter was significantly overestimated by QCA in comparison to 3D IVUS ($3.0±0.5$ mm versus $2.6±0.4$ mm, respectively; $P< 0.01$). In four out of 41 lesions (10%) strut protrusion within the vessel lumen and/or asymmetrical stent expansion caused by a large eccentric underlying plaque was present.

A residual plaque burden more than 50% in the segments adjacent to stent endings was found in eight patients (19%).

Impact on revascularization strategy

The revascularization strategy was modified in two of eight cases, in which an additional lesion, not recognized by QCA, was identified and two sequential stents were placed. After stent implantation, 3D IVUS triggered further high-pressure balloon dilatations within the stent in 15 patients (37%) in order to correct asymmetric stent expansion or increase the intrastent lumen area. Additional stent implantation was carried out in eight patients (19%) to cover diseased segments adjacent to stent endings with plaque burden more than 50% by 3D IVUS evaluation. On the whole, after stenting, the management strategy was modified in 23 of 41 patients (56%).

Clinical outcome

A subacute stent thrombosis occurred in one patient (2%) who received a Gianturco–Roubin implantation in the left anterior descending artery as a bail-out procedure for real acute vessel occlusion.

Discussion

Feasibility of on-line 3D reconstruction

A reliable on-line 3D reconstruction was obtained in 80% of cases. The presence of plaque calcifications and of side-branches was the main cause of failure of the system algorithm properly to identify the vessel lumen, before and after catheter-based revascularizations.

Similar findings were reported in a previous study performed on a smaller population in which the three-dimensional reconstruction of IVUS was attempted in 10 coronary segments during coronary interventions. The study was designed to compare the on-line automated measurements of lumen cross-sections with the measurements obtained off-line after manual correction performed by an experienced analyst. Of the 1710 on-line cross-sections obtained, 232 (13.6%) could not be properly identified by the system algorithm due to the presence of side-branches, shadowing of calcium interpreted as lumen, and lack of sharpness of the lumen–wall interface.[13]

Assessment of preintervention target lesion

Unlike angiography, IVUS permits direct visualization of plaque characteristics and dimensions and can reveal significant stenoses that were not suspected angiographically.[14–16] For this reason the use of IVUS has been proposed for guidance of interventional procedures.[17,18]

The accurate definition of longitudinal vessel architecture that can be obtained with 3D IVUS offers consistent advantages over 2D IVUS. The evaluation of the lesion length and distance between lesion and coronary ostium or large side-branches obviates the risk of angiographic vessel foreshortening and is a prerequisite for an appropriate selection of the stent length.

In this study 3D IVUS evaluation before stenting was rarely performed but altered the treatment strategy in two out of eight patients (25%) in which two additional significant lesions, underestimated by QCA, were stented.

It should be noted that in two cases 3D IVUS also supported the decision to avoid revascularizations planned on QCA evaluations. Similarly, in a recent study by Mintz et al.[19] on IVUS assessment of ambiguous and intermediate angiographic lesions, planned revascularizations were aborted in a high percentage of cases and only 10% of these patients required target lesion revascularization at a one-year follow-up.

Assessment of stent expansion

Further trials are needed to clarify whether the use of IVUS reduces stent subacute thrombosis and late restenosis to a larger extent than angiography.[6,20,21] However, for an IVUS-guided application, the use of three-dimensional reconstruction after stenting

offers advantages over conventional IVUS assessment since the on-line longitudinal view of the entire stent length and of the adjacent segments provides a quick overview of the adequacy of stent deployment and of the unstented vessel architecture.[10,11]

Only a few reports on the use of 3D IVUS for the evaluation of stent positioning are available. Mintz et al.[22] performed the three-dimensional reconstruction of 10 stents in vitro and 37 in vivo, using a thresholding-based algorithm. Three-dimensional reconstruction offered clear details on the geometry of the endovascular stent designs.

Other reports documented the usefulness of 3D reconstruction for treatment of coronary dissections with stent deployment. Three-dimensional IVUS measured accurately the length of the coronary lesions to be stented and as a consequence facilitated stent selection. Furthermore, after stent deployment 3D IVUS documented the adequacy of stent expansion.[23,24]

IVUS evaluation of residual lesions adjacent to stent provides valuable information, since previous studies documented that a significant atherosclerotic involvement and the presence of dissection in the unstented segment may impair the inflow or outflow of the stented segment and lead to early thrombotic events.[25,26] Three-dimensional IVUS was significantly instrumental in interrogating residual lesions after stent deployment and triggered additional stent implantations in 19% of cases in which residual lesions in coronary segments either proximal or distal to stent endings (with cross-sectional stenosis greater than 50%) were documented (Fig. 31.3).

Despite the use of multiple stents and long Wallstent in a substantial percentage of cases for treatment of long lesions (> 15 mm) and of dissections occurring after stent positioning, a plaque burden greater than 50% was found in a high percentage of cases, indicating that a complete restoration of the original vessel lumen cannot be achieved in all cases. The routine use of 3D IVUS before interventions might significantly reduce the incidence of residual lesions adjacent to stents. In fact, based on the assessment of the longitudinal extension of target lesions an accurate selection of stent length is possible.

Furthermore, despite the achievement of optimal QCA results in all cases, residual stent underexpansion was often identified by 3D IVUS and triggered additional inflation within the stented segments in 35% of cases (Figs 31.4–31.6). Stent underexpansion seems to be detected more

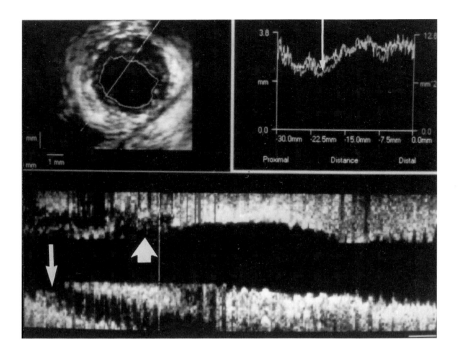

Figure 31.3 The 3D IVUS reconstruction, obtained after positioning of a 15-mm long Palmaz–Schatz stent in the mid-left anterior descending artery, clearly shows a large residual plaque proximal to the stent. The longitudinal view in the lower panel shows the residual plaque (arrowhead) starting immediately after the take-off of a large diagonal branch (arrowhead). The presence of a residual plaque is also documented by the corresponding transverse view (left upper panel) and by the measurement diagram (right upper panel) exhibiting a reduction of lumen area due to plaque protrusion (arrowhead).

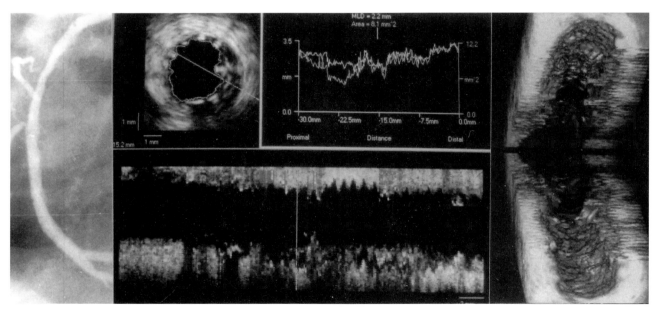

Figure 31.4 Despite a satisfactory angiographic appearance of the right coronary artery after the deployment of three AVE stents, 3D IVUS reveals the underexpansion of the mid AVE stent. The longitudinal view in the lower panel shows a clear stent strut protrusion within the lumen corresponding to an abrupt reduction of minimal lumen area in the measurement diagram (right upper panel). The protrusion of the stent struts within the lumen is also visible in the transverse view (left upper panel) and in the 'clam shell' view.

accurately and objectively by 3D than 2D IVUS since the combined use of a longitudinal display and of a measurement diagram leads to a precise evaluation of the stent minimal lumen cross-sectional area. In a previous report on the comparison between 2D and 3D IVUS measurements after

stent deployment, 3D IVUS was more sensitive in the evaluation of inadequate stent expansion.[27]

The low incidence of subacute stent thrombosis reported in this study confirms the utility of 3D IVUS guidance during stenting.

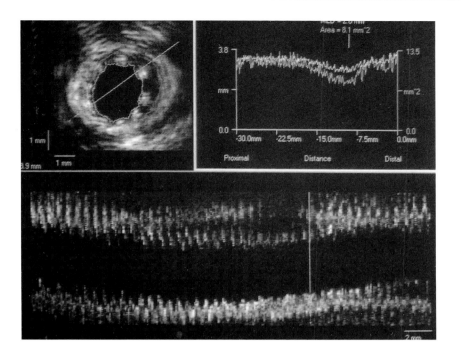

Figure 31.5 The figure illustrates a case with nonadequate Wallstent deployment in a left anterior descending artery. Three-dimensional IVUS clearly reveals stent underexpansion. The longitudinal view in the lower panel shows a residual plaque, indicated by a vertical line, that corresponds to a reduction of minimal lumen area in the measurement diagram (right upper panel).

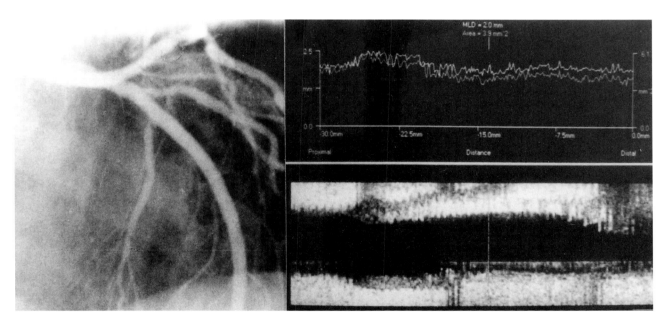

Figure 31.6 Wallstent deployment in a left anterior descending artery. Despite a satisfactory evaluation of stent deployment by angiography (left panel), the 3D longitudinal view in the lower panel shows a residual plaque. A corresponding reduction of minimal lumen area and of minimal lumen diameter can be appreciated in the measurement diagram (right upper panel).

Limitations

Since there is not a clear consensus on the IVUS criteria of adequate stent expansion to be used, the authors only attempted to maximize stent minimal

lumen area to approximate the reference artery lumen.

Some factors can interfere with a correct acquisition of the sequence of IVUS images and limit the quality of three-dimensional reconstruction. In particular, curvature of the vessel also induces a distortion of the 3D image which is reconstructed on a straight line through the center of successive cross-sections. Since an ECG-triggered (electrocardiogram) acquisition was not performed, the accuracy of quantitative measurements was limited by the systolic expansion of the coronary vessel lumen and the movement artifact of the ultrasound catheter.[10,11,28]

Conclusions

Three-dimensional reconstruction of IVUS is a feasible technique for the guidance of stent deployment procedures which facilitates stent selection and strongly affects the revascularization strategy by accurately detecting stent underexpansion and the presence of uncovered lesions.

References

1 Nakamura S, Colombo A, Gaglione A et al. Intracoronary ultrasound observations during stent implantation. *Circulation* 1994; **89**: 2026–34.

2 Goldberg SL, Colombo A, Nakamura S, Almagor Y, Maiello L, Tobis JM. The benefit of intracoronary ultrasound in the deployment of Palmaz–Schatz stents. *J Am Coll Cardiol* 1994; **24**: 996–1003.

3 Mudra H, Klauss V, Blasini R et al. Ultrasound guidance of Palmaz–Schatz intracoronary stenting with a combined intravascular ultrasound balloon catheter. *Circulation* 1994; **90**: 1252–61.

4 Russo RR, Schatz RA, Sklar MA, Johnson AD, Tobis JM, Teirstein PS. Ultrasound guided coronary stent placement without prolonged systemic anticoagulation. *J Am Coll Cardiol* 1995; **25**: 50A (abst).

5 Hall P, Nakamura S, Maiello L et al. Factors associated with late angiographic outcome after intravascular ultrasound guided Palmaz–Schatz coronary stent implantation: a multivariate analysis. *J Am Coll Cardiol* 1995; **25**: 36A (abst).

6 Serruys PW, Di Mario C. Who was thrombogenic: the stent or the doctor? *Circulation* 1995; **91**: 1891–3.

7 Colombo A, Hall P, Nakamura S et al. Intracoronary stenting without anticoagulation accomplished with intravascular ultrasound guidance. *Circulation* 1995; **91**: 1676–88.

8 Serruys PW, de Jaegere P, Kiemeneij F et al. for the BENESTENT Study Group. A comparison of balloon-expandable stent implantation with balloon angioplasty in patients with coronary artery disease. *N Engl J Med* 1994; **331**: 489–95.

9 Fischman DL, Leon MB, Baim DS et al. for the Stent Restenosis Study Investigators. A randomized comparison of coronary stent placement and balloon angioplasty in the treatment of coronary artery disease. *N Engl J Med* 1994; **331**: 496–501.

10 Roelandt JRTC, Di Mario C, Pandian NG et al. Three-dimensional reconstruction of intracoronary ultrasound images: rationale, approaches, problems and directions. *Circulation* 1994; **90**: 1044–55.

11 Di Mario C, von Birgelen C, Prati F et al. Three-dimensional reconstruction of two-dimensional intracoronary ultrasound: clinical or research tool? *Br Heart J* 1995; **73(suppl 2)**: 26–32.

12 Hausmann D, Friedrich G, Sudhir K et al. 3-D intravascular ultrasound imaging with automated border detection using 2.9 F catheters. *J Am Coll Cardiol* 1994; **23**: 174A (abst).

13 Prati F, Di Mario C, von Birgelen C et al. On-line automated lumen volume measurements with 3-D intracoronary ultrasound during coronary interventions. *J Am Coll Cardiol* 1995; **25**: 345A (abst).

14 Nissen SE, Gurley JC, Grines CL et al. Intravascular ultrasound assessment of lumen size and wall morphology in normal subjects and patients with coronary artery disease. *Circulation* 1991; **84**: 1087–99.

15 White CJ, Ramee RS, Collins TJ, Jain A, Mesa JE. Ambiguous coronary angiography: clinical utility of intravascular ultrasound. *Cathet Cardiovasc Diagn* 1992; **26**: 200–3.

16 Ehrlich S, Honye J, Mahon D, Bernstein R, Tobis J. Unrecognized stenosis by angiography documented by intracoronary ultrasound imaging. *Cathet Cardiovasc Diagn* 1991; **23**: 198–201.

17 Mintz GS, Pichard AD, Kovach JA et al. Impact of preintervention intravascular ultrasound imaging on transcatheter treatment strategies in coronary artery disease. *Am J Cardiol* 1994; **73**: 423–30.

18 Yock PG, Fitzgerald PJ, Linker DT, Angelsen BAJ. Intravascular ultrasound guidance for catheter-based coronary interventions. *J Am Coll Cardiol* 1991; **17**: 39B–45B.

19 Mintz GS, Bucher TA, Kent KM et al. Clinical outcomes of patients not undergoing coronary artery revascularization as a result of intravascular ultrasound imaging. *J Am Coll Cardiol* 1995; **25**: 61A (abst).

20 Emanuelsson H, Serruys PW, Belardi J et al. Clinical experience with heparin-coated stents. The BENESTENT II pilot phase 1. *J Am Coll Cardiol* 1995; **25**: 181A (abst).

21 Morice MC, Bouronnec C, Lefevre T. Coronary stenting without Coumadin. Phase III. *Circulation* 1994; **90-I**: 127 (abst).

22 Mintz GS, Pichard AD, Satler LF, Popma JJ, Kent KM, Leon MB. Three-dimensional intravascular ultrasonography: reconstruction of endovascular stents in vitro and in vivo. *J Clin Ultrasound* 1993; **21**: 609–15.

23 Schryver TE, Popma JJ, Kent KM, Leon MB, Eldredge S, Mintz GS. Use of intracoronary ultrasound to identify the 'true' coronary lumen in chronic coronary dissections treated with intracoronary stenting. *Am J Cardiol* 1992; **69**: 1107–8.

24 Prati F, Di Mario C, Hamburger JN, Gil R, von Birgelen C, Serruys PW. Guidance of multiple stent deployment in a chronic totally occluded coronary artery using three-dimensional reconstruction of intracoronary ultrasound. *Am Heart J* 1995; **130**: 1285–9.

25 Roubin SS, Cannon AD, Agrawal SK et al. Intracoronary stenting for acute and threatened closure complicating percutaneous transluminal coronary angioplasty. *Circulation* 1992; **85**: 916–27.

26 Schuhlen H, Blasini R, Mufra H et al. Stenting for progressive dissection during PTCA: clinical, angiographic and intravascular ultrasound criteria to define a low-risk group not requiring subsequent anticoagulation. *J Am Coll Cardiol* 1995; **25**: 123A (abst).

27 Prati F, Di Mario C, Gil R et al. 3-D intracoronary ultrasound reconstruction in the assessment of stent deployment after angiographic optimization. Comparison with 2-D intracoronary ultrasound. *Eur Heart J* 1995; **16**: 427 (abst).

28 Dhavale PJ, Wilson DL, Hodgson J. Optimal data acquisition for volumetric intracoronary ultrasound. *Cathet Cardiovasc Diagn* 1994; **32**: 288–99.

32 Intravascular ultrasound in aortic dissection

Günter Görge, Thomas Buck, Junbo Ge and Raimund Erbel

Introduction

Aortic dissections and aortic aneurysms are diseases with high mortality. Therefore early diagnosis is crucial for correct patient management. Angiography was the only available diagnostic tool for over two decades before computed tomography added significantly to the diagnosis and understanding of aortic diseases.[1] However, both techniques have limitations. Angiography is invasive, usually requires large amounts of contrast material and is still often inconclusive, especially in the abdominal organs. Computed tomography (CT) is noninvasive, but also requires large amounts of contrast material. Its sensitivity and specificity is largely operator-dependent. The most important limitation of CT scanning is that the technique is not always available, especially for patients in an unstable condition, where rapid diagnosis and institution of appropriate care is crucial.[2,3]

Transesophageal echocardiography (TEE) made it possible for the first time to assess patients with aortic dissection at the bedside. TEE proved to be very sensitive and specific in the diagnosis of aortic aneurysms and dissections.[1] Additionally, TEE increased our understanding of the pathophysiology of aortic dissections, leading to a modification of previous grading systems. But TEE also has limitations, such as the inferior image quality in the aortic arch and the ability to scan only the proximal half of the descending aorta. Therefore the distal extension of the dissection membrane cannot be assessed in a significant number of patients.

Role of intravascular ultrasound (IVUS) in aortic disease

Pandian et al. and Roelandt et al. first suggested the potential role of IVUS in aortic diseases.[4,5] Gerber et al. assessed the feasibility and safety of aortic imaging by IVUS.[6] Görge et al. were the first to report on a larger series of patients with aortic abnormalities studied with IVUS, angiography and CT scans.[2] IVUS could be performed in all patients, but image quality in the ascending aorta, the aortic arch, and aneurysmatic parts of the aorta was inferior due to limitations in far field penetration (Fig. 32.1). However, the dissection membrane could be imaged in all patients and the distal extension could be identified. Weintraub et al. reported on IVUS in 28 patients with suspected aortic dissection.[3] All patients underwent contrast angiography; seven had computed tomography and 22 had TEE. Imaging of the aorta from the root level to its bifurcation was performed in all patients in an average of 10 minutes. No IVUS-related complications occurred. Dissection was present in 23 patients and absent in five. In all patients with dissection, IVUS demonstrated the intimal flap and the true and false lumens. The longitudinal and circumferential extent of aortic dissection, contents of the false lumen, involvement of branch vessels and the presence of intramural hematoma in the aortic wall could also be identified. In all cases where aortography could not define the distal extent of the dissection, intravascular ultrasound was able to do so (Figs 32.2 and 32.3).

Yamada et al. were able to confirm these results in studying 15 patients with aortic dissection, imaging by IVUS and angiography, TEE, computed tomography, or magnetic resonance imaging. The detection rate of the intimal flap was 100% on all segments of the aorta, and the detection rate of the intimal tear was 0%, 50%, 50%, and 77.8% in the ascending, arch, descending, and abdominal aorta, respectively, reflecting the limitations of present IVUS technology in larger vessels.[7] In the study by Yamada et al., IVUS demonstrated in all cases the celiac and renal arteries, and in 80% of patients the superior mesenteric arteries and their relation to dissection. Good correlation between IVUS and

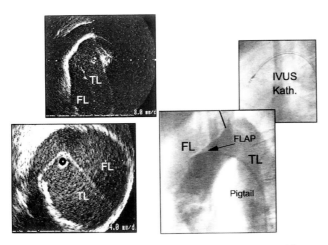

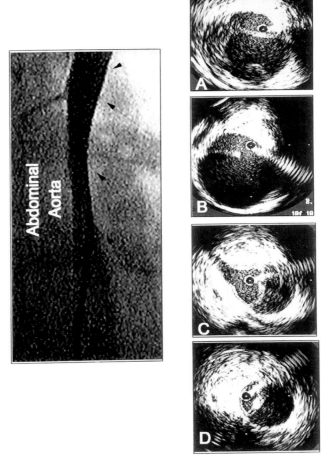

Figure 32.1. Intravascular ultrasound in a 28-year-old patient with Marfan's syndrome and aortic dissection. The lower right image shows the angiogram obtained in a 60° LAO angulation. The true (TL), the false (FL) lumen, and the dissection membrane are clearly visible. A flap prolapsed into the left subclavian artery, and is indicated by the black line. The right upper image shows the position of a 10 F. 10 MHz catheter (CVIS system). In the ascending aorta, the elasticity of the IVUS catheter stretches the dissection membrane and the true and false lumen are clearly visible. In the aortic arch, a large entry with a free floating 'flap' was visualized by IVUS. This flap protruded into the left subclavian artery causing variable symptoms in this patient. However, in the aortic arch, no complete, circumferential image could be obtained in this position. In the upper image, distance between two spots represents 8.0 mm, and 4.0 mm in the left lower image.

Figure 32.3. Same patient as in Fig. 32.2 in images A and B. In the abdominal aorta, a side-branch originating from the true lumen (arrow, image C) could be imaged by IVUS. During further pullback (image D), the true lumen became very small (distance between two spots equals 8.0 mm).

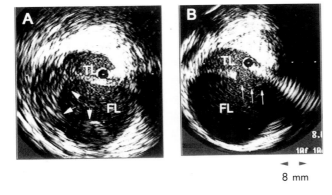

Figure 32.2. Image A: the IVUS catheter is in the true lumen (TL). The much larger false lumen (FL) can be imaged. At 6 o'clock and from 8–10 o'clock, thrombotic material can be imaged by the 10 F. 10 MHz IVUS catheter. Image B: during pullback of the IVUS catheter, the communication of the true and false lumen, a relatively wide gap, could be imaged. The structure at 4 o'clock represents the guide-wire artefact.

computed tomographic values for vessel diameter (r = 0.98, $P < 0.01$) was found. IVUS accurately demonstrated thrombus or spontaneous echo contrast in the false lumen. It was especially useful in evaluating the abdominal aorta with regard to determining the size of the vessel, the extent of dissection, the relation of the branches to the false lumen, and the detection of intimal tears. This additional information allows the cardiologist to examine the entire aorta and to plan further treatment (Fig. 32.4).

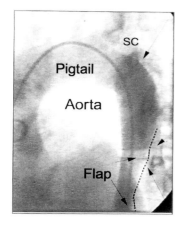
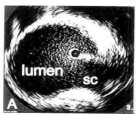
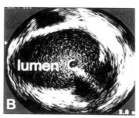
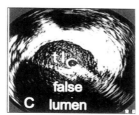

Figure 32.4. Patient with aortic dissection starting from his left subclavian artery (image A). Image B shows a large re-entry. Image C the true (TL) and false lumen. The pigtail is in the true lumen. All IVUS images obtained with a 10 F. 10 MHz IVUS catheter (CVIS system). Transesophageal echocardiography showed another communication just above the diaphragm not imaged by IVUS.

Present role of IVUS and outlook

Unfortunately, in all studies limited far field penetration and steerability led to inferior image quality in the ascending aortic and the aortic arch, especially in patients with ectatic vessels or aneurysms. Therefore IVUS is of limited value in patients with aneurysms. Despite this, IVUS is at present the only echo-based technique to allow the complete scanning of the aorta and its side-branches. It has a significant impact on the diagnosis of aortic diseases and guidance of intra-aortic interventions such as dilatation of aortic coarctation or fenestration of dissection membrane in ischemic

syndromes. Further technical developments such as forward-viewing catheters, steerable catheters or multifrequency transducers, and combined devices, will, it is hoped, facilitate these procedures.[8–10] Finally, the addition of color and Doppler flow and of three-dimensional reconstruction will further facilitate the understanding of the often complex diseases of the aorta.[11]

References

1 Erbel R, Engberding R, Daniel W, Roelandt J, Visser C, Rennollet H. Echocardiography in diagnosis of aortic dissection. *Lancet* 1989; **i**: 457–61.

2 Görge G, Erbel R, Gerber T et al. Intravascular ultrasound in patients with suspected aortic dissection: comparison with transesophageal echocardiography. *Z Kardiol* 1992; **81**: 37–43.

3 Weintraub AR, Erbel R, Görge G et al. Intravascular ultrasound imaging in acute aortic dissection. *J Am Coll Cardiol* 1994; **24**: 495–503.

4 Roelandt J, Serruys PW, Tuccillo B, Gussenhoven WJ. Clinical perspectives of intravascular ultrasound. *Echocardiography* 1990; **7**: 503–14.

5 Pandian NG, Kreis A, Weintraub A et al. Real-time intravascular ultrasound imaging in humans. *Am J Cardiol* 1990; **65**: 1392–6.

6 Gerber T, Erbel R, Görge G, Ge J, Meyer J. Comparison of aortic diameter and area as determined by angiography and intravascular ultrasound. *Herz Kreisl* 1991; **23**: 403–8.

7 Yamada E, Matsumura M, Kyo S, Omoto R. Usefulness of a prototype intravascular ultrasound imaging in evaluation of aortic dissection and comparison with angiographic study, transesophageal echocardiography, computed tomography, and magnetic resonance imaging. *Am J Cardiol* 1995; **75**: 161–5.

8 Görge G, Ge J, Haude M, Baumgart D, Buck T, Erbel R. Initial experience with a steerable intravascular ultrasound catheter in the aorta and pulmonary artery. *Am J Card Imaging* 1995; **9**: 180–4.

9 Evans JL, Ng KH, Vonesh MJ et al. Arterial imaging with a new forward-viewing intravascular ultrasound catheter. I. Initial studies. *Circulation* 1994; **89**: 712–17.

10 Ng KH, Evans JL, Vonesh MJ et al. Arterial imaging with a new forward-viewing intravascular ultrasound catheter. II. Three-dimensional reconstruction and display of data. *Circulation* 1994; **89**: 718–23.

11 Roelandt JR, di Mario C, Pandian NG et al. Three-dimensional reconstruction of intracoronary ultrasound images. Rationale, approaches, problems, and directions. *Circulation* 1994; **90**: 1044–55.

33 Three-dimensional reconstruction of transesophageal and intravascular imaging in aortic disease using IVUS catheters

Thomas Buck, Günter Görge, Junbo Ge and Raimund Erbel

Introduction

The previous chapters have shown the feasibility of the IVUS technique for the diagnosis of aortic diseases. The IVUS technique described, with an ultrasound (US) catheter placed intra-aortally, provides a 360°, panoramic cross-sectional image of the aortic inner wall via a 360° fast rotation of the US element at the tip of the catheter. Similar to intra-coronary imaging with cross-sections of coronary vessels, the intra-aortal two-dimensional images show the morphologic changes in the respective aortic cross-sections. However, to obtain information about the extension of any aortic wall disease along the aorta, the IVUS catheter has to be pulled back slowly with on-line image registration. During that procedure the two-dimensional cross-sectional images change, corresponding to the catheter position, and the observer mentally composes the single images to form a three-dimensional impression. The interpretation of that kind of 3-dimensional impression is strongly observer-dependent, and therefore subjective, and not available for documentation.

By a new technical solution it is possible to perform dynamic, three-dimensional reconstructions of the thoracic aorta on the basis of tomographic two-dimensional images. The technique of a tomographic 3D reconstruction of an echocardiographic B-mode image was introduced in 1989 by Wollschläger et al.[1]

and already used for making clinical decisions. Now, practical experiences of 3D imaging of cardiac valve disease,[2,3] intracardiac masses,[4] ventricular shape and size,[5] and myocardial function[6,7] are available. In particular, the accurate detection of asymmetric volumes such as ventricles with aneurysms allows a volume quantification, which is more precise compared with conventional 2D methods.[8,9]

Three-dimensional reconstruction of the thoracic aorta is a very new diagnostic opportunity and previously only a few preliminary experiences existed. For the present study, 3D reconstruction and 2D ultrasound imaging of the aorta were performed, from a transesophageal (TEUS) and an intra-aortic (IAUS)[10] position using an IVUS catheter, respectively (Fig. 33.1). The 3D reconstructions will be compared with 3D reconstructions of conventional transesophageal echocardiographic (TEE) images.[11] Subsequently, the principles, practice, advantages, and limitations of 3D imaging of the thoracic aorta using these methods will be described.

Different techniques of aortic imaging using ultrasound

Intravascular ultrasound (IVUS) catheters provide 360° images from a high frequency rotating tip of the probe. Besides intravascular scanning of the aorta

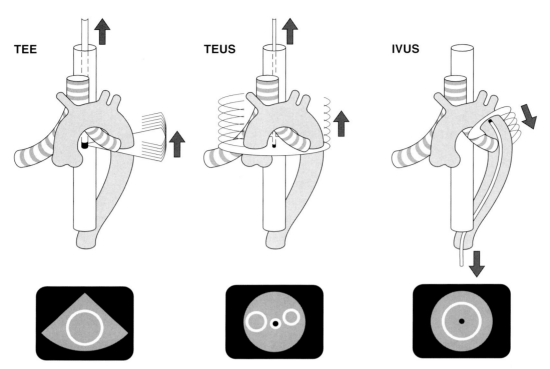

Figure 33.1. Different methods of echocardiographic imaging of the thoracic aorta. Left: conventional transesophageal echocardiography using a TEE probe with an ultrasound frequency of 5–7.5 MHz and an image sector of 90°. The arrows indicate the pullback movement. The figure shows the necessity of scanning the ascending and descending aortae separately using a sector of 90°. The simplified anatomy of the thoracic aorta represents the anticlockwise rotation around the esophagus. The lower picture shows the corresponding image on the screen of the ultrasound unit. Centre: using an IVUS catheter with a sector of 360° transesophageal scanning of the thoracic aorta provides a simultaneous visualization of the ascending and descending aortae as a prerequisite for 3D reconstruction of the entire thoracic aorta. Right: intravascular scanning of the thoracic aorta provides images depicting the aorta without any topographic orientation and 3D reconstruction will be absolutely straight.

(IAUS) using an 8 F. 20 MHz catheter as described in the previous contributions, transesophageal scanning of the thoracic aorta using a 10 F. 10 MHz catheter is possible also, as first described for 2D imaging by Görge et al. in 1993.[12] A thin IVUS catheter is inserted into the esophagus transnasally or transorally. The procedure of insertion affects patients less compared with a conventional TEE probe. The contact between the thin IVUS catheter and the wall of the esophagus is mostly sufficient so that a fluid-filled balloon around the tip of the probe seems unnecessary. The idea of this technique was to obtain more image data from the distal ascending aorta and the aortic arch. Imaging of these regions is limited using conventional TEE as described by Konstadt et al. who documented a visualization of only 42% of the length of the ascending aorta.[13] Nienaber et al. reported that reliability of TEE

decreased significantly from the ascending segment to the arch ($P < 0.05$) and to the distal descending aorta ($P < 0.005$).[14] In addition, this technique offered the possibility for the first time of obtaining ultrasonic tomographic images of the mediastinum including the entire thoracic aorta, similar to magnetic resonance imaging or computed tomography. Now, using 3D reconstruction, this technique has the potential to provide an unlimited 3D visualization of the complex shape of the thoracic aorta including the entire aortic arch.

Conventional transesophageal echocardiography, using the phased array scan technique, transducers with up to 96 crystals, and a frequency of usually 5 MHz, provides 2D B-Mode images of a very high resolution.[15–17] But the TEE technique, as well as the transthoracic technique, is limited by the fact that the scan area uses a transducer with 90° sectors. In fact, due to the anatomy of the thoracic aorta, with an angle of 170–180° between ascending and descending aortae relative to the esophagus, using a 90° TEE probe requires separate scanning of ascending and descending aortae. This leads to a loss of topographic resolution of the aortic wall. Moreover, from cranial to caudal the aorta winds anticlockwise around the esophagus, requiring a compensatory rotation of the TEE probe during pullback scanning.[18] This maneuver yields an absolutely straight 3D reconstruction of the aorta. A real topographic 3D reconstruction of the thoracic aorta would require a 270 or 360° sector imaging probe. Transesophageal examination using a monoplane probe with a sector of 270° (Esaote Medica, Genoa,

Italy) was performed by Hsu et al.[19] and showed, for 2D 270° images, an increase of topographic orientation. However, due to a limited performance the monoplane probe is rarely used.

Principle and practice of 3D reconstruction

Three-dimensional reconstruction of the aorta is performed on the basis of multiple tomographic cross-sectional images (Fig. 33.2). The tomographic images are acquired by pulling back the IVUS catheter thus obtaining a quantity of 360° sector images in a parallel arrangement leading to a

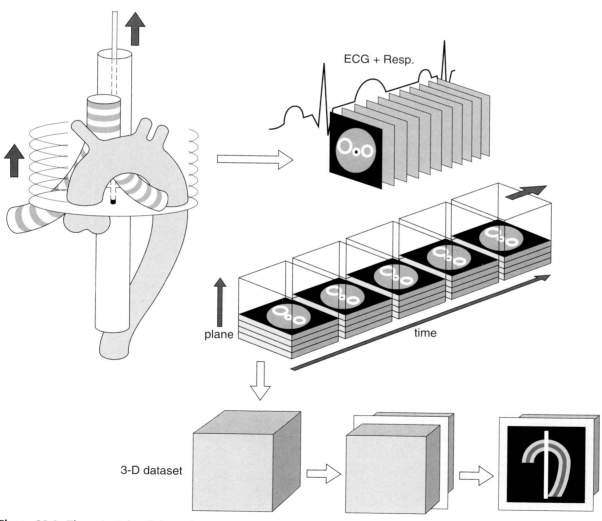

Figure 33.2. The principle of dynamic tomographic 3D reconstruction. At each slice of the pullback single 2D images are acquired at the same ECG intervals and end-expiratory. After postprocessing as many 3D datasets of the scanned space are generated as frames of the R–R interval were indicated. A high processing capability provides dynamic visualization of 3D reconstructions of arbitrary perspectives in a cine loop motion.

cylindrical 3D dataset. The pullback of the IVUS catheter as well as of the TEE probe is performed continuously either by hand or using an automatic pullback device. For the acquisition and storing of the 2D images an external, personal-computer-based system for 3D reconstruction of ultrasound images (Echoscan, TomTec, Unterschleißheim, Germany) is used. The 3D reconstructions, shown in this chapter, are performed with a preset of 15 cm for pullback distance and a total number of 99 equidistant images with a resulting distance of 1.5 mm between the images. For preparing dynamic 3D reconstructions in a cine loop motion, acquisition of the 2D images is ECG (electrocardiogram) and respiration-triggered (Fig. 33.2). After acquisition the 2D image data were prepared by a postprocessing procedure including 'conversion' of the data to a cubical order of pixels (256 × 256 × 256 pixels) and 'gap filling' to complete the 3D dataset. Thus, average image information from the two slices bordering the gap is used as infill. The resulting 3D dataset can be moved (rotated) freely and arbitrary cross-sections with various interesting perspectives are possible (Fig. 33.2). Surfaces of the 3D voxel images — mainly aortic inner wall in this study — are visualized by a rendering procedure and individual surface shading.

Quality and content of information of 3D reconstructions

Quality and content of information of the 3D reconstruction strongly depends on the 2D image quality of each of the scanning techniques previously described, but also on the ability to depict the complete object of interest. The performance of an intravasal pullback scanning of the aortae has the potential to provide cross-sectional images of the complete thoracic aorta with ascending and descending aortae and aortic arch. To achieve a central intraluminal position of the IVUS catheter, especially in the ascending aorta and the aortic arch, it would be necessary to use a steerable IVUS catheter as introduced by Görge et al. for the examination of pulmonary arteries and the thoracic aorta.[20] But 3D reconstruction of the thoracic aorta on the basis of cross-sectional images scanned intraluminally provides a totally straight shape of the aorta without any topographic orientation due to the intraluminal pullback (Figs 33.3 and 33.4). As regards image quality, intra-aortic scanning has the advantage that all parts of the aortic wall are depicted with the same good quality due to its orthogonal orientation to the US beam (Figs 33.4 and 33.5).

Transesophageal scanning and 3D reconstruction of the thoracic aorta using a 360° sector IVUS catheter

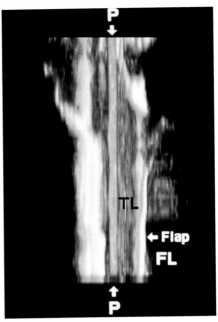

Figure 33.3. The same patient as in Figs 33.6 and 33.14–33.15. Intravascular 3D reconstruction using an 8 F. 20 MHz IVUS catheter. The 3D reconstruction also represents the dissection of the descending aorta with the intimal flap (Flap) and true (TL) and false lumen (FL) but the image quality and the capability of identifying morphological details are reduced compared with TEE and TEUS 3D reconstruction. P: IVUS probe.

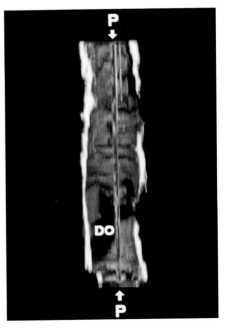

Figure 33.4. Intravascular 3D reconstruction of the descending aorta using an 8 F. 20 MHz IVUS catheter in a 20-year-old patient sent for occlusion of a persistent ductus arteriosus botulli. The long-axis perspective represents a view into the lumen of the descending aorta with the probe (P) in the middle of the vessel. Using this technique only a few echo dropout phenomena occur. The visible inner aortic wall is smooth without signs of atherosclerosis.

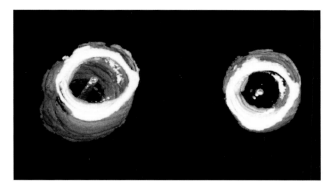

Figure 33.5. The same 3D dataset as in Fig. 33.4. The 3D reconstruction shows a short-axis view through the descending aorta from caudal to cranial. The view on the right is a long-axis view with the probe in the middle of the vessel. The view on the left with an angle deviating from the long axis shows, on the right, the smooth aortic inner wall and the probe running along the middle of the vessel.

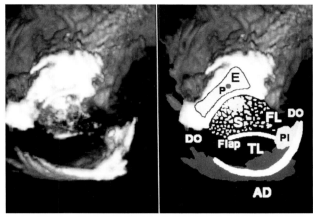

Figure 33.6. The same patient as in Figs 33.14 and 33.15. Transesophageal 3D reconstruction using a 10 F. 10 MHz IVUS catheter (TEUS) with an image sector of 360°. The short-axis 3D reconstruction represents the same morphology as shown by TEE 3D reconstruction (Fig. 33.14). Owing to the image generation by a fast rotation of a single-crystal ultrasound element, the echo dropout phenomenon (DO) at the parts parallel to the ultrasound beam is more prevalent compared with TEE 3D reconstruction. At the left part of the aortic inner wall an intimal plaque is detected (see also Fig. 33.8). E: esophagus: P: ultrasound probe; FL: false lumen; TL: true lumen; Pl: intimal plaque; AD: descending aorta.

has the advantage of being the only method to detect all parts of the thoracic aorta in a real topographic orientation (Figs 33.1, 33.6–33.12). However, the use of an IVUS catheter with an US frequency of 10 MHz for transesophageal scanning of the aorta provides a limited image quality with marked echo dropouts on the two parts of the aortic wall parallel to the US beam (Figs 33.6, 33.7, 33.9, 33.12, 33.13) and a poor penetration intensity. As a consequence with 10 MHz not all parts of the aorta are detected and surface reconstruction is incomplete.

Compared with the IVUS techniques described, 3D reconstructions of TEE pullback examination of the thoracic aorta have a superior image quality due to the more complex US probe technique with a higher resolution and an adequate US frequency of 5–7.5 MHz (Figs 33.14 and 33.15). Therefore, 3D reconstruction on the basis of TEE images is actually the best choice for detecting morphologic details of the aortic inner wall such as plaques and the flaps of dissections (Figs 33.14 and 33.15). In addition, 2D TEE imaging and consequently 3D reconstruction is limited, but only moderately by echo dropouts on the parts of the aortic wall parallel to the US beam. Moreover, and more relevantly, the topographic orientation is lost due to the fact that the ascending and descending aortae have to be scanned separately.

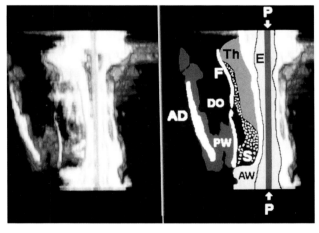

Figure 33.7. The same 3D dataset as in Fig. 33.6. The long-axis 3D reconstruction shows the same morphology as in Fig. 33.15 even more clearly than in TEE 3D reconstruction. Additionally the esophagus with the probe is depicted using this technique. True and false lumen are not indicated but can be identified from Fig. 33.6. PW: posterior aortic inner wall; AW: anterior aortic wall; Th: thrombotic occlusion; S: sludge phenomenon; F: intimal flap. (For other abbreviations see Fig. 33.6.)

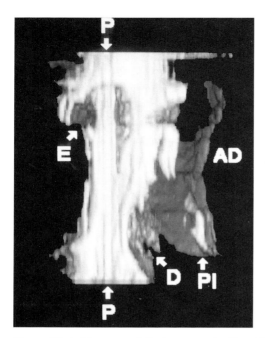

Figure 33.8. The same 3D dataset as in Figs 33.6 and 33.7. Compared with Fig. 33.7 the long-axis 3D reconstruction represents the view after a clockwise rotation of 100° of the dataset. This view represents the dissection (D) with the distal end of the sludge phenomenon and the intimal plaque depicted as before in Fig. 33.6. (For other abbreviations see Figs 33.6 and 33.7.)

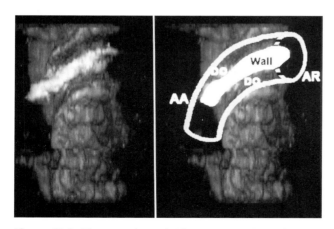

Figure 33.9. Transesophageal 3D reconstruction using an IVUS catheter (TEUS) in a controled respirated patient in an intensive care unit without known aortic disease. The 3D reconstruction represents the thoracic aorta from the mid ascending aorta (AA) to the mid aortic arch (AR) in its natural topographic course around the esophagus which was not possible before with other techniques. Due to the type of IVUS catheter, echo dropout phenomena (DO) are apparent. In the foreground of the 3D reconstruction the anterior wall of the aorta is represented more brightly.

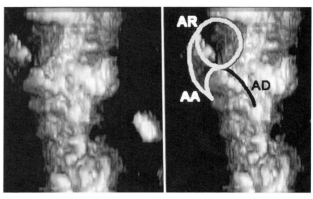

Figure 33.10. The same 3D dataset as in Fig. 33.9. Compared with Fig. 33.9 with a long-axis perspective of the aortic arch the 3D reconstruction is rotated 90° clockwise and now represents a short-axis view of the aortic arch (AR). In the rear the ascending aorta (AA) is winding around the esophagus and in the foreground the course of the descending aorta (AD) is hinted at. The free lateral wall (Wall) and the echo dropout phenomena (DO) depicted in Fig. 33.9 are also visible.

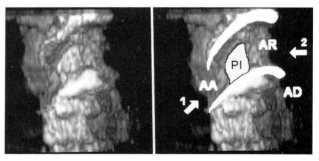

Figure 33.11. The same 3D dataset as in Figs 33.9 and 33.10. The 3D reconstruction from a plane closer to the middle of the dataset gives a view of a large intimal plaque (PI) at the medial aortic inner wall. (For other abbreviations see Figs 33.9 and 33.10.) Arrow 1: perspective of Fig. 33.13; arrow 2: perspective of Fig. 33.12.

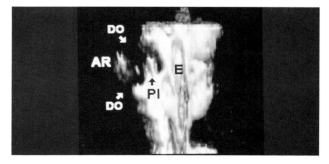

Figure 33.12. The same 3D dataset as in Figs 33.9–33.11 and 33.13. The 3D reconstruction depicts the intimal plaque (PI) in a short-axis view from the aortic arch (AR) to the distal ascending aorta as indicated in Fig. 33.11 (arrow 2). (For other abbreviations see Fig. 33.13.)

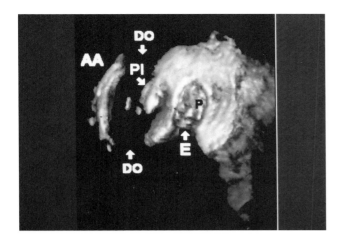

Figure 33.13. The same 3D dataset as in Figs 33.9–33.11. The 3D reconstruction depicts the intimal plaque (Pl) in a short-axis view from the proximal to the distal ascending aorta (AA) as indicated in Fig. 33.11 (arrow 1). P: IVUS probe; E: esophagus; DO: echo dropout.

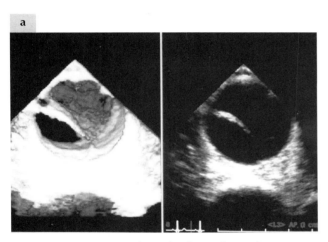

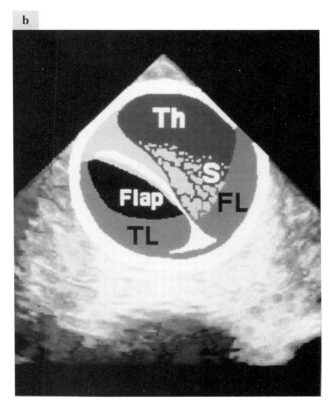

Figure 33.14. Transesophageal echocardiographic (TEE) 3D reconstruction of a 7-day-old dissection of the descending aorta with a progressive clotting of the false lumen (FL) from proximal to distal and a sludge phenomenon (S) at the distal part. It is a short-axis view from caudal to cranial. Th: occlusion by thrombotic clot; TL: true lumen; Flap: flap of dissection. The image information of the 3D reconstruction is opposed to the 2D image which is identical to the nearest slice of the 3D reconstruction.

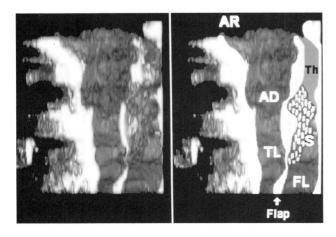

Figure 33.15. The same 3D dataset as in Fig. 33.14. Three-dimensional reconstruction of the descending aorta depicting the intimal flap (Flap) of the dissection from a longitudinal view with the beginning of the aortic arch (AR) at the top. The 3D reconstruction identifies very clearly the progressive occlusion of the false lumen (FL) from proximal to distal with the sludge phenomenon (S) at the transition from completely occluded to free lumen. Th: thrombotic occlusion; TL: true lumen; AD: descending aorta.

Conclusions and perspectives

To obtain an echocardiographic 3D reconstruction of the thoracic aorta noninvasively, with a complete surface representation of all parts of the aortic wall combined with high resolution for the assessment of details of the aortic wall and the potential for 3D reconstruction with real topographic representation, is possible but not with only one technique. Each of the three techniques described above fulfills one or more of these criteria, but not all. Transesophageal scanning of the thoracic aorta and 3D reconstruction using an IVUS catheter was introduced as a new and promising method. By further development, including an improvement in the performance of the transducer and a more appropriate frequency, this method has the potential to fulfill all the important criteria. A further advantage is the easy and fast applicability of the thin IVUS probe without any complex steering mechanism, which is obsolete when 3D reconstruction is performed.

References

1   Wollschläger H, Zeiher AM, Klein HP, Kasper W, Geibel A, Wollschläger S. Transesophageal echo computer tomography: a new method for dynamic 3-D imaging of the heart. *Circulation* 1989; **80**: II569 (abst).

2   Levine RA, Handschumacher MD, Sanfilippo AJ et al. Three-dimensional echocardiographic reconstruction of the mitral valve, with implications for the diagnosis of mitral vale prolapse. *Circulation* 1989; **80**: 589–98.

3   Roelandt JRTC, ten Cate FJ, Vletter WB, Taams MA. Ultrasonic dynamic three-dimensional visualization of the heart with a multiplane transesophageal imaging transducer. *J Am Soc Echocardiogr* 1994; **7**: 217–19.

4   Kupferwasser I, Mohr-Kahaly S, Erbel R et al. Three-dimensional imaging of cardiac mass lesions by transesophageal echocardiographic computed tomography. *J Am Soc Echocardiogr* 1994; **7**: 561–70.

5   Kupferwasser I, Mohr-Kahaly S, Wittlich N, Erbel R, Meyer J. Volumetry in three-dimensional echocardiography using echo-CT. *Eur Heart J* 1994; **18**: 441 (abst).

6   Buck T, Erbel R. Diagnosis of coronary heart disease by echocardiographic 3-dimensional reconstruction — analysis of regional and global left ventricular function. *Hertz* 1995; **4**: 252–62.

7   Buck T, Hunold P, Erbel R. Dynamic 3-dimensional stress echocardiography — a new insight into ischemia induced regional left ventricular dysfunction. *Circulation* 1995; **92 (suppl)**: I799 (abst).

8   Buck T, Schön F, Baumgart D et al. Tomographic left ventricular volume determination in presence of aneurysm by three-dimensional echocardiographic imaging. *J Am Soc Echocardiogr* 1996; **5**: 488–500.

9   Buck T, Hunold P, Wentz KU, Tkalec W, Niel J, Nesser HJ. Comparison of dynamic 3-dimensional echocardiographic and magnetic resonance image reconstruction for the quantification of left ventricular function in presence of aneurysm. *Circulation* 1995; **92 (suppl)**: I70 (abst).

10 Yamada E, Matsumura M, Kyo S, Omoto R. Usefulness of a prototype intravascular ultrasound imaging in evaluation of aortic dissection and comparison with angiographic study, transesophageal echocardiography, computed tomography, and magnet resonance imaging. *Am J Cardiol* 1995; **75**: 161–5.

11 von Hehn A. Initial experiences with echocardiography 3D reconstruction of the thoracic aorta. *Bildgebung* 1994; **192**: 645–50.

12 Görge G,. Erbel R. Intra-vascular ultrasound catheters for transesophageal echocardiography: lighthouse transesophageal echocardiography. *Eur Heart J* 1994; **15 (suppl)**: 101 (abst).

13 Konstadt SN, Reich DL, Quintana C, Levy M. The ascending aorta: how much does transesophageal echocardiography see? *Anesth Analg* 1994; **78**: 240–4.

14 Nienaber CA, von Kodolitsch Y, Brockhoff CJ, Koschyk DH, Spielmann RP. Comparison of conventional and transesophageal echocardiography with magnetic resonance imaging for anatomical mapping of thoracic aortic dissection. A dual noninvasive imaging study with anatomical and/or angiographic validation. *Int J Card Imaging* 1994; **10**: 1–14.

15 Erbel R, Engberding R, Daniel W, Roelandt JRTC. Visser C, Rennollet H. Echocardiography in diagnosis of aortic dissection. *Lancet* 1989; **i**: 457–61.

16. Blanchard DG, Kimura BJ, Dittrich HC, DeMaria AN. Transesophageal echocardiography of the aorta. *JAMA* 1994; **272**: 546–51.

17 Goldstein SA, Mintz GS, Lindsay J Jr. Aorta: comprehensive evaluation by echocardiography and transesophageal echocardiography. *J Am Soc Echocardiogr* 1993; **6**: 634–59.

18 Seward JB, Khanderia BK, Oh JK et al. Transesophageal echocardiography: technique, anatomic correlations, implementation, and clinical applications. *Mayo Clin Proc* 1988; **63**: 649–80.

19 Hsu TL, Weintraub AR, Ritter SB, Pandian NG. Panoramic transesophageal echocardiography. *Echocardiography* 1991; **8**: 677–85.

20 Görge G, Ge J, Haude M, Baumgart D, Buck T, Erbel R. Initial experience with a steerable intravascular ultrasound catheter in the aorta and pulmonary artery. *Am J Card Imaging* 1995; **9**: 180–4.

34 Intravascular ultrasound in the pulmonary circulation

Günter Görge and Raimund Erbel

Introduction

Acute massive pulmonary embolism is an often missed but significant disease, with an estimated 500 000 cases per year in the United States. The diagnostic approach has changed greatly over the last two decades, mainly due to the introduction of noninvasive tests such as ventilation-perfusion scans and transthoracic and transesophageal echocardiography.[1–3] Transthoracic echocardiography usually enables us to determine noninvasively the pulmonary artery pressure and the right ventricular volumes and function, that is, the hemodynamic consequences of a pulmonary embolus. Transesophageal echocardiography has the additional advantage of identifying proximal pulmonary artery embolism in a high percentage of patients.[4] Thus, echocardiography, as a bedside technique, makes the diagnosis of a pulmonary embolism easier and faster, so that patients identified as having hemodynamically relevant embolic events can be treated earlier.[5,6]

Potential role of IVUS in the pulmonary circulation

Angiography is an invasive method that gives a rapid and complete image of the entire pulmonary circulation, yet it need not be performed in all patients. While the value of angiography in the detection of a complete obstruction is uniformly accepted, the imaging of partially occluded vessel segments has been prone to misinterpretation.[7] As a contour method, angiography cannot be adequate in the visualization of soft, wall-adherent thrombus formation; furthermore, cross-sectional imaging of the entire vessel wall is impossible. Intravascular ultra-

sound (IVUS) is, in contrast, a technique which allows imaging of the lumen and the vessel wall. Roelandt et al. and Pandian et al. both realized the diagnostic potential of IVUS in the pulmonary circulation.[8,9] It should therefore serve as a diagnostic tool in examinations of the pulmonary circulation. IVUS could help to identify the various causes of pulmonary hypertension. In patients with acute pulmonary hypertension without failure of the left ventricle, the cause is often acute massive pulmonary embolism. In patients with chronic pulmonary hypertension, the main reasons are either functional impairment of the left ventricle, mitral valve abnormalities or pulmonary diseases, with low oxygen saturation leading to pulmonary hypertension. But, in a minority of patients, the causes of pulmonary hypertension are unclear. A significant percentage of these patients have precapillary, pulmonary-artery-located reasons for chronic pulmonary hypertension, for example, chronic thromboembolic events. Many patients can undergo successful surgery (pulmonary thrombectomy) with complete restoration of normal cardiac function. Unfortunately, the diagnosis of recurrent thromboembolic events is often difficult and there is often a long delay between the onset of symptoms and diagnosis.[10]

The potential role of IVUS as a tomographic method in addition to angiography and other tomographic techniques would include the following:

a) Assessment of vessel wall motion
b) Imaging of small pulmonary arteries (diameter 1.5–3 mm) to assess the vessel wall changes in patients with pulmonary hypertension without thromboembolic events
c) Visualization of thin, wall-adherent or 'soft' thrombus, not visible by angiography
d) Imaging of venous vessels for occurrence of thrombi

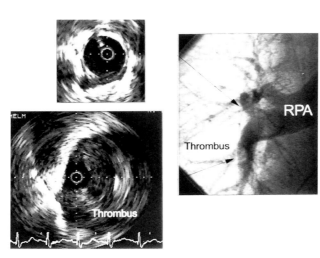

Figure 34.1. Intravascular ultrasound (IVUS) in a 56-year-old patient with recurrent events of acute pulmonary embolism. A 3.5 F. 30 MHz IVUS probe was positioned into the right pulmonary artery (RPA) and its side-branches. The IVUS probe could be advanced into the thrombus (lower left). A small lumen and a large, 'soft' thrombus with signs of thrombotic 'layering' were found. A smaller side-branch (top left) showed normal pulmonary artery anatomy.

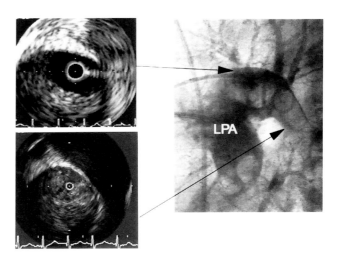

Figure 34.2. Same patient as in Fig. 34.1. Left lateral view during angiography of the left pulmonary artery (LPA). The upper image shows a partial obstruction, the lower image an almost complete occlusion in the left lower lobe. The image shows a 'solid' part and very 'soft' thrombus around the IVUS catheter, suggesting multiple embolic events. A tiny free lumen is visible. This patient had evidence of recurrent embolic events.

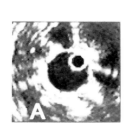 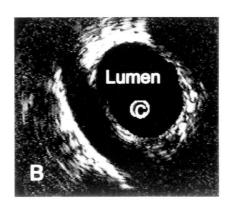 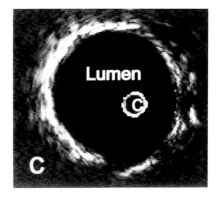

Figure 34.3. Examples of normal pulmonary artery anatomy. All images were obtained by a 3.5 F. 20 MHz IVUS catheter. In image A, the catheter had been advanced into the peripheral pulmonary artery circulation. A thin, 'monolayer' appearance was found.

Image B shows a larger side-branch. Another vessel crosses the pulmonary artery. The vessel walls are very thin, with almost no visible echo contrast of the vessel wall. Image C shows the right pulmonary artery in the same patient. No signs of thrombosis. (C: IVUS catheter.)

Results of IVUS studies in pulmonary circulation

Pandian et al. and Porter et al. described the role of IVUS in patients with various pulmonary artery diseases and the response of the pulmonary circulation in patients with chronic heart failure.[8,11–13] Kravitz examined a patient with pulmonary atherosclerosis, not visualized by angiography.[14] A detailed description of pulmonary anatomy has been reported recently by Kawano.[15] In patients with different degrees of pulmonary hypertension, he found a three-layered appearance of the pulmonary vessels in comparison with the monolayer appearance found normally.

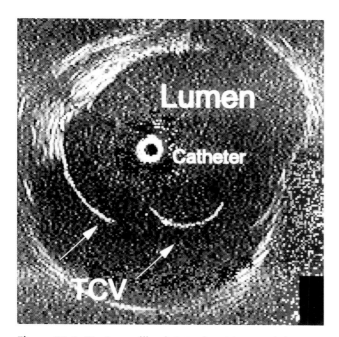

Figure 34.4. During pullback into the right ventricle (10 F. 10 MHz IVUS catheter) a tangential view of the tricuspid valve (TCV) could be obtained. Limited steerability in this position did not allow a cross-sectional image of the valve.

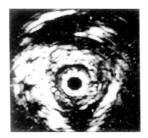
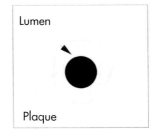

Pulmonary Hypertension

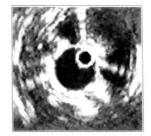
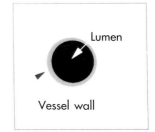

Normal Pulmonary Artery

Figure 34.5. Comparison of the pulmonary artery wall anatomy in a patient with severe pulmonary hypertension (pulmonary artery pressures 95/40 mmHg) (top) and a patient with normal hemodynamics (bottom). In the patient with pulmonary hypertension, a marked intimal thickening could be found. In contrast patients with normal pulmonary artery pressures show only a thin monolayer appearance.

Additionally, he also found evidence of a plaque-like structure in one patient.

The first report on IVUS findings in acute pulmonary embolism was published in 1991 (Figs 34.1 and 34.2).[16] It was possible to cross total obstructions and to identify both wall-adherent and free-floating thrombi. Tapson et al. reported their initial experience with IVUS in a canine model of pulmonary embolism, and found a higher sensitivity of IVUS for detection of residual thrombus in comparison with angiography.[17] Scott et al. and Tapson et al. reported their initial experiences with IVUS in three patients with acute massive pulmonary embolism.[18,19] We reported on a larger series of patients with IVUS after acute massive pulmonary embolism.[20] IVUS was superior to angiography for the identification of residual thrombus formation. Ricou et al. were the first to report on a larger series of IVUS in patients with recurrent thromboembolic disease.[10] Again, IVUS was superior to angiography in revealing wall-adherent thrombus formation. However, besides these interesting findings, IVUS in the pulmonary circulation has still significant shortcomings:

a) IVUS is an invasive method and the positioning of IVUS catheters in the pulmonary circulation is often cumbersome.
b) IVUS catheters with small crystals and high frequencies are not designed for use in the larger pulmonary arteries. Therefore, far field is limited and assessment of the proximal circulation is difficult (Fig. 34.3).
c) Present IVUS catheters are not steerable. Thus, their position cannot be controled in the pulmonary circulation (Fig. 34.4).
d) Because of difficulties in steering the catheter, only a limited number of vessels in the pulmonary circulation can be examined.

Outlook

Despite these shortcomings, IVUS has already proved to be useful in the diagnosis of acute and chronic thromboembolic disease in animal models and patients (Fig. 34.5). Sensitivity in the detection of thrombi seems to be superior to angiography (Fig. 34.6), and is therefore important because pulmonary

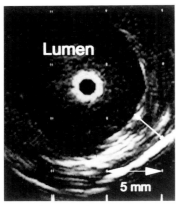

Pulmonary hypertension
Recurrent thromboembolism

Normal pulmonary artery

＞ Wall thickness

Figure 34.6. First-level pulmonary arteries in a patient with recurrent thromboembolic events (left, diagnosis confirmed at post mortem) and a patient with normal pulmonary artery hemodynamics and anatomy. In the patient with recurrent thromboembolic events, the authors obtained a marked increase in vessel wall thickness. However, pulmonary angiography had been normal in this segment.

thrombectomy has become an important new choice for treatment. Demonstration of mural thrombi in these patients is therefore essential.

The limitations in far field penetration and steerability could be overcome by steerable IVUS catheters, and forward-viewing catheters will allow for orientation within the venous circulation with less fluoroscopy.[21-23] If in-dwelling IVUS catheters similar to Swan–Ganz catheters become available, IVUS-based examination of the pulmonary circulation could potentially be a bedside technique.

References

1   Stein PD, Coleman RE, Gottschalk A, Saltzman HA, Terrin ML, Weg JG. Diagnostic utility of ventilation/perfusion lung scans in acute pulmonary embolism is not diminished by pre-existing cardiac or pulmonary disease. *Chest* 1991; **100**: 604–6.

2   McIntyre KM, Sasahara AA. The hemodynamic response to pulmonary embolism in patients without prior cardiopulmonary disease. *Am J Cardiol* 1974; **28**: 288–94.

3   Coates G. Isotope lung imaging. *Curr Opin Radiol* 1992; **4**: 79–86.

4   Wittlich N, Erbel R, Eichler A et al. Detection of central pulmonary artery thromboemboli by transesophageal echocardiography in patients with severe pulmonary embolism. *J Am Soc Echocardiogr* 1992; **5**: 515–24.

5   Kasper W, Meinertz T, Kersting F, Löllgen H, Limbourg P, Just H. Echocardiography in assessing acute pulmonary hypertension due to pulmonary embolism. *Am J Cardiol* 1980; **45**: 567–72.

6   Yock PG, Popp RL. Noninvasive estimation of right ventricular systolic pressure by Doppler ultrasound in patients with tricuspid regurgitation. *Circulation* 1984; **70**: 657–62.

7   Benotti JR, Grossmann W. Pulmonary angiography. In: Grossmann W, ed. *Cardiac Catheterization and Angiography*, third edition. Philadelphia, PA: Lea and Febiger, 1985: 213–26.

8   Pandian NG, Weintraub A, Kreis A, Schwartz SL, Konstam MA, Salem DN. Intracardiac, intravascular, two-dimensional, high-frequency ultrasound imaging of pulmonary artery and its branches in humans and animals. *Circulation* 1990; **81**: 2007–12.

9   Roelandt J, Serruys PW, Tuccillo B, Gussenhoven WJ. Clinical perspectives of intravascular ultrasound. *Echocardiography* 1990; **7**: 503–14.

10 Ricou F, Nicod PH, Moser KM, Peterson KL. Catheter-based intravascular ultrasound imaging of chronic thromboembolic pulmonary disease. *Am J Cardiol* 1991; **67**: 749–52.

11 Pandian NG, Hsu TL. Intravascular ultrasound and intracardiac echocardiography: concepts for the future. *Am J Cardiol* 1992; **69**(20): 6H–17H.

12 Porter TR, Taylor DO, Fields J et al. Direct in vivo evaluation of pulmonary arterial pathology in chronic congestive heart failure with catheter-based

intravascular ultrasound imaging. *Am J Cardiol* 1993; **71**: 754–7.

13 Porter TR, Taylor DO, Cycan A et al. Endothelium-dependent pulmonary artery responses in chronic heart failure: influence of pulmonary hypertension. *J Am Coll Cardiol* 1993; **22**: 1418–24.

14 Kravitz KD, Scharf GR, Chandrasekaran K. In vivo diagnosis of pulmonary atherosclerosis. Role of intravascular ultrasound. *Chest* 1994; **106**: 632–4.

15 Kawano T. Wall morphology of the pulmonary artery—intravascular ultrasound imaging and pathological evaluations. *Kurume Med J* 1994; **41**: 221–32.

16 Görge G, Erbel R, Schuster S, Ge J, Meyer J. Intravascular ultrasound in diagnosis of acute pulmonary embolism. *Lancet* 1991; **337**: 623–4 (letter).

17 Tapson VF, Davidson CJ, Gurbel PA, Sheikh KH, Kisslo KB, Stack RS. Rapid and accurate diagnosis of pulmonary emboli in a canine model using intravascular ultrasound imaging. *Chest* 1991; **100**: 1410–13.

18 Scott PJ, Essop AR, al Ashab W, Deaner A, Parsons J, Williams G. Imaging of pulmonary vascular disease by intravascular ultrasound. *Int J Card Imaging* 1993; **9**: 179–84.

19 Tapson VF, Davidson CJ, Kisslo KB, Stack RS. Rapid visualization of massive pulmonary emboli utilizing intravascular ultrasound. *Chest* 1994; **105**: 888–90.

20 Görge G, Schuster S, Ge J et al. Intravascular ultrasound in patients with acute pulmonary embolism after treatment with intravenous urokinase and high-dose heparin. *Heart* 1996 (in press).

21 Evans JL, Ng KH, Vonesh MJ et al. Arterial imaging with a new forward-viewing intravascular ultrasound catheter. I. Initial studies. *Circulation* 1994; **89**: 712–17.

22 Ng KH, Evans JL, Vonesh MJ et al. Arterial imaging with a new forward-viewing intravascular ultrasound catheter. II. Three-dimensional reconstruction and display of data. *Circulation* 1994; **89**: 718–23.

23 Görge G, Ge J, Haude M, Baumgart D, Buck T, Erbel R. Initial experience with a steerable intravascular ultrasound catheter in the aorta and pulmonary artery. *Am J Card Imaging* 1995; **9**: 180–4.

35 Intravascular ultrasound imaging of angiographically normal coronary arteries

Junbo Ge and Raimund Erbel

Evaluation of vascular morphology and architecture in patients with coronary heart disease has previously depended on contrast coronary angiography. Reports have shown, however, that angiography can only define the contour of the vessel lumen and major structural alterations or abnormalities of the vessels.[1-3] Little information regarding arterial wall thickness and the true three-dimensional configuration of the vessel lumen is available from angiography, despite biplane imaging. Furthermore, other reports have shown considerable discrepancies between cineangiographic and post mortem findings, demonstrating that complex and eccentric coronary atherosclerotic lesions are frequently not identified by angiography.[4,5] To establish the range of normal coronary artery is very important for interpreting coronary abnormalities. Although normal values have been established in histopathologic examinations, they do not represent the physiologic status.

Intravascular ultrasound imaging (IVUS), a catheter-based ultrasound technique, has elicited considerable interest because it offers in-vivo information concerning vascular anatomy, physiology, and pathology that has previously not been available.[6-10] Preliminary in-vitro and in-vivo studies have shown that IVUS is a safe, feasible and accurate method for evaluating vascular morphology.[11-14] Excellent correlations have been obtained in assessing vessel wall thickness, lumen area, lumen diameter and perimeter in vitro;[11-14] controversies still exist with regard to in-vivo research.[9-11] Therefore normal values based on IVUS seem to represent the physiologic status of the coronary arteries.

Normal values of coronary arteries

Coronary arteries taper from proximal to distal in their course. The authors evaluated 55 consecutive patients (28 men, 27 women) who underwent diagnostic coronary angiography for suspected ischemic heart disease and were found to have angiographically normal coronary arteries with intracoronary ultrasound imaging. The patients range in age from 42 to 70 years.[15]

Morphological observations

A total of 413 sites in the 55 patients were analyzed. The lumen of the normal coronary segment portrayed by IVUS was circular or elliptical with a smooth surface (Fig. 35.1). Among the 413 sites examined, atherosclerotic plaques were identified by IVUS in 72 (17%) sites in 25 (45%) patients. The plaque area was 5.55 ± 3.56 mm^2 (2–26 mm^2), which occupied $28.8 \pm 9.6\%$ (13–70%) of the coronary cross-sectional area. In 24/72 (33%) sites of nine patients, calcific deposits were detected (Fig. 35.2). Most of the plaques (84%) were eccentric (Fig. 35.3). In all patients, no obvious stenoses were documented by coronary angiography. Because of the remodeling process in the development of atherosclerosis, the early stage of plaque formation cannot be detected by coronary angiography (Figs 35.4 and 35.5).

267

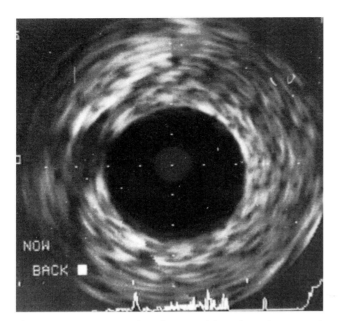

Figure 35.1. Intravascular ultrasound imaging of a normal coronary artery. The arterial wall shows a mono-layer appearance. 3.5 F catheter, 30 MHz transducer, 1 mm calibration.

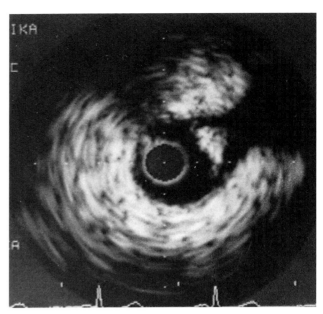

Figure 35.2. A small eccentric plaque with calcification which is characterized by an acoustic shadow behind (2–4 o'clock). 3.5 F catheter, 30 MHz transducer, 1 mm calibration.

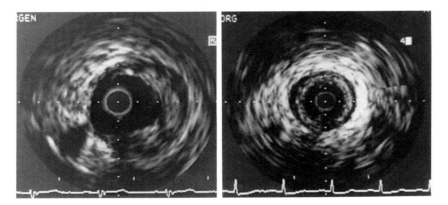

Figure 35.3. Two angiographically normal coronary arteries. Intravascular ultrasound shows eccentric plaque (left) and concentric plaque (right). Because of the compensatory enlargement, no obvious lumen reduction was found by coronary angiography. 3.5 F catheter, 20 MHz transducer, 1 mm calibration.

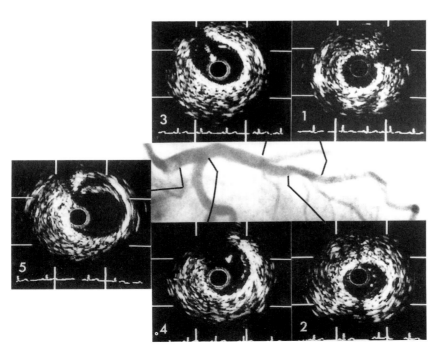

Figure 35.4. Angiogram and IVUS images at corresponding sites of LCA. No abnormalities were documented by angiography while IVUS shows plaque formation in the left main coronary artery. (From Ge et al.,[15] with permission.) 4.8 F catheter, 20 MHz transducer, 1 mm calibration.

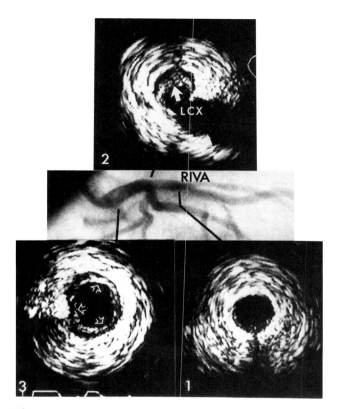

Figure 35.5. Angiogram and intravascular ultrasound images at corresponding sites of LCA. No abnormalities were detected by angiography. An eccentric plaque at the bifurcation of the circumflex coronary artery and a concentric plaque in the LMCA are clearly visualized by intravascular ultrasound. (From Erbel et al.,[16] with permission.) 4.8 F catheter, 20 MHz transducer, 1 mm calibration. RIVA = romus interventricular anterior; LCX = left circumflex coronary artery.

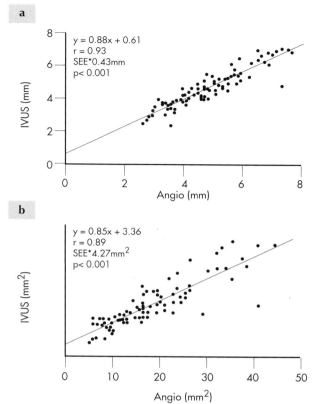

Figure 35.6. The relationship of lumen dimensions between angiographic and ultrasonic measurements in normal sites. **a** indicates lumen diameter. **b** indicates lumen area.

Dimensional correlation with angiography

For vessel diameter, the intraobserver correlation of 30 IVUS images was $r = 0.99$, SEE = 0.16 mm; interobserver correlation was $r = 0.99$, SEE = 0.17 mm. For vessel area, the intraobserver correlation was $T = 0.99$, SEE = 1.39 mm²; interobserver correlation was $r = 0.98$, SEE = 1.81 mm².

Of the 341 normal sites, the lumen diameter ranged from 2.7 to 7.6 mm measured by IVUS, and 2.6 to 7.3 mm measured by angiography. Linear regression of the lumen dimensions of 100 randomly selected sites was performed. Close correlations were obtained between IVUS and angiography for lumen diameter and area (Fig. 35.6).

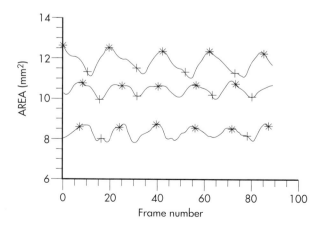

Figure 35.7. Pulsatile variation of the cross-sectional area of LMCA (**a**), of the proximal LAD (**b**), and of the mid LAD (**c**) in 90 consecutive frames. +: beginning of QRS complex, *: end of T-wave.

Table 35.1 **Cross-sectional areas of normal LCA during cardiac cycle.**

	Maximum area (mm²)	Minimum area (mm²)	End-diastole (mm²)	Pulsation (%)
LMCA	18.33 ± 8.18	16.49 ± 6.77*	17.33 ± 7.98*	10.2 ± 4.0
Range	9.74–36.02	8.83–29.95	9.12–30.71	
Proximal LAD	14.01 ± 5.54	12.95 ± 5.08*	13.56 ± 5.85**	8.3 ± 4.7
Range	6.91–26.21	6.34–23.61	6.42–26.10	
Mid LAD	10.70 ± 4 47	9.78 ± 4.24*	9.75 ± 4.67*	9.8 ± 4.0
Range	4.78–22.74	4.49–21.47	4.53–22.01	

Note: Values are in mean ± standard deviation.
*$P < 0.001$, **$P < 0.005$.
LMCA: left main coronary artery; LCA: left coronary artery.

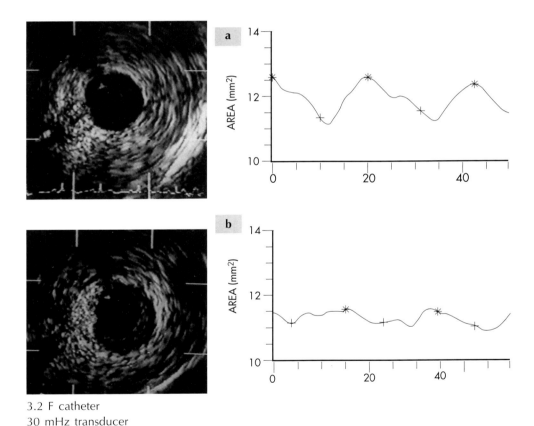

3.2 F catheter
30 mHz transducer
5 mm calibration

Figure 35.8.
Comparison of the pulsatile variation of the cross-sectional area of a normal (**a**) coronary artery and a coronary artery with an eccentric plaque (**b**).

Normal values of the left coronary artery (LCA)

Of the 30 patients without IVUS-detected plaques in the LCA, 16 patients (8 male, 8 female, ranging in age from 42 to 68 years, mean 53.6 ± 7.4 years) who were free of risk factors for coronary artery disease including systemic hypertension, cigarette smoking, hypercholesterolemia, and diabetes mellitus were regarded as being truly normal subjects following

their negative IVUS examination. Table 35.1 lists the cross-sectional areas of left main coronary artery (LMCA), proximal LAD (left anterior descending artery), and mid LAD at end-diastole (at the beginning of QRS complex); these were 17.33 ± 7.98 mm² (range 9.12–30.71), 13.56 ± 5.85 mm² (range 6.42–20.05) and 9.75 ± 4.67 mm² (range 4.53–22.01). Significant differences were found between the maximum areas and the end-diastolic areas.

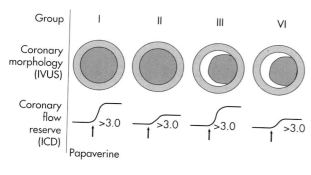

Figure 35.9. Classification of coronary arteries based on coronary morphology (IVUS) and coronary flow reserve (intracoronary Doppler).

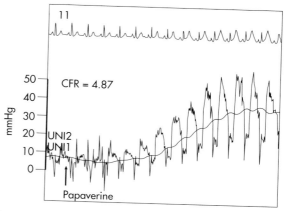

Figure 35.10. Intracoronary Doppler flow recording of a patient with normal coronary flow reserve. The mean coronary flow velocity increased nearly fivefold after the intracoronary injection of 10 mg papaverine. CFR: coronary flow reserve.

Pulsatile variation of the cross-sectional lumen area

The pulsatile variations during the cardiac cycle of the normal patients were 10.2 ± 4.0% in LMCA, 8.3 ± 4.7% in the proximal LAD, and 9.8 ± 4.0% in mid LAD. The cross-sectional area changes on 90 consecutive frames incorporating three to five cardiac cycles of the LMCA, the proximal LAD, and the mid LAD are shown in Fig. 35.7. The pulsatile variation of 11 patients with plaques was 5.8 ± 3.1%, significantly decreased compared with the normal group ($P < 0.001$) (Fig. 35.8).

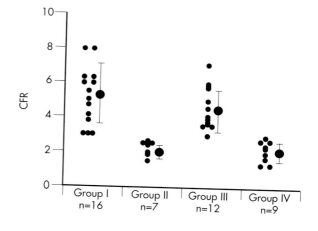

Figure 35.11. Coronary flow reserve in different groups. CFR: coronary flow reserve.

Coronary flow measurement

To date, no normal values have been established for coronary flow velocity and coronary flow reserve. Erbel et al. studied a group of patients who had angina pectoris but had angiographically normal coronary arteries.[16] Based on intravascular ultrasound and Doppler studies, they divided the patients into four groups (Fig. 35.9). They considered a coronary flow reserve of over 3 as normal (Fig 35.10). However, nearly one-third of the patients had a coronary flow reserve of over 3 but with plaque formation (Fig. 35.11). Only 36% of the patients were truly normal. Because atherosclerosis is a long-term, slowly progressing process which starts in childhood, it is difficult to find absolutely normal coronary arteries in adult patients who come for diagnostic catheterization. Based on current diagnostic techniques such as intravascular ultrasound and Doppler, we can detect only relatively normal coronary arteries.

Conclusion

Intracoronary Doppler and ultrasound are new important techniques which can be used to further classify patients with normal coronary artery bedding to a better discrimination and hopefully to a better patient arrangement.

References

1   Grondin CM, Dyrada I, Pasternac A, Campeu L, Bourassa MG, Lesperance J. Discrepancies between cineangiographic and postmortem findings in patients with coronary artery disease and recent myocardial revascularization. *Circulation* 1974; **49**: 703–13.

2   Eusterman JH, Achor RWP, Kincaid OW, Brown AL Jr. Atherosclerotic disease of the coronary arteries: a pathologic–radiologic study. *Circulation* 1962; **26**: 1288–95.

3   White CW, Wright CB, Doty DB et al. Does visual interpretation of the coronary angiograms predict the physiologic importance of the coronary stenosis? *New Engl J Med* 1984; **310**: 819–24.

4   Vlodaver Z, French R, van Tassel RA, Edwards JE. Correlation of the antemortem coronary angiogram and the postmortem specimen. *Circulation* 1973; **47**: 162–8.

5   Isner JM, Kishel J, Kent KM. Accuracy of angiographic determination of the left main coronary arterial narrowing. *Circulation* 1981; **63**: 1056–61.

6   Hodgson JM, Graham SP, Savakus AD et al. Clinical percutaneous imaging of coronary anatomy using an over-the-wire ultrasound catheter system. *Int J Card Imaging* 1989; **4**: 187–93.

7   Bartorelli AL, Potkin BN, Almagor Y, Keren G, Roberts WC, Leon MB. Plaque characterization of atherosclerotic coronary arteries by intravascular ultrasound. *Echocardiography* 1990; **7**: 389–95.

8   Siegel RJ, Chae JS, Forrester JM, Ruiz CE. Angiography, angioscopy, and ultrasound imaging before and after percutaneous balloon angioplasty. *Am Heart J* 1990; **120**: 1086–90.

9   Tobis JM, Mallery J, Mahon D et al. Intravascular ultrasound imaging of human coronary arteries in vivo. *Circulation* 1991; **83**: 913–26.

10   Nissen SE, Gurley JC, Grines CL et al. Intravascular ultrasound assessment of lumen size and wall morphology in normal subjects and patients with coronary artery disease. *Circulation* 1991; **84**: 1087–99.

11   Davidson CJ, Sheikh KH, Harrison JK et al. Intravascular ultrasonography versus digital subtraction angiography. *Am J Coll Cardiol* 1990; **16**: 633–66.

12   Ge J, Erbel R, Seidel I et al. Experimental evaluation of accuracy and safety of intraluminal ultrasound. *Z Kardiol* 1991; **80**: 595–601.

13   Nishimura RA, Edwards WD, Warnes CA et al. Intravascular ultrasound imaging: in vitro validation and pathologic correlation. *Am J Coll Cardiol* 1990; **16**: 145–54.

14   Pandian NG, Kreis A. Brokway B et al. Ultrasound angioscopy: real-time, two-dimensional, intraluminal ultrasound imaging of blood vessels. *Am J Coll Cardiol* 1988; **62**: 493–4.

15   Ge J, Erbel R, Gerber T et al. Intravascular ultrasound imaging of angiographically normal coronary arteries: a prospective study in vivo. *Br Heart J* 1994; **71**: 572–8.

16   Erbel R, Ge J, Kearney P et al. Value of intracoronary ultrasound and Doppler in the differentiation of angiographically normal coronary arteries: a prospective study in patients with angina pectoris. *Eur Heart J* 1996; **17**: 880–9.

36 Safety of intravascular ultrasound examination

Junbo Ge

Introduction

In the intensive use of intravascular ultrasound (IVUS) in coronary diagnosis cardiologists encountered the challenge of various complications of advancing an IVUS catheter into the coronary artery. Like other interventional coronary catheters IVUS catheters may also induce common complications such as coronary spasm, coronary dissection, acute coronary closure, thrombus formation, arrhythmia,

Table 36.1 Incidence of complications with certain or uncertain relation to intravascular ultrasound imaging: correlation to demographic, clinical and procedural variables (from Hausmann et al).

		Complications			
		Spasm		Acute + major	
Procedural	No.	No.	(%)	No.	(%)
All patients*	2120	63	(3.0)	23	(1.1)
Male patients	1657	52	(3.1)	21	(1.3)
Age, y (mean ± SD)	56.2 ± 11.3	53.7 ± 13.1		56.0 ± 11.5	
Presentation					
Unstable angina/acute MI	717	22	(3.0)	15	(2.1)§
Stable angina	608	13	(2.1)	5	(0.8)
Asymptomatic/other	795	28	(3.5)	3	(0.4)
Indication for ICUS study					
Diagnostic in transplants	495	15	(3.0)	0	(0)
Diagnostic in nontransplants	650	21	(3.2)	4	(0.6)
Interventions	975	27	(2.8)	19	(1.9)§
Coronary vessel imaged†					
Left anterior descending artery	1360	43	(3.2)	11	(0.8)
Left circumflex artery	288	5	(1.7)	2	(0.7)
Right coronary artery	452	14	(3.1)	8	(1.8)
Other	139	2	(1.4)	2	(1.4)
Size of ICUS catheter					
<4.0F	734	20	(2.7)	10	(1.2)
4.0F to 4.5F	855	26	(3.0)	10	(1.2)
>4.5F	531	17	(3.2)	3	(0.6)
Center experience (No. of cases)‡					
1 to 19	499	14	(2.8)	8	(1.6)
20 to 100	1074	28	(2.6)	12	(1.1)
>100	547	21	(3.8)	3	(0.5)

MI indicates myocardial infarction; ICUS, intracoronary ultrasound.
*Eighty-seven patients with complications unrelated to ICUS imaging were excluded for this analysis; †including patients with >1 vessel imaged; ‡complications are categorized according to the number of cases done by the center at the time the complication occurred; §$P<.01$.

Table 36.2 Complications judged to have a certain relation or an uncertain relation to intracoronary ultrasound imaging (from Hausmann et al).

	Certain/uncertain: complications			
	Diagnostic ICUS in transplant patients (n = 503)	Diagnostic ICUS in nontransplant patients (n = 656)	ICUS during interventions (n = 1048)	All patients (n = 2207)
Spasm	15/0	21/0	27/0	63 (2.9%)/0
Acute procedural complications				
Acute occlusion	0/0	1/0	2/5	3/5
Dissection	0/0	0/0	1/3	1/3
Thrombus	0/0	1/0	0/0	1/0
Embolism	0/0	0/0	1/0	1/0
Arrhythmia	0/0	1/0	0/0	0/1
Total	0/0	2/1	4/8	6 (0.3%)/9 (0.4%)
Major complications				
Nonfatal MI	0/0	0/0	3/2	3/2
Emergency CABG	0/0	0/1	0/2	0/3
Death	0/0	0/0	0/0	0/0
Total	0/0	0/1	3/4	3 (0.1%)/5 (0.2%)

ICUS indicates intracoronary ultrasound; MI, myocardial infarction; and CABG, coronary artery bypass graft.

and myocardial infarction. In a multicenter study of 2207 intracoronary examinations complications occurred during 7.8% of interventional procedures, of which 3.9% were judged to be not related to intracoronary ultrasound imaging.[1] Tables 36.1 and 36.2 show the complications during IVUS examination. In 229 consecutive intravascular ultrasound procedures the present author and colleagues found an incidence of 4.8%.[2]

Coronary spasm

Coronary spasm is the most frequent complication during IVUS examination. In the above-mentioned multicenter IVUS study the overall incidence of coronary spasm was found in 2.9%.[1] In the author's center it was found that the incidence of coronary spasm is lower if intracoronary nitroglycerin and heparin are given before the examination.[3] Figure 36.1 shows an example of coronary spasm during IVUS examination, which was released after intracoronary administration of 0.2 mg nitroglycerin. In the presence of coronary spasm the IVUS images mimic intimal thickening or plaque formation (Fig. 36.2). After the spasm had been released the intima presented with a monolayer appearance (Fig. 36.3).

Therefore, close attention should be paid when interpreting IVUS images. The operator must be sure that no spasm exists. Clinically, patients with coronary spasm may present ischemic ECG changes and experience angina pectoris. These manifestations improve when the spasm has released. Bory et al. found that atherosclerotic plaque is always present at the site of focal vasospasm and that atherosclerosis plays an important role in the occurrence of vasospasm.[4]

Acute coronary closure

Acute closure of the coronary artery is a severe complication of IVUS examination. In the multicenter registry acute closure of the coronary artery was documented in 14/2207 patients (0.6%) of which 3/2207 (0.1%) were considered to be related to IVUS examination.[1] The present author studied 550 IVUS procedures and found that 2/550 patients suffered acute closure of coronary arteries during IVUS procedure.[3] Figure 36.4 shows an acute closure of the left anterior descending coronary artery (LAD) during IVUS examination with a 4.8 F. monorail ultrasound catheter before coronary intervention. After withdrawal of the IVUS catheter it appeared

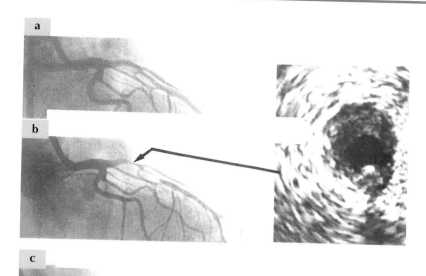

Figure 36.1. Coronary artery spasm in LAD during IVUS imaging. Left panel shows the coronary angiogram before (**a**) and after (**b**) IVUS examination. After intracoronary administration of 0.2 mg nitroglycerin the spasm released (**c**). IVUS shows no free lumen around the catheter and an eccentric plaque with a Starry IV lesion and an opposite normal vessel wall responsible for the spasm.

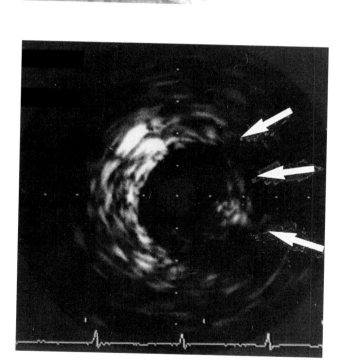

Figure 36.2. IVUS image of a right coronary artery during spasm. A 'plaque' which caused a percentage stenosis of about 50% can be visualized.

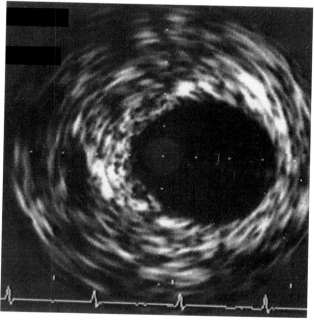

Figure 36.3. IVUS image of the same cross-section as in Fig. 36.2 after intracoronary administration of nitroglycerin. No plaque is visualized, indicating the plaque in Fig. 36.2 might actually be squeezed intima.

that an intimal dissection and thrombus formation with subtotal occlusion of the proximal LAD was present (Fig. 36.4c) followed by a total occlusion (Fig. 36.4d). The occluded coronary artery was successfully recanalized by percutaneous transluminal coronary angioplasty (PTCA). However, thrombotic debris caused side-branch embolization (Fig.

36.5). Figure 36.6 shows a right coronary artery occlusion during IVUS examination. The cause was an intimal dissection of the distal segment by a 2.9 F. over-the-wire ultrasound catheter sheath. The vessel was recanalized with an over-the-wire balloon catheter but the two side-branches distal to the crux cordis still showed filling defects. The

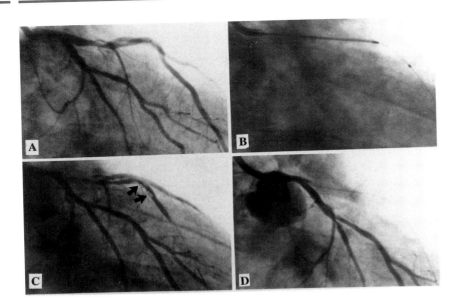

Figure 36.4. Coronary angiogram of left coronary artery in right anterior oblique (RAO) projection. (A) An 80% stenosis is seen in the proximal LAD. (B) The IVUS catheter is advanced into the LAD with a 0.014-inch (0.36-mm) guide wire in the distal segment. (C) The distal LAD is occluded with signs of intimal dissection and thrombus formation in the proximal LAD (arrows). (D) The whole LAD is occluded at the proximal part with the guide wire positioned in the distal LAD. (From Ge et al.,[3] with

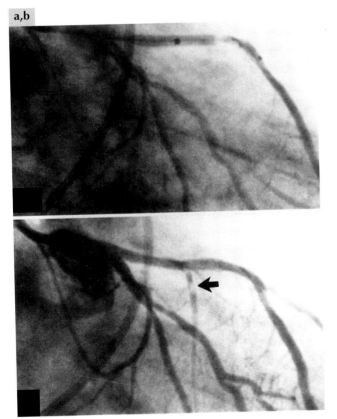

Figure 36.5. The same patient as in Fig. 36.4. The vessel was successfully recanalized and dilated with a 3.0 mm continuous perfusion catheter. (A) The whole LAD is open with antegrade blood flow of TIMI 3. (B) Residual thrombi can still be seen in the first septal branch (arrow). (From Ge et al.,[3] with permission.)

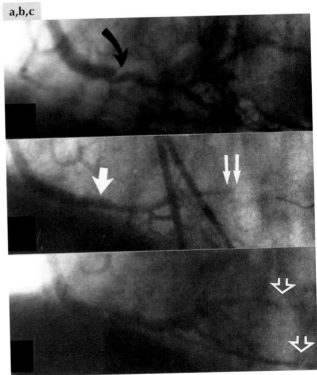

Figure 36.6. Distal part of right coronary artery in left anterior oblique (LAO) projection. A high-degree stenosis is seen angiographically (A, arrow). (B) Intimal dissection (single white arrow) with the guide wire in the right coronary artery. (C) After recanalization and PTCA the vessel is open but two small branches distal to the crus cordis remain as contrast-filling defects. (From Ge et al.,[3] with permission.)

patient had a CK value of 432 U/l after returning to the ward compared with 50 U/l pre-examination. In the above-mentioned multicenter survey, all the acute closures were also successfully managed by PTCA or thrombolytic therapy.[1]

Coronary dissection and thrombus formation

Coronary dissection and thrombus formation may occur during IVUS examination. In the author's study,[3] both patients with acute coronary closure had first intimal dissection followed by thrombus formation which led to coronary occlusion. In the multicenter study one instance of dissection occurred and was treated with PTCA. One patient with thrombus formation was successfully treated with thrombolysis. Although these complications are rare, they are serious and great attention should be paid during IVUS procedure to avoiding them.

Other complications

Apart from ischemic electrocardiogram (ECG) changes caused by coronary spasm, the IVUS catheter may cause obstruction when crossing a severe stenosis and lead to ischemic changes. In this situation patients normally presented with angina pectoris in accordance with ST-elevation. In cases of left main coronary stenosis, bradycardia or asystole may occur when the ultrasound catheter is placed in the left main coronary artery (Fig. 36.7). Extrasystoles and other arrhythmias such as ventricular tachycardia may also occur when the ultrasound catheter is advanced.

Because the IVUS catheters currently used are often monorail catheters it is sometimes very difficult to guide the catheter into a tortuous coronary artery or a steep angle of the circumflex coronary artery. The author found that, with the use of an Amplatz (Cordis, Miami, FL) guiding catheter, nonuniform rotating of the mechanical rotating catheter often occurred because of the acute course of the catheter (Fig. 36.8); moreover, a guide wire artifact exists in every monorail IVUS catheter.

Another common complication during IVUS examination is guide wire winding (Fig. 36.9). This is due to the monorail of the IVUS catheter being too short. When pulling the IVUS catheter back and then advancing again, the soft guide wire could be advanced together with the ultrasound catheter, forming a loop just proximal to the monorail. When pulling the IVUS catheter into the guiding catheter, the looped wire and IVUS catheter tip at the site of

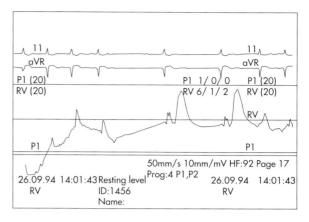

Figure 36.7. A patient with left main coronary artery stenosis and ostium stenosis. A systole occurred during IVUS examination.

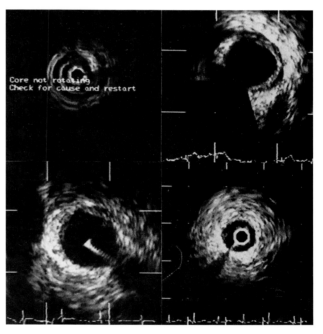

Figure 36.8. Nonuniform rotation of the mechanically rotated catheter because of the acute course of the guiding catheter. Typical guidewire artifact, 3.5 F catheter, 20 MHz.

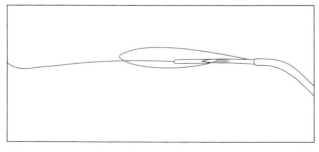

Figure 36.9. Guide wire winding on the tip of the guiding catheter.

the monorail will be stacked at the tip of the guiding catheter (Fig. 36.9). This is more common when using FloWire (Cardiometrics, Mountain View, CA) as guide wire because the long distal part of the FloWire is very soft. Thus, when the coronary artery is repeatedly scanned, the IVUS catheter and FloWire should be withdrawn together and then advanced together again. When a normal floppy wire is used it should be advanced as far as possible to the distal part of the target coronary artery to prevent the occurrence of this complication. When guide wire winding occurs the whole system (guiding catheter, together with the IVUS catheter and guide wire) should be removed. One should always avoid pulling the IVUS catheter with force!

IVUS is a useful tool in interventional cardiology today. Concerning the long-term effects of this procedure, no angiographically quantifiable changes in previously instrumented segments were found with regard to acceleration of atherosclerosis.[5] Therefore the technique can be safely used for the evaluation of coronary artery disease, for diagnostic purposes and for follow-up studies.

References

1   Hausmann D, Erbel R, Alibelli-Chemarin MJ et al. The safety of intracoronary ultrasound: a multicenter survery of 2207 examinations. *Circulation* 1995; **91**: 623–30.

2   Erbel R, Ge J, Gerber T, Görge G, Rupprecht HJ, Meyer J. Safety and limitations of intravascular ultrasound. *Circulation* 1992; **86**: I195.

3   Ge J, Liu F, Kearney P, Görge G, Haude M, Erbel R. Acute coronary artery closure following intracoronary ultrasound examination. *Cathet Cardiovasc Diagn* 1995; **35**: 232–5.

4   Bory M, Panagides D, Yvorra S, Colin R, Fourcade L, Bonnet JL. Intravascular ultrasound detection of atherosclerosis at the site of vasospasm in angiographically normal or mild narrowed coronary arteries. *Eur Heart J* 1995; **16**: 205A.

5   Pinto FJ, St Goar FG, Gao SZ et al. Immediate and one-year safety of intracoronary ultrasonic imaging: evaluation with serial quantative angiography. *Circulation* 1993; **88**: 1709–14.

Index